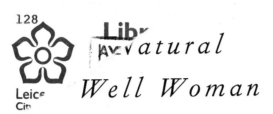

Natural
Well Woman

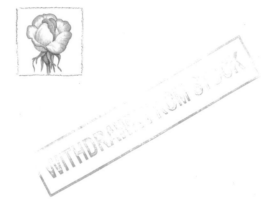

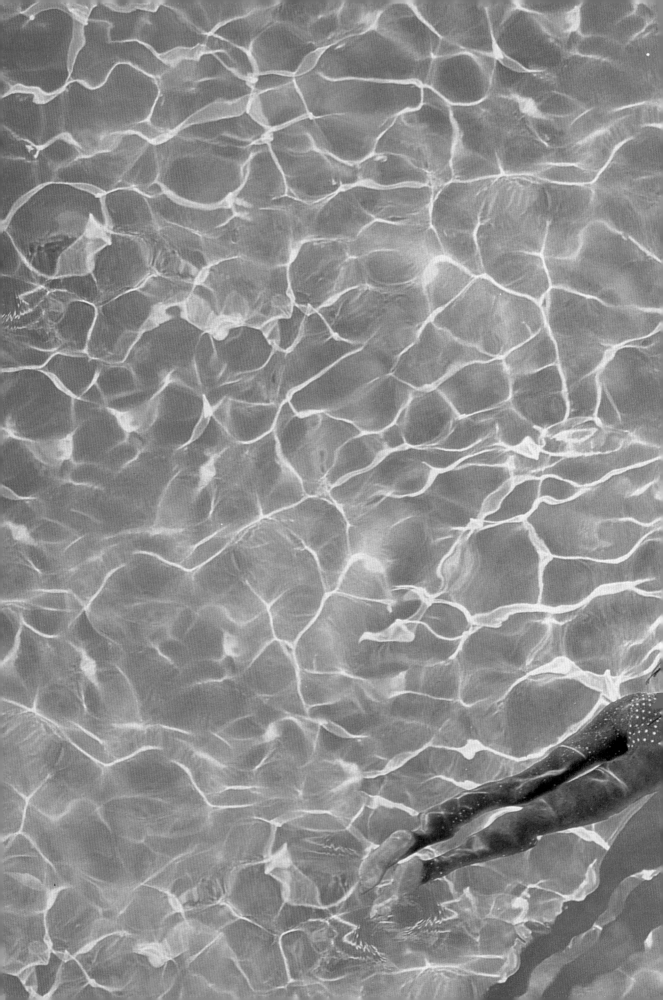

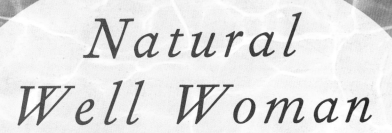

Natural Well Woman

A PRACTICAL GUIDE TO HEALTH AND WELLBEING FOR LIFE

Penny Stanway MD

ELEMENT

Element
An Imprint of HarperCollinsPublishers
77-85 Fulham Palace Road
Hammersmith, London W6 8JB

The website address is: www.elementbooks.co.uk

First published in Great Britain in 2001 by Element

M 10 9 8 7 6 5 4 3 2 1

A catalogue record for this book is available from the British Library

ISBN 1 86 204791 X

Printed and bound in Italy.

Designed and created with The Bridgewater Book Company Limited

THE BRIDGEWATER BOOK COMPANY
Art Director Terry Jeavons
Editorial Director Fiona Biggs
Designer John Grain
Project Editors Mari Roberts, Sarah Doughty
Picture Research Caroline Thomas
Illustrations Rhian Nest James, MTG, Debbie Hinks, Coral Mula, Nadine Faye James
Three-dimensional Models Mark Jamieson
Photographer Guy Ryecart

Special thanks go to
Maria Anderson, Claire Bayes, Kimberley Bunn, Carla Carrington, Dina Christie, Juliet Cox,
Jennifer Dean, Sarah Dean, Tana Dean, Angela Enahoro, Charlotte Fordyce, Sarah Fordyce, Tara Gould,
Betty Green, Sally Hardy, Tara Harley, Joan Ironside, Karel Ironside, Maria Lloyd, Kay Macmullan,
Shanade McClelland, A Norman, Marigold Norman, Sara McGowan, Donna Poplett, Francesca Selkirk,
Ruben Simmons, Tania Simmons, Sheila Sword, Joan Whittaker, Emilie Woodman.
For help with photography

With thanks to
Armadillo, Brighton; Bright Ideas, Lewes; C&E Sports, Seaford; Dollywood, Brighton;
King's Farmers, Lewes; Plate Expectations, Brighton; Starfish, Brighton; Tie Rack, Brighton
For the kind loan of props

CONTENTS

Disclaimer: The information in this book is not intended to replace advice from your physician. Whenever worrying or persistent symptoms occur, consult your doctor.

INTRODUCTION

When writing this book I built on the concept that life is full of experiences and circumstances that can affect how well our bodies perform and how well we feel. The various stages of life have wide-ranging effects on our body, mind, and spirit. In addition, we may inherit a high risk of certain illnesses, live in a way that encourages certain diseases, or fall prey to accidents or infections. So it's hardly surprising that our physical and mental state can vary from day to day, month to month, and year to year.

Being sensitive to how we feel enables us to spot disease early. This early state of "dis-ease" is when we first notice that our health or wellbeing isn't quite right. We can then intervene to help ourselves, perhaps with advice and support from a doctor or other health-care practitioner.

As an experienced doctor I'm well aware that medical diagnosis and treatment can be extremely helpful and sometimes life-saving. I'm also conscious that using sophisticated medical or surgical techniques for treating most common ailments is like using a sledgehammer to crack a nut. It often isn't necessary and sometimes it is undesirable. Many medical drugs, for example, have side effects, and some operations lead to complications. Medical treatments tend to be expensive and may be covered only partially by insurance. They also require a visit to the doctor and, perhaps, to the drugstore. Given that four out of five common ailments are self-limiting – they get better naturally – it's in everyone's interest to do what you can to help your body heal itself.

Our age and stage of life can have important bearings on our health. But we don't necessarily move from one stage of life to another in any order. And a woman's apparent age may be different from her chronological age. While you can easily measure your chronological age (the number of years you have been around), your biological age (the degree of aging of your cells) may be more or less, depending on your genes, health, and lifestyle. And there's even more to how we feel and perform than this. Each of us, whatever our actual or biological age or stage, has in our mind a range of what Jungian psychologists call "archetypes." These are patterns for our thinking and behavior, and they are partly inborn and partly based on what we have learned from others. You may, for example, be pregnant and 30, yet able to access the know-how of your "wise woman," "young virgin," or "adventurous warrior" archetypes. And these archetypes will influence the way you look after your health.

The lifestyle changes and natural remedies and therapies outlined in this book are often effective for common ailments. They may also help prevent or treat some more serious health problems. They are usually relatively cheap and have few or no side effects and they are easy and quick to use at home or alongside medical treatment. I don't see medical treatment and complementary remedies and therapies as mutually exclusive. And an increasing majority of lay people, and medical and other health practitioners, feel the same way.

What we all want for our health and wellbeing is a system of healing that gives us the best of both worlds. That is what this book is all about.

Penny Stanway

HOW TO USE THIS BOOK

Feeling well and full of energy means we can live our lives to the full. I hope this book will help you with both, because encouraging good health is not only my profession, but also my passion. Yet we are all unwell sometimes. And when we are, we want to be able to treat ailments with sensitivity and skill so we get better sooner, or minimize the effects of long-term illness.

The book's aim is to help you use lifestyle changes and, when necessary, natural remedies and therapies to make the most of your health and wellbeing. It is as up-to-date as possible. The content draws on a wide variety of sources, both scientific and lay, and from orthodox, complementary, and alternative medicine. The book is divided into four parts.

PART 1

Good health starts by looking at how the environment affects our lives and health, and what it means to live a healthy lifestyle. There is information on food and drink; exercise and movement; relaxing, playing, and managing stress; and sleep. The last section invites you to look more closely at who you are, and includes a brief discussion of relationships, fulfilling your potential, and the concepts of soul and spirit.

How lifestyle can affect a woman's health

Information on each food and the nutrients they contain

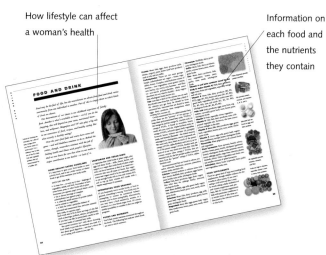

Part 1 teaches you about lifestyle, and environment and how they affect a woman's health and wellbeing.

PART 2

Health in a lifetime builds on Part 1 by outlining specific measures that can help balance your lifestyle, maintain good health, and prevent illness during each stage of life. Its sections focus, in turn, on growing girls and teenagers, young women, pregnancy, mothers, mature women, women around their menopause, and "seniors."

How your requirements change as you grow older

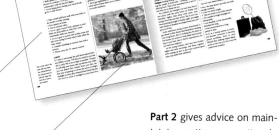

Specific advice for all ages from teens through to seniors

How to manage the joys and pressures of career and motherhood

Part 2 gives advice on maintaining optimum emotional and physical health during each stage of a woman's life.

PART 3

Complementary therapies and remedies first examines the exciting topic of integrated medicine. It continues with practical ways of using this concept when necessary. Finally, it discusses 16 types of natural remedies or therapies you might like to consider using at home.

Part 3 explains the concept of integrated medicine and examines a wide range of complementary remedies and therapies.

Detailed explanation of each therapy

Cross-references to other therapies and warnings where it is inadvisable to use a particular therapy

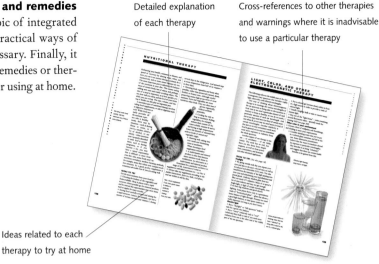

Ideas related to each therapy to try at home

PART 4

Common ailments begins by looking at how the various parts and systems of the body interrelate. This is followed by some guidelines on using natural treatments at home. The bulk of this part of the book is about how to treat common ailments. Under each heading there's an explanation of what the ailment is and what causes it (and, therefore, how you might go about preventing it). Various appropriate remedies and therapies are suggested, usually accompanied by reasons why or how they may help. There is also a short section on what else doctors may suggest, since doctors today often recommend natural remedies and therapies as well as more "medical" treatments.

Explanation and symptoms of each ailment

Treatment advice includes lifestyle changes, therapies, and remedies to use at home

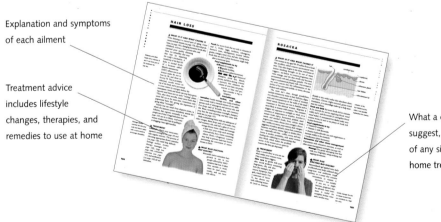

What a doctor may suggest, plus warnings of any side effects of home treatment

Part 4 contains comprehensive information on common ailments and lists a wide range of complementary treatments as well as advice on what doctors may suggest.

Finally, the book closes with an afterword, a glossary, further reading, useful addresses, and websites.

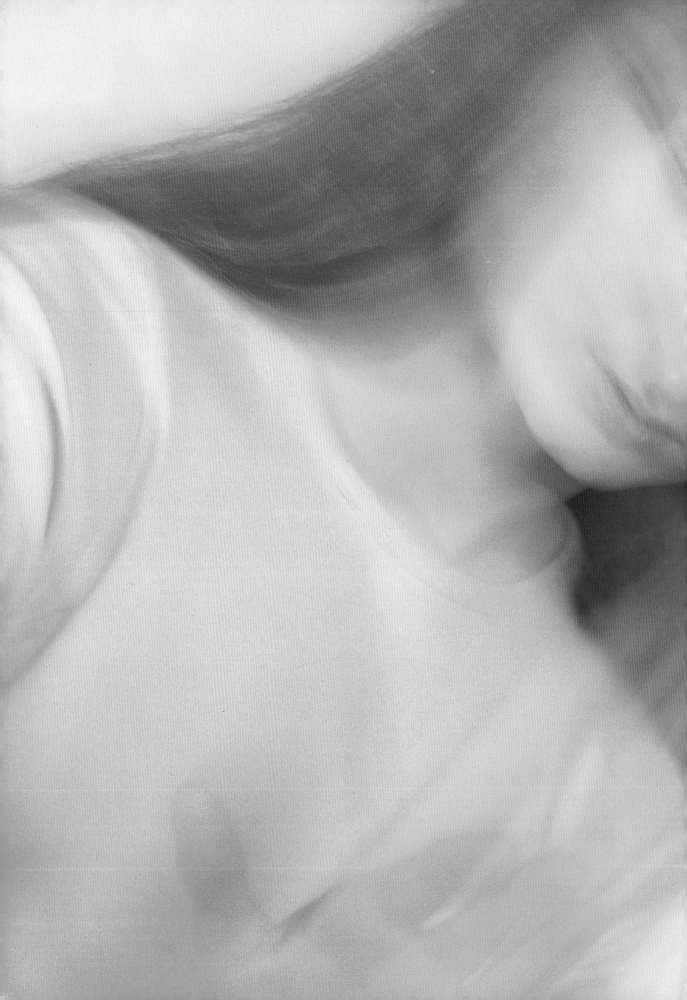

PART 1

Good Health

YOUR SURROUNDINGS, YOUR LIFESTYLE AND WHO YOU ARE.

AIR AND BREATHING

Breathing has a very special significance. Not only does it supply the oxygen we need and get rid of carbon dioxide, but it also enlivens and enriches us in other ways.

Ancient philosophers and physicians, and many alternative medical therapists today, see breath as the very "spirit" of our souls. Most people, when asked to say where they think their soul is, lay their hands on their chest. In fact, the two meanings of the word "inspiration" – what we do when we breathe in, and the experience of having a new idea – come from the concept of "–in–spirit–ation".

This "taking in of the spirit" makes breathing a symbolic activity that goes way beyond its physiological functions. And this is probably why it is so central to good health.

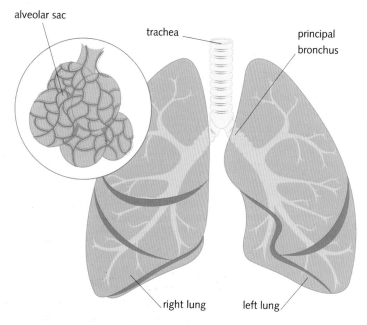

alveolar sac
trachea
principal bronchus
right lung
left lung

Air goes down the throat into the trachea, and from there into the lungs, through the bronchial tubes. Each of the tiny air sacs, or alveoli, is like a balloon surrounded by blood vessels. Blood extracts oxygen from the air and then carries it all around the body.

HOW YOU BREATHE

When you inhale, your chest expands and your diaphragm descends. Deep in your lungs, at the ends of the breathing passages, lie 800 million air sacs known as alveoli, each surrounded by a network of tiny blood vessels called capillaries. As each breath fills the sacs, oxygen passes into the bloodstream and then on to the heart, where it's pumped around the body. At the same time, carbon dioxide passes from the blood into the air sacs, ready to be exhaled.

When you breathe out, your chest and diaphragm return to their resting states, emptying carbon-dioxide-laden air from the sacs. Then the inspiration–expiration cycle starts again.

YOUR "BREATHING SIGNATURE"

A woman's basic breathing style can be thought of as her "breathing signature". Its nature depends on her health, emotional state, and behavioral habits. It can also be altered at will. You can identify your breathing signature by estimating how fast and how deeply you breathe.

Breathing rate Your breathing rate is simply the number of breaths you take each minute. One whole breath is one inhalation and one exhalation. The average young woman, breathing normally, takes 13–17 breaths a minute at rest. Some healthy people take as few as 11–12 breaths, and others ten or even fewer.

Several things make breathing faster, including exercise, emotion, pain, lung or heart disease, severe anemia, and shallow breathing. Excessively rapid breathing can result in hyperventilation (*see opposite page*).

Depth of breathing The average young woman, breathing normally, inhales approximately 400 milliliters (nearly three-quarters of a pint) of air with each breath. To estimate how deeply you breathe, put one hand on your upper chest and the other on your stomach:

◆ If you are breathing normally, with abdominal breathing (breathing "into your belly," *see opposite page*), your stomach hand moves slightly more than the chest one.

◆ If you are breathing deeply, the stomach hand moves much more than the chest one.

◆ If your breathing is shallow, the chest hand moves but the stomach one stays still.

BREATHING STYLE AND HEALTH

Inefficient breathing means you are breathing in a style inappropriate for your activity level and state of health. This can cause low spirits and poor health. And various states of health and emotional conditions can, in turn, influence breathing. So if you feel down or unwell, or simply want more energy, it may well be worth altering your breathing signature. You can override the autopilot in your brain's breathing control center and breathe more deeply or slowly whenever you want.

Breathing "into the belly" (abdominal breathing) This is what to aim for. It involves breathing relatively deeply so you expand the upper and lower parts of your lungs. Your diaphragm then presses on your abdominal organs and pushes out your stomach. All this encourages a healthy turnover of gases and stimulates good digestion. Deeper breaths allow you to inhale

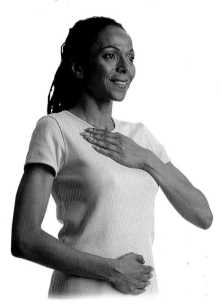

more oxygen and exhale more carbon dioxide when necessary. Indeed, vigorous exercise and strong emotion can trigger breaths up to ten times their size at rest.

Shallow breathing This is generally second best. Shallow breaths expand only the upper parts of the lungs. So in order to get enough oxygen, you have to breathe more rapidly. Emotion (especially anxiety and panic), wearing a tight bra or belt, pregnancy, indigestion, and lung or heart disease can all trigger shallow breathing. Breathing that is both shallow and rapid can cause problems because you may exhale too much carbon dioxide (*see Hyperventilation*).

HYPERVENTILATION

Feeling anxious, panicky, angry or otherwise emotional can make breathing excessively rapid and shallow (or, less often, excessively deep). This is known as hyperventilation. Less-common causes include untreated or poorly controlled diabetes (*see page 180*), kidney and lung disease, and the air hunger people experience at high altitudes.

You might think hyperventilation would guarantee plenty of oxygen, but it does the opposite. When we breathe very rapidly, we puff out so much carbon dioxide that our blood becomes alkaline. Being too alkaline isn't good because it means the cells can't get enough oxygen.

HYPERVENTILATION CAN LEAD TO ANY COMBINATION OF:

- Dizziness.
- Disorientation.
- Diarrhea.
- Pins and needles.
- Numb fingers or toes.
- Faintness.
- Chest pain.
- A racing heart.
- Stomachache.
- Headache.
- Fatigue.
- Tense, twitchy muscles.
- Gasping for air.
- Yawning.
- A feeling of dread.
- Panic attacks.
- Anxiety.

These feelings can be so worrying that they encourage even faster breathing. And it's suggested, though not proven, that hyperventilating encourages infections, allergies, obesity, arthritis, and nasal polyps. Practice breathing from the abdomen to improve your general wellbeing.

Inhale more oxygen with abdominal breathing.

WHAT TO DO IF YOU SUSPECT YOU ARE HYPERVENTILATING

1 Concentrate on breathing more slowly, through your nose, not your mouth.

2 Breathe into a paper bag, or your cupped hands, for two minutes. This increases your body's carbon-dioxide level.

3 Do some exercise so your muscles produce more carbon dioxide. Warning: Don't do this if you feel faint, as you might fall over! Later, practice breathing exercises and other effective ways of managing stress (*see page 141*).

POLLUTION

Despite legislation to control emissions from motor vehicles, this view over a polluted city indicates the problem caused when pollutants are kept close to the ground by atmospheric ozone.

Unless we live in the mountains, we all breathe air that is somewhat soiled by vehicle-exhaust and industrial fumes. Vehicle-exhaust pollutants include carbon monoxide, nitrogen oxides, lead, and particulates (tiny particles of hydrocarbons from diesel fuel). On sunny days, atmospheric ozone combines with these pollutants to form a "photochemical smog" that can make lung disease or heart disease worse.

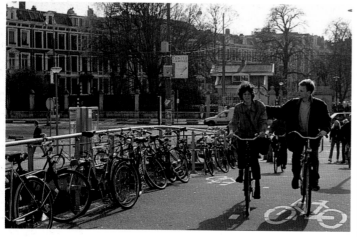

Smoke-free zones and car-free town centers are much less harmful to health. If more people abandoned four wheels in favor of two, the air around us would be much less polluted.

Fortunately, some countries are trying to clean up their polluted air. Laws can prohibit factories and power plants from belching filthy smoke, prevent drivers from running vehicles that generate excessive exhaust fumes, and limit the use of certain types of fuel.

But the bad news is that polluted air from nations that haven't yet curbed pollution are blown by the wind to other countries. The wind can also spread pesticides from farmers' sprays, and dioxins from incinerators that increase the risk of cancer and genetic mutation.

One of the prime indoor pollutants is cigarette smoke. Smoking pollutes air not just for smokers but also for those around them – the "passive smokers." Another source of indoor pollution is "out-gassing" (vaporization) from chemicals such as formaldehyde, wood preservatives, and anti-fungal pesticides in the materials from which buildings are made. This can continue for some weeks, months, or, in the case of certain chemicals, much longer.

HOW TO BREATHE CLEANER AIR:

◆ Live somewhere with cleaner air, even if this means commuting (ideally by public transport).
◆ Wear a mask outside when the air quality is poor if you have lung or heart disease, or have had a stroke or mini-stroke, or a blood clot in a leg vein (deep vein thrombosis) or in the lungs (pulmonary embolism).
◆ Close windows if the outside air is unpleasant.
◆ Open windows when cooking, painting, paint-stripping, sandpapering, gluing, soldering, welding, or heating with a kerosene heater.
◆ If you live on a busy road, consider growing a hedge or erecting a high fence, if possible, to exclude traffic fumes. Use curtains at windows to keep out airborne particles.
◆ Don't smoke – and try to avoid smoky environments. For example, when you fly, don't just choose a flight with a no-smoking section, because smoke readily travels all through the aircraft in the air-conditioning system. Instead, go for one with no smoking at all.
◆ Have some indoor plants. These can absorb pollutants and improve air quality a little bit. Among the most efficient are the coconut palm, weeping fig (*Ficus benjamina*), dracaena, spathiphyllum, gerbera, spider plants, and chrysanthemums.
◆ Support anti-pollution legislation.

AIR TEMPERATURE

Hot air Living in a hot climate and breathing warm air make asthma, bronchitis, and joint pain less likely. However, overheating can lead to nausea, headaches, convulsions and, at worst, a heart attack or stroke.

PROTECT YOURSELF BY:

◆ Going somewhere cooler (if possible).
◆ Drinking plenty.
◆ Taking in salt when lost by perspiration.
◆ Dressing appropriately.

Cold air Being inadequately protected from cold air encourages high blood pressure, heart attacks, strokes, asthma, chilblains, hypothermia, and frostbite. However, many people find cold air invigorating.

PROTECT YOURSELF BY:

◆ Dressing appropriately, with several layers.
◆ Remembering a hat, scarf, gloves, and good, insulating footwear when going out, even for a minute. Wind the scarf around your mouth and nose to warm the air you breathe.
◆ Having hot food and hot drinks.
◆ Asking friends, neighbors, community or governmental organizations for help if heating costs are a problem.

AIR HUMIDITY

Wet air Breathing cold, humid air exacerbates bronchitis, whereas breathing hot, humid air makes some people exhausted, though it often reduces asthma and croup.

PROTECT YOURSELF FROM BRONCHITIS BY:

◆ Staying in on cold, foggy, or misty days.
◆ If it's hot and humid, going somewhere with a bit of breeze (such as coastal or high land), or using a fan or air conditioning.

Dry air Breathing dry air encourages hay fever and pollen-sensitive asthma (*see Allergens below*). Hot, dry air promotes ozone formation, which irritates the lungs. Air conditioning dehumidifies hot moist air. When you breathe dried air, you lose more moisture from your lungs. This means you must drink more to combat dehydration. You can help your exposed skin retain its moisture by smoothing in a little oil or cream.

A potential hazard of breathing air cooled by a poorly maintained air-conditioning system is the (extremely low) risk of contracting the unusual bacterial pneumonia Legionnaires' Disease.

PROTECT YOURSELF INDOORS WITH:

◆ An electric humidifier.
◆ Bowls of water near heaters.
◆ Plenty of well-watered houseplants.

AIR PRESSURE

Low pressure A sudden fall in barometric pressure can trigger asthma. It can also make accidents more likely by slowing reaction times. And in-flight pressure changes can trigger earache, especially if you have a cold.

If you do have a cold, and have to fly, protect yourself from cabin-pressure changes by swallowing frequently, and sniffing the decongestant vapor from a couple of drops of eucalyptus and peppermint oils on a tissue. If you feel your ears blocking, breathe in, pinch your nose and close your mouth, then, while attempting to exhale press your tongue hard against the back of your palate. This will make your ears "pop" as your congested Eustachian tubes open and allow the air pressures in your middle ear and throat to equalize. As an aircraft climbs, the air pressure inside the cabin falls. Pressurization helps counteract this fall, but the pressure is still relatively low.

If you suffer from heart disease or from a lung disease such as chronic bronchitis, you may find that you need to breathe faster or more deeply when you are flying, so that you get enough oxygen and feel comfortable.

High altitude Traveling from a low-lying area to a mountainous area can cause nausea and breathlessness. This unpleasant condition is called altitude sickness.

Avoid altitude sickness by taking plenty of time over your climb. This allows your bone marrow to make extra red blood cells so the blood can extract oxygen more efficiently from the thin air.

POSITIVE AND NEGATIVE IONS

Air contains tiny particles called ions that carry positive or negative electrical charges. Inhaling too many positive ions can make you tired, nauseated and headachy. Several things encourage a high positive-ion concentration. These include dry, hot, stale air; air conditioning; central heating; cigarette smoke and other air pollutants; dust; thunderstorms; natural hot winds; and electromagnetic fields from electrical appliances.

GUARD AGAINST POSITIVE-ION ATTACK BY:

◆ Getting fresh air – for example, by opening windows whenever possible.
◆ Keeping air as dust-free as possible, because floating dust attracts positive ions.
◆ Using an electrical ionizer to raise the negative-ion concentration.

ALLERGENS

There are certain airborne substances, such as house dust mites' droppings and pollen, which can trigger an allergic reaction when inhaled by susceptible individuals. (*See page 167 for ways of minimizing exposure.*)

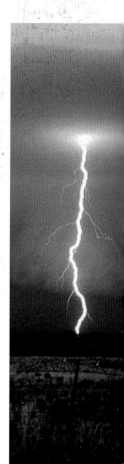

Air contains particles with positive or negative electrical charges. Lightning is a massive electrical discharge.

LIGHT, COLOR, AND OTHER ELECTROMAGNETIC INPUTS

The range of rays of different wavelengths that comes from the sun, outer space, and some man-made equipment is called the electromagnetic spectrum.

This spectrum includes cosmic rays, gamma rays, X-rays, ultraviolet (UV) rays, visible light rays, infrared rays, microwaves, radio waves, and certain very long waves. These rays can be either good or bad for us depending on their intensity and balance.

The seven colors of visible light are clear in the rainbow in the photograph on the right and in the diagram below. The diagram also shows invisible light rays.

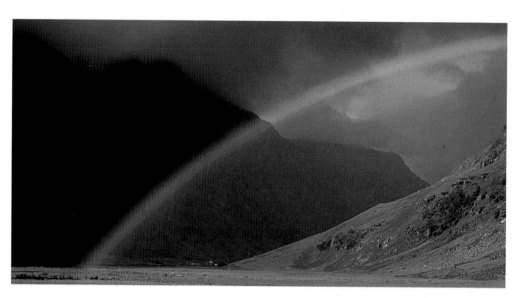

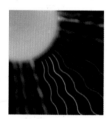

INVISIBLE LIGHT:

- cosmic rays
- gamma rays
- X-rays
- far ultraviolet
- mid and near ultraviolet
- shortwave infrared
- infrared
- radio waves
- power frequency waves

BENEFITS OF VISIBLE LIGHT, UV LIGHT, AND INFRARED RADIATION

Visible light Light consists of red, orange, yellow, green, blue, indigo, and violet rays. It can come from electricity, explosions, lightning, fire, and far-flung stars. But most, of course, comes from our nearest star – the sun.

Daylight (white or "full-spectrum" light) has healing powers, as do its colored and UV rays *(see below)*. Light acts both on the skin and, via eye exposure, on the brain.

Intense white light, whether from sunlight or an artificial source, affects hormones, emotions, behavior, and appetite. Light helps the body produce estrogen, encourages fertility, and discourages SAD (Seasonal Affective Disorder or winter depression, *see page 202*). The different colors of the rays that make up the "white" light from the sun have particular benefits *(see page 18)*. Indeed, so powerful and far-reaching are the effects of light on our health and wellbeing that it's sometimes called "the medicine of the future."

BENEFIT FROM DAYLIGHT BY:

◆ Going outside for half an hour or so each day. There is no need to uncover your body – the light on your face and in your eyes is enough.

◆ In winter in relatively northerly locations, going outside around noon, when the light is most intense.

◆ Taking a whole-body light bath sometimes (though don't get burnt in direct sunlight).

◆ Being outside as much of the day as possible when you've traveled across time zones. Daylight helps reset your body clock which, in turn, helps prevent jet lag.

Ultraviolet (UV) rays Maximum UV-light exposure comes from being outside on sunny, cloud-free days in summer around noon, although we do get some UV even on cloudy days.

UV light enables the skin to manufacture vitamin D, needed for calcium to enter bones. This is why people who don't get enough daylight on their skin (or vitamin D in their diet) may develop rickets. Dark-skinned children living in very

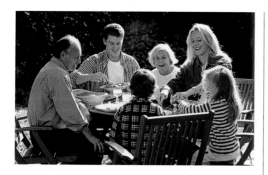

northerly (or southerly) climes are particularly at risk, and may need vitamin D supplements.

Ultraviolet light has other benefits too. For example, UV therapy reduces jaundice in newborns. And dermatologists use light-sensitizing psoralen drugs together with UV therapy for severe psoriasis (*see page 150*) and eczema (*see page 149*). You can gently copy this at home by eating natural psoralens (found in many vegetables and fruits, especially celery, parsnips, peas, parsley, and citrus fruits), and going outside to expose yourself carefully to unfiltered daylight (light that hasn't had to pass through window glass, which blocks out some UV rays).

Infrared rays This sort of radiation provides heat, which is why sunlight warms us during the day, and helps to prevent aching muscles. An infrared lamp can also ease sore, aching muscles.

SUNLIGHT AND THE SKIN – CAUTIONS AND PROTECTION

Clouds, fog, and air pollution diminish the amount of white and UV light, and alter the color balance (proportions of different colors) of white light.

The angle of the sun changes with the time of day and your distance from the equator. This alters the nature of the sunlight you receive. The further you are from the equator, the more slanted are the sun's rays, the further they have to travel through the atmosphere, and the more blue and UV light is lost. This is why the nearer the equator you are, the more likely you are to burn.

Excessive UV exposure causes sunburn, speeds skin aging, and increases the risk of skin cancer. Both malignant melanoma and non-melanoma cancers (squamous cell carcinomas, and rodent ulcers – or basal cell carcinomas) are becoming more common.

SEE YOUR DOCTOR IF A MOLE:

◆ Enlarges.
◆ Develops an irregular border.

◆ Measures more than 7mm (¼in) across.
◆ Darkens or becomes multicolored.
◆ Itches.
◆ Becomes inflamed.
◆ Bleeds.
◆ Crusts or scabs.
◆ Develops satellite moles.

If you notice any of these symptoms, visit a dermatologist, have the mole removed, and receive further treatment if required.

Protecting your skin from outside Most experts agree that any sunburn is bad (and some say it's safer not to tan at all). So it makes sense to protect your skin from too much sun. Even if you tan carefully, brown skin gives little protection against UV. Tanned skin is thick and colored, but not particularly UV-resistant.

Better, then, to avoid sun exposure between 11a.m. and 3p.m.; to use any available shade; to cover up with a sun hat, sunglasses, and clothing; and to buy a suitable sunscreen (factor 15 or higher). Choose a sunscreen containing beta carotene and vitamin E as these antioxidants help protect against the damaging effects of UV light. Surprisingly, white or other light-colored cotton clothing is less protective than navy or red clothing made of polyester or nylon, with Lycra. You can now buy clothes with a scientifically validated sun-protection factor.

CAUTION

◆ Don't rely on a sunscreen to protect you. Even if you don't burn, certain UV rays (UVA) can encourage aging and other skin damage.
◆ Avoid sun-beds; studies show that UVA encourages skin cancer and premature aging.

Protecting your skin from within Eating fruit and vegetables helps counteract sun damage because they contain naturally occurring antioxidants such as vitamins C and E, and beta carotene. Antioxidants are useful because they protect the skin against UV-triggered chemical reactions called oxidation. This oxidation produces substances called free radicals that can disrupt genes, burn the skin, and damage the collagen in the elastic fibers that make skin resilient and strong and keep it looking young. Taking an antioxidant supplement may provide additional protection.

FAR LEFT: Good food, good company, and warm sunlight all contribute to wellbeing.

Always take care not to burn your skin, especially if you are fair. The fairer you are the more vigilance is required.

Blueberries – like most other berries – are rich in antioxidant properties.

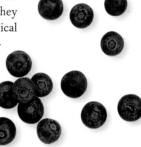

COLOR AND HEALTH

Light varies enormously in its color balance. For example, bright sunlight on a clear day at the equator is virtually pure white light. Cloud-filtered sunlight leans toward the red end of the spectrum, because cloud filters out some blue and UV light . Electric light from standard household (incandescent) bulbs comes in various color balances. The light from most fluorescent tubes is relatively blue, though you can buy tubes that give off "warmer" – redder – light, as well as "full-spectrum" tubes whose color balance is closer to that of mid-day sunlight on a clear day.

The color balance of light can affect our health and wellbeing (*see also page 129*).

Laser light Lasers are artificially induced intense beams of colored light from irradiated gas, colored liquid, or crystals such as rubies. They are used medically as scalpels in cosmetic surgery and in operations for cataracts, short sight, snoring, fibroids, and cervical cancer.

In the treatment known as photodynamic therapy, a person with cancer is treated with a light-sensitive dye that is preferentially taken up by their cancer cells. The dye-soaked cancer is sensitive to red light, so can be destroyed with a red laser beam directed through a fiber-optic tube inserted into the body. This has echoes of PUVA treatment for psoriasis (*see page 150*), and signals the possibility that eating combinations of various

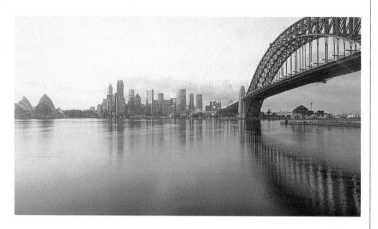

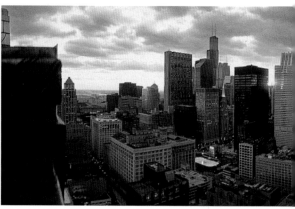

Exposure to light affects our moods. Early morning light is a warm, stimulating light. Evening light (above right) is a blue, calming light and thought to promote relaxation.

Red light This is "warm" and scientists say it raises low blood pressure, quickens the heart rate, and may promote energy. For this reason, exposure to early morning light, which is relatively red, may help prepare you to start the day. Red light therapy can also help relieve the symptoms of the premenstrual syndrome (*see page 186*). However, red light makes some people feel irritable.

Blue and green light These "cool" colors have been shown to be calming and to reduce the blood pressure. Because evening light is bluish, the twilight of the day tends to be a calming time – a time for winding down and relaxing before the night.

Spectacle lenses Researchers have found that wearing glasses with lenses of a particular color sometimes helps counteract dyslexia, epilepsy, behavioral problems, and migraine. This, they suggest, is due to changes in the type of stimulation received by the brain when colored lenses filter out certain colors from light. The color needed varies from one person to another, and each individual needs to choose the precise hue that helps them most.

flavonoids (plant pigments) in fruit and vegetables, plus exposing our body to light of a particular color, could have as yet unknown healing effects.

Colors in the environment Of course most things in the world around us are colored. Simply looking at them means we receive colored light. This may explain why certain items and their color can have such profound effects on how we feel.

Some people wear spectacles with red-tinted lenses to improve mood and treat certain physical and psychological conditions.

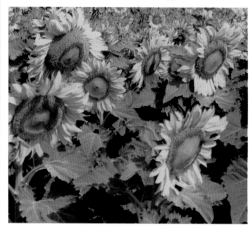

ELECTROMAGNETIC FIELDS

The Earth acts as a magnet and is surrounded by its own weak electro magnetic field. Particles in magnetizable substances align themselves within the Earth's field so their north poles point to the Earth's South Pole, and vice versa. Moving such a substance generates an electric current.

There are many other electromagnetic fields (emfs) around us, including those generated by TVs, computers, halogen light transformers, electric wiring, radiators, blankets and clocks. Outdoor electrical installations, including high-voltage power lines, also create emfs. Household electrical appliances and wiring sometimes produce emfs whose magnitude is comparable

your face the positive ones. This can encourage skin and eye irritation.

Until the effects of emfs are clearer, you might like to take some precautions.

AVOIDING EMFS

◆ Sit further than 2m (6ft) from your TV screen, because the strength of an emf decreases rapidly the further away you are from its source.
◆ Work at a computer screen in shorter rather than longer bursts.

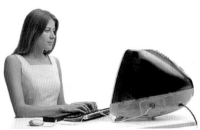

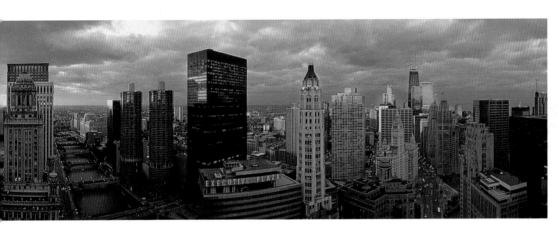

ABOVE: If you cannot avoid sitting at your computer for long periods of time, at least make sure you take a five-minute break every hour.

to those formed in the surrounding area by high-voltage power lines.

We are all exposed to the Earth's emf, and this and other emfs around us create small currents in our bodies by affecting our iron and other magnetizable substances. Within limits this is normal. But overexposure to certain emfs may prove harmful. Researchers continue to investigate the suspicion that headaches, depression, fatigue, leukemia, and lowered fertility and immunity can result from living within the emf created by a nearby high-voltage power line, or from spending too much time within the fields from electrical appliances indoors.

One problem that is fully accepted comes from the large positive charge (20,000 volts) on the inside of a TV or computer screen. Your body's electrical charge as you sit at the screen is virtually nil. So the difference between your charge and that of the screen creates a large field of static electricity. Dust particles in the air can be positively or negatively charged. And because of the field of static, the screen attracts the negative ions, and

◆ Splash your face with water between sessions at the screen in order to discourage positive ions from settling.
◆ Discourage positive ions by opening windows, clearing away dust from your work area, and using a negative ionizer (*see page 15*).
◆ Don't be fooled into buying a "low radiation" monitor; this doesn't reduce the levels of extremely low and very low frequency emfs.
◆ When working in an office with several computers, don't sit close to the side of any monitor or processor as the emf is more intense here.
◆ Turn off electrical appliances when not in use.
◆ Don't keep an electric blanket on all night.
◆ Don't sleep with an electric clock too close to you.
◆ Consider measuring the emfs where you spend a lot of time, such as at your desk, where you sit in the sitting room, and in bed. In some countries you can buy or hire an emf monitor. Alternatively, ask someone from an electricity company to do the measuring.

YOUR HOME ENVIRONMENT

Try to create surroundings that make you comfortable, happy, and well.

You may have a whole house or workplace to decorate, or simply one room. Or you may need to share the decision-making about your surroundings with someone else. But however much input you have, choosing furniture and furnishings to make the place more attractive and comfortable can lift your spirits and be a joy to you and others. Another pleasure is the creativity involved in making your surroundings fit your needs and reflect your personality, aspirations, and interests.

Collect swatches and try out paint samples before decorating, to be sure you choose colors that set the desired mood in each room.

DECOR

Have you ever wondered why, when entering a room for the first time, you might fall in love with it? One reason may be that the style and colors of the walls, furniture, floor covering, and soft furnishings evoke memories of times that were happy in some way. Another is that you instinctively like the color scheme because the colors meet some physical or mental need. On the other hand, it may evoke negative emotions.

When you enter a room one of several things can happen, depending on your physical and emotional state.

WARM-COLORED ROOMS IN RED, ORANGE, OR TERRACOTTA

◆ If you feel tired, dull, and energy-sapped, these colors might energize and excite you and make you feel brighter and better, because they have a generally stimulating effect on the heart, arteries, and brain.

◆ However, if you feel overwrought, stressed out, irritable, or angry, you could feel worse, because warm colors can foster feelings of irritation, tension, and aggression.

◆ If you are unconsciously angry or anxious deep inside, you might be attracted by the color because it seems to fit your state. Or it might bring your feelings to the surface. This could be beneficial because an emotion out in the open is no longer as likely to lead to displacement behavior such as binge-eating, drinking too much, or blaming others for what's really only to do with you.

COOL-COLORED ROOMS DECORATED IN GREEN, BLUE, OR GRAY

◆ If you feel excited, anxious, stressed, irritable, or angry, these colors might be calming, because they tend to have relaxing effects on the heart, arteries, and brain.

◆ However, if you feel tired and lethargic, these colors might make you feel worse still, because they sometimes encourage sleepiness, depression and fatigue.

◆ If you're depressed without knowing it, cool colors might attract you. Or they might bring your feelings to the surface. This could be beneficial because once out in the open, an emotion is no longer as likely to lead to negative thoughts or behaviors.

HEATING, VENTILATION, AND HUMIDITY

We all have to adjust the temperatures of our indoor living and working environments sometimes, depending on the climate, prevailing weather conditions, and our health and activity levels. Heating advisers – motivated by a desire to save money – always recommend preventing heat loss by using good insulation. However, draft-proofing too efficiently can also harm your health. We all need fresh air, but the air inside a well-insulated modern home can become stale, lacking in oxygen and over-filled with carbon dioxide.

Ventilation You can avoid this problem with adequate ventilation. Window vents are one possibility, or you can open the windows to allow fresh air to circulate. Another idea is to have plenty of indoor plants. These use up carbon dioxide as they photosynthesize. Ventilation is especially vital in kitchens and bathrooms. If you have a warm room that isn't ventilated properly, then besides breathing stale air, you lay yourself open to two potentially serious problems.

The first is that moist, warm air encourages molds to grow. This includes molds on walls, as well as wet and dry rot in the building's structural woodwork. Fungal growth can be treated with antifungal products, such as those in various wood preservatives. But then the chemical vaporizes or "out-gasses." This means you breathe pesticide-contaminated air which, depending on the particular product, may not be too healthy (*see page 22*). It is far better to ventilate your home more effectively than to save money on heating and run the risk of illness, unless you are able to leave home for several days when the out-gassing is at its worst.

The second problem is that warm, moist air creates ideal conditions for house dust mites to breed. These can trigger asthma (*see page 167*) and eczema (*see page 149*).

Heating Electric heating appliances create electromagnetic fields that extend a foot or so around each one. And there is now some concern that sleeping, sitting, or working within range of one of these emfs for too long could be risky (*see page 14*).

Have your gas-fired central heating or individual gas fires serviced each year. Otherwise there is the chance that faulty combustion will release carbon monoxide. This can be fatal – the risk is greater if your accommodation is poorly ventilated. Put your mind at rest by buying a carbon-monoxide monitor that indicates unsafe levels. Paraffin fires are rarely used these days, but if you do have one, always check that it can't be tipped over.

Lastly, an open coal or log fire is attractive and cheering, but a guard is essential if you are out of the room even for a very short time, or if you have young children or anyone frail around.

Leafy, green plants may be useful for improving the quality of air in the home.

BELOW LEFT: The easiest way to introduce ventilation into a room is to open the window and let in fresh air.

BELOW: A well-ventilated open fire creates a cozy glow and is less drying than electric or even gas central heating.

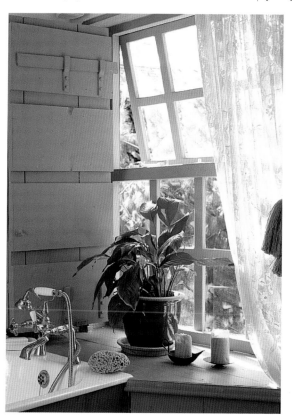

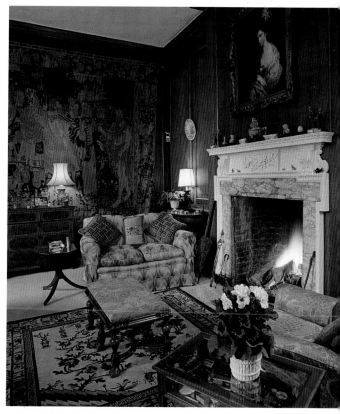

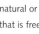

Avoid hazardous chemicals and use a natural or organic paint that is free from PCPs.

AVOIDABLE HAZARDS

Increasing numbers of women are becoming involved in large-scale home-improvement projects to enhance or maintain their homes. But before beginning, it's worth taking steps to avoid the potential health hazards.

Paints Chemicals such as vinyl molecules and fungicides vaporize ("out-gas") from dry paint for weeks. One fungicide in paint, an organochlorine called pentachlorophenol (PCP), is banned from indoor use in the USA and some other countries, as it has been linked with cancer and damage to liver, nerves, and immunity. Keep windows open while painting and for several days afterward. Don't put fresh paint in rooms a baby or young child uses. Consider using a natural or organic paint that is free from potentially hazardous chemicals, especially in children's rooms.

Particle boards Chipboard and medium-density fiber-board (MDF) can contain urea formaldehyde resin which vaporizes for years. With prolonged or excessive exposure, one in five people develops problems such as a rash, sore eyes, respiratory irritation, headaches, depression, memory loss, and dizziness. This resin is banned in some countries (including Canada and many US states). If available, consider using wood or some other material instead. If you must use particle board, wear a mask when cutting, drilling, or sanding.

Wood preservatives Many wood preservatives contain pesticides – insecticides (for woodworm and death-watch beetle) and fungicides (for wet and dry rot). These out-gas for a long time. Some – lindane, tributyltin oxide, and PCP – are banned in many countries because of possible links with asthma and cancer. If they aren't banned where you live, check the label so you can avoid them. Alternatives to pesticides, such

Goggles and a mask protect the face from the resins in particle boards.

as improving ventilation in a loft that has fungal rot, are very successful.

Floor tile or carpet glue Having floor tiles stuck down with a petroleum-based or other synthetic adhesive means you will inhale toxic vapor for months. This has echoes of glue sniffing and has been linked with sudden death and cancer. Choose white, latex-based adhesives instead.

Asbestos This must be professionally removed because inhaled fibers can cause lung cancer.

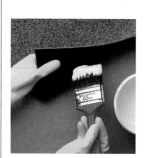

Latex-based adhesives are the safest choice when carrying out such jobs as gluing carpet tiles. Using petroleum-based adhesive means you inhale toxic vapor.

COMMON
PREVENTABLE SAFETY HAZARDS
Take yourself on a home inspection tour
to check for these:
◆ Trailing electric appliance cords (buy
curled ones instead).
◆ Unsecured rugs, especially at the
bottom of the stairs
(add a non-slip backing).
◆ Loose or frayed stair carpet
(repair or replace).
◆ Too high a setting for hot water,
especially with someone very old, young,
or frail around (turn down the
thermostat).
◆ Loose plugs or damaged wiring to
electric appliances (repair or replace).
◆ Overloaded sockets (disconnect some
appliances, or use a plug board).
◆ A slippery kitchen or bathroom floor
(use a non-slip mat or install a
non-slip floor).
◆ The absence of smoke alarms and a
fire extinguisher or blanket (get your
home prepared).
◆ Time-expired medicines, natural
remedies, and vitamins and other
supplements (throw them away).

HOSPITALITY AND SOLITUDE

Having visitors Welcoming others into your home promotes a feeling of wellbeing. It offers opportunities for shared meals, conversation, empathic listening, challenges, and encouragement. It can bring excitement and vitality, the sharing of irritations, woes and other difficulties, the exchange of ideas and energy, and increased levels of friendship and intimacy.

Good hospitality is more about making visitors feel welcome and warm inside than filling them with food and drink, though these too play their part. Aim for guests to leave feeling better than when they arrived. If you think about what makes you feel happy and at ease when you visit someone, you'll probably find it's about being listened to and encouraged, as much as having your creature comforts catered for.

Being alone Home should also provide a sanctuary – somewhere you can do what you want and find opportunities for relaxation and inspiration. Of course, if you share your home with others, they need sanctuary too, in which case your special place may simply be a room, such as your bedroom or even part of a room. Some people make their beds their sanctuaries. But if even this is impossible because you share your bed, consider arranging a "time-share;" somewhere in your home you can have to yourself for a while each day.

Having said all this, some people who live in overcrowded conditions may be able to do without physical solitude. Instead, they find ways of contacting a still, quiet place in their minds, far away from the noise and bustle around them. This is a valuable skill for us all, whatever our domestic circumstances. If you'd like to learn how to do this, there are some tips on *page 142*.

Solitude provides time to think of the past, present, and future. Some people concentrate so hard on the past or present that they never look ahead; others think only of what they hope to do one day, and so can't enjoy the present. Next time you're alone and quiet, think for a while about the balance of the past, present, and future in your thoughts and daydreams.

CONSIDER, FOR EXAMPLE, WHETHER YOU NEED TO USE YOUR QUIET TIME TO:

◆ Reflect and learn from the events of the day. This can seal precious memories into your mind and lets you begin to find ways of dealing with problems or challenges.

◆ Be aware of the present moment – especially if you feel stressed and want to relax body, mind, or spirit. Many relaxation exercises (*see page 141*) encourage awareness of the here-and-now as an essential part of recognizing physical and emotional tension.

◆ Think about the future – about enhancing relationships, building on new ideas, meeting challenges, or simply enjoying the prospect of things to come.

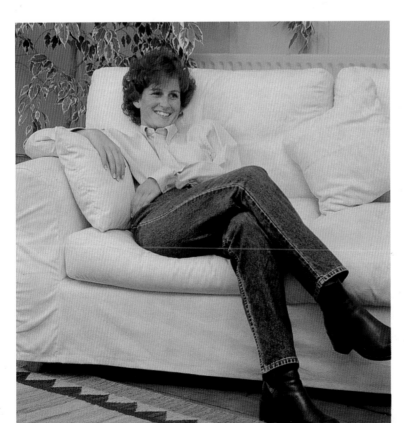

Your home should be a comfortable and peaceful place where you can feel at ease either when relaxing on your own or when entertaining visitors.

FOOD AND DRINK

Food may be the fuel of life, but the nourishment we obtain from food and drink varies enormously from one individual to another. Part of this is simply down to which kinds of foods we choose.

One determinant of our choice is our childhood experience of family food. Another is what's available at home – and if you do the shopping, this will depend on your taste, nutritional know-how, and willpower. Magazines and TV also play a big role in our awareness of food, recipes, and healthy eating. But what exactly is healthy eating?

Over the years food fads and scares have come and gone – and will doubtless continue to do so. Behind the scenes, though, researchers continue with the job of linking health and illness with people's lifestyles. And we now know for sure that what we eat makes a major contribution to our health – or lack of it.

Instead of reaching for chocolate, try a slice of juicy mango when you feel in need of a sweet snack. It is a delicious way to take one of the five daily fruit and vegetable portions that are recommended for a healthy diet.

SOME HEALTHY EATING GUIDELINES

It's important to gear your food intake to your activity level, and to eat a wide variety of wholefoods to get all the nutrients your body needs.

EACH DAY AIM FOR:

◆ At least five – or even up to nine – helpings of vegetables, salads, and fruit. Remember to have some beans, peas, or other foods rich in plant hormones (*see opposite page*) several times a week.
◆ Six to eleven servings of complex carbohydrates (*see opposite page*).
◆ A relatively small amount of protein (which can be animal or vegetable).
◆ A little fat (with a particular balance of saturated and unsaturated fats, and some essential fatty acids, *see opposite page*).
Each week aim to fit in three servings of oily fish (such as herrings, sardines, salmon, and pilchards). If you don't eat fish, be particularly careful to balance your intake of essential fatty acids.

But good nutrition isn't only about choosing food wisely to provide the nutrients you need. It's also about good digestion – and that's where the art of eating well comes in (*see page 26*).

VEGETARIAN AND VEGAN DIETS

A vegetarian diet (with foods of plant origin, plus eggs and dairy foods – milk, cheese, butter, and yogurt) or a vegan diet (with foods of plant origin only) can be as nutritious as that of an omnivore – someone who eats all types of foods. But vegetarians and vegans need to be be especially careful to eat enough foods rich in iron and vitamin B12, and to top up their vitamin B12 intake with a regular supplement if necessary.

INTERPRETING FOOD CRAVINGS

If you frequently crave certain foods, or food in general, something is wrong. Your body may be attempting to correct its nutritional balance because you've been eating badly. Alternatively, you may have a food sensitivity, anemia, or a tendency to a low blood-sugar level. Of course, another possibility to consider is that you might be pregnant.

FOODS AND NUTRIENTS

You'll find certain nutrients mentioned throughout the book. The following lists indicate which foods are rich in which nutrients:

Protein Meat; fish; eggs; dairy products (milk, cheese, yogurt); peas; beans (and bean products such as tofu and soy milk).

Carbohydrates There are two main groups. Simple carbohydrates are sugars – fruits; vegetables; honey. Complex carbohydrates consist of starches – root vegetables; cereal grains (wheat, oats, barley, rye, corn); rice; bananas – and fiber (or non-starch polysaccharides, which aren't absorbed, but are vital for health) – fruit; vegetables; wholegrain foods; brown rice.

Fats Less than a third of the calories you eat each day should come from fats. And less than a third of the calories you get from fat should be from saturated fats. Saturated fats are found in meat; eggs; dairy products; most margarines; white cooking fats; coconut oil.

Certain unsaturated fats are called essential fatty acids; these are the "parents" of two groups of long-chain polyunsaturated fatty acids, "PUFAs," the omega-6s and the omega-3s. Linoleic acid, an omega-6 PUFA, is found in avocados; beans; seeds; all corn; seed oils. Alpha-linolenic acid, an omega-3 PUFA, is found in green leafy vegetables; broccoli; beans; walnuts and their oil; pumpkin seeds, and linseeds (flaxseeds – the richest source); wheatgerm in wholegrains; canola (rapeseed) oil. We need only three times as much of the parent omega-6 PUFA, alpha-linolenic acid (ALA), as we do of the parent omega-3 PUFA, linoleic acid, yet most of us eat very much more than this. Oily fish contain certain other omega-3 PUFAs that are essential only for the few people unable to produce them from the "parent" omega-3 PUFA, alpha-linolenic acid.

Monounsaturated fats are found in olives; avocados; almonds; hazelnuts; peanuts; pistachios; sesame seeds; and their oils.

Calcium Canned sardines or salmon eaten with their bones; shellfish; dairy products; eggs; beans; peas; lentils; nuts; seeds; wholegrain foods.

Iodine Fish; dairy products; eggs; fruit; vegetables other than the cabbage family; seaweed; wholegrain foods.

Iron Meat; shellfish; egg yolk; green leafy vegetables; elderberries; beans; peas; nuts; seeds; wholegrain foods.

Selenium Meat; fish; dairy products; egg yolk; green leafy vegetables; mushrooms; garlic; beans; peas; wholegrain foods.

Magnesium Meat; fish; eggs; green leafy vegetables; mushrooms; beans; peas; nuts; seeds; wholegrain foods.

Chromium Shellfish; dairy products; wholegrain foods.

Sulfur Meat; fish; dairy products; garlic; onions; beans; peas; wholegrain foods.

Zinc Meat; dairy products; fish; root vegetables; beans; peas; garlic; nuts; seeds; wholegrain foods.

Vitamin A and beta carotene (used by the body to make vitamin A) Fish; dairy products; eggs; many fruits and vegetables, especially orange and red ones.

Vitamin B Meat; fish; dairy products (B2, B3, B12); eggs (B1, B2); beans and peas (B1, B3, B6); green leafy vegetables (B2, B6); mushrooms (B1, B2, B3, B6); nuts and seeds (B1, B2, B3, B6); wholegrain foods (B1, B2, B3, B6).

Folic acid Dairy products; eggs; nuts; fruit; vegetables, especially green leafy ones; beans; peas; wholegrain foods.

Vitamin C Fruit, especially citrus; vegetables.

Vitamin D Oily fish; dairy products; nuts; cold-pressed vegetable oils. However, the main source is from sunlight on the skin.

Vitamin E Meat; fish; dairy products; eggs; green leafy vegetables; beans; peas; nuts; seeds; wholegrain foods.

Vitamin K Liver; egg yolk; green leafy vegetables; cauliflower; turnips; beans; wholegrain foods.

Flavonoids Plant pigments in all colored fruits and vegetables.

Plant hormones Bean sprouts; fennel; celery; parsley; beans; peas; lentils; chickpeas (garbanzo beans); wholegrain foods; seeds; potatoes; carrots; beets; cabbage; garlic; sage; beer; cherries; plums; rhubarb; olives. Other vegetables and fruits contain smaller amounts of plant hormones.

Salicylates Many fruits (especially their peels) and vegetables; seeds; nuts.

FOOD SUPPLEMENTS

There is a great deal of hype surrounding food supplements, though reliable evidence for the benefits is often scanty. If you aren't eating a well-balanced diet, it may be worth taking a daily multimineral and vitamin supplement and, perhaps, fish oil. Certain supplements help with particular conditions or at certain times of life; these are discussed in the relevant sections of this book.

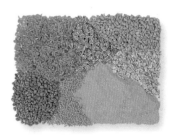

Pulses (legumes) provide protein and fiber.

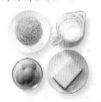

Fish provide protein, minerals, and vitamins A, B, D, and E.

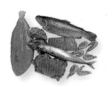

Saturated fats are found in eggs and dairy produce.

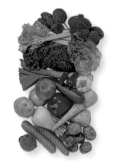

All vegetables provide vitamins, minerals, and fiber.

Fruits are high in vitamins, especially vitamin C and, in many, beta carotene.

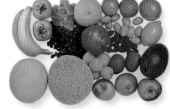

25

FOOD SHOPPING

There are two golden guidelines to consider when shopping for food:

◆ Try not to shop when you're very hungry unless you have plenty of willpower. Many women find it all too easy to load candy, cookies, or chips into their cart when they're hungry. If they then snack on the way home, they may not have enough room for a more nutritious meal later.

◆ Help yourself choose a balanced diet by selecting vegetables, salad, and fruit first. Progress to the bakery counter for bread, and to the home-baking or other aisle for nuts, seeds, and dried fruit. Then look for dried or canned beans. Choose your meat and fish, eggs, and dairy food. Add some frozen food if you want. And only then select less nutritious "extras."

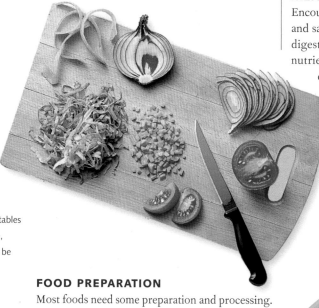

Buy fruit and vegetables as fresh as possible, preferably daily, to be sure of the highest possible nutritional value. Even better, grow your own.

FOOD PREPARATION

Most foods need some preparation and processing. Even something as simple as an apple, for example, is best washed first. Nowadays many of us buy ready-to-cook or even precooked, chilled dishes some of the time. And a few people live off them. However, there can be a lot of pleasure in peeling, chopping, and mixing food if you have the time and inclination. Preparing food for yourself and your family or friends also means you know what you're getting.

Choose fresh vegetables when possible; canning destroys up to half their folic acid, and vegetables blanched before being frozen can lose a quarter of their vitamin C. Aim to eat some raw vegetables in a salad or as vegetable stick nibbles every day. When you cook vegetables or fruit, peel them only just

A seasonal salad of mixed raw vegetables and greens is filling and healthy.

beforehand. This prevents enzymes released by cutting from destroying too much vitamin C. Cook them for as short a time as possible to preserve their vitamins B12 and C, and folic acid. Use the water in which you've cooked vegetables for making sauce, gravy, or soup.

It's best to deep-fry only infrequently, and not to reuse fat. Overheating produces trans fats — ones that behave like saturated fats.

EATING WELL

Eating can be one of life's great pleasures, but if you stuff yourself on the run because you're stressed or busy, you'll lose out on a lot of benefits. Respect your body and food by making time to prepare nourishing meals and to enjoy eating well.

MEALTIMES

Encourage relaxed mealtimes so you can eat slowly and savor the taste of your food. This encourages digestive juices to flow and helps you absorb nutrients. Mealtimes are not the best of times to discuss stressful topics, but can be excellent occasions to share news with family and friends and relax together. Children who eat meals sitting down at the table with their family are more likely to eat better and develop better manners and social skills. It also gives you all a chance to talk and to be listened to.

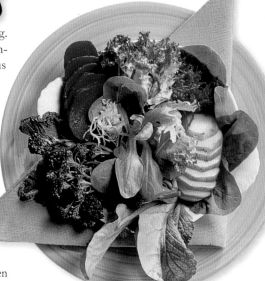

BODY WEIGHT

Fashions in body weight come and go. The developed world is currently experiencing an "anti-fat" era. Ironically, though, being fat is increasingly common, with one in two people now classed as overweight or even obese. But is being fat really bad for your health?

WHAT SHOULD YOU WEIGH?

One way of discovering whether your weight is hazardous is to calculate your Body Mass Index (BMI). This method is approved by health authorities in the USA, UK, and many other countries, as well as by the World Health Organization.

TO WORK OUT YOUR BMI:

1. Take your weight in pounds, and multiply by 703.
2. Multiply your height, in inches, by itself.
3. Divide your weight-number by the "height-squared" number.

Alternatively, if you prefer metric:

1. Take your weight in kilograms.
2. Multiply your height, in meters, by itself.
3. Divide your weight by this "height-squared" number.

A BMI of 20–25 represents a normal weight; one of 25–30, a slight degree of overweight. If your BMI is 30–35, you are said to be obese; and over 35, very obese.

The risk of weight-induced health problems is only very slightly increased if a person's BMI is 25–30. However, if it's 30–35, problems become more likely. And if it's over 35, they are very much more likely.

YOUR WAIST MEASUREMENT

Another indication that excess weight is a health risk is your waist measurement. This is because being overweight is more risky if there's a lot of fat in the abdomen.

If you are over 40, and your waist measures less than 80cm (31in), there isn't enough fat around your middle to endanger your health. However, if your waist is bigger than 88cm (34in), you need to take more exercise and adjust what you eat (*see page 165*) so as to shrink your abdominal fat stores.

If you are under 40, your waist measurement is a health risk only if it's over 89cm (35in).

Being either overweight or obese encourages back pain, osteoarthritis, diabetes, high blood pressure, heart attacks, strokes, some cancers, indigestion, snoring, and varicose veins. You can lower your risk of all of these, reduce their symptoms, or maybe even cure some of them, just by losing weight.

THE BEST WAY TO SHED UNWANTED WEIGHT IS USUALLY WITH A COMBINATION OF:

◆ Doing more daily exercise.
◆ Eating a healthier balance of foods.
◆ Eating moderately and regularly.
◆ Seeking solutions for stress that don't involve comfort eating (*see page 34*).

THE BEST WAY OF STAYING SLIM

Researchers say that only 1 slimmer in 20 keeps off her shed pounds. However, successful slimmers learn to keep their weight as they want it by cutting back their food intake – particularly carbohydrates and fat – as soon as they gain a couple of pounds or so. They recognize this because of a tight waistband, from the scales, or simply because they know they've eaten more than usual. They don't think of such a cutback as being a "slimming diet," so they never come to the attention of researchers.

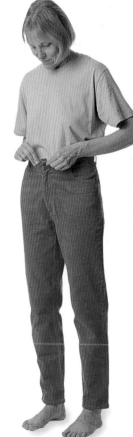

When your clothes feel tight, cut back on your calorie intake until you feel more comfortable.

EXERCISE AND MOVEMENT

Our bodies are designed to move all day, every day. Some movement is involuntary. The heartbeat, for example, continues automatically, day and night. We also have no direct control over our body movements when asleep, or over the contractions of our blood vessels and intestines. And at a microscopic level we have little direct power over the ceaseless movement of the millions of ions and molecules in our bodies.

However, it is possible to control our "voluntary" muscles. These move the face, pelvic floor, voicebox, chest, back, limbs, and other joints. Keeping these well exercised has several benefits.

Moving your face (with exercises, talking, and lively expressions) keeps you looking young. Doing pelvic floor exercises (see page 136) is the best way of helping to prevent the urine leaks that sometimes occur after a difficult childbirth experience, or with aging. These also reduce the risk of the womb sagging ("prolapsing"). Last but not least, they make sex more pleasurable. Training the muscles that adjust the vocal cords and alter the resonance of mouth and throat allows you to use your voice more expressively and with greater confidence.

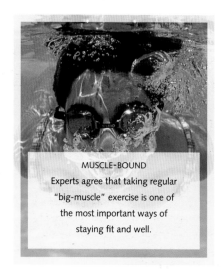

MUSCLE-BOUND
Experts agree that taking regular "big-muscle" exercise is one of the most important ways of staying fit and well.

Regular aerobic exercise will keep you energized and in good shape. Remember to warm up and cool down before and after your exercise session.

BIG-MUSCLE EXERCISE

When we think about exercise, most of us really mean exercise of the big muscles that move (or stabilize) the joints of the limbs, shoulders, hips, and back. All movements, even small ones such as brushing our teeth or lifting a cup of tea, exercise these muscles. And "big-muscle" exercise, however little, has several important health benefits. One is that it raises the body's metabolic rate – the rate at which cells burn energy. The extent of this rise depends on the intensity of the exercise. Another is that it increases the amount of joint lubricating fluid, which helps keep joints flexible and enables us to look and feel good when we walk, sit, and stand. Even gentle forms of exercise, such as walking, slow swimming, and t'ai chi, have health benefits.

However, the biggest benefits of all come from aerobic, muscle-strengthening ("strength" or "endurance"), and stretching ("flexibility") exercises.

AEROBIC EXERCISE

This is movement that is brisk enough to boost the blood-flow and get you breathing faster and taking in more air. It's called "aerobic" because the muscle cells receive all the oxygen they need. This means you could continue for hours.

For cardiovascular (heart and circulation) benefits, you need to exercise hard enough to increase your heart rate to within a certain range. This sort of exercise is called cardiovascular or "cardio" work.

Athletes in training may need to undertake high-intensity cardio work. But most of us should be aiming for aerobic cardio work of only moderate intensity. This means exercising vigorously enough to raise the heart rate to between 50 and 75 percent of its safe maximum.

TO CALCULATE YOUR CARDIO RANGE:

◆ Subtract your age from 220 (the maximum safe human heart rate). The result indicates the maximum possible rate at which your age of heart should beat.

◆ Multiply this figure by 0.75 to get the upper limit of the range for cardio work.

◆ Multiply the same figure by 0.5 to get the lower limit of this range.

If you're relatively unfit, start cardio work with your heart-rate at the lower end of this range. As you become fitter over the next few weeks, gradually increase your heart-rate toward the upper limit of this range. *Warning:* If ever your heartbeat exceeds the upper limit, slow down; if it falls below the lower limit, speed up.

Examples of aerobic exercise include fast walking (not a gentle stroll that doesn't make you breathe faster or feel warmer); washing the floor; running (a gentle, low-impact jog or a short-lived sprint); and brisk swimming (a gentle breaststroke up and down the pool isn't the same at all).

PROS

Aerobic exercise speeds the blood-flow and supplies more oxygen and nutrients not only to your muscles but also to every other cell. This increases your body's metabolic rate – the rate at which your cells burn energy – more than other types of exercise. It also raises the blood levels of endorphins, natural hormone-like substances that lift the spirits and increase the pain threshold. All this means regular aerobic exercise can:

◆ Benefit the whole body, including the heart and blood vessels.

◆ Burn an extra 200–300 calories for 24–48 hours afterward by raising your metabolic rate. This "afterburn" helps you shed excess fat, or lets you eat more without putting on weight.

◆ Increase vitality, wellbeing, and *joie de vivre*.

◆ Boost brain-power, memory, and creativity.

◆ Aid good quality sleep.

◆ Make you look and feel healthier.

◆ Reduce the risk of several types of cancer, including breast cancer.

◆ Ease fibromyalgia (*see page 200*).

◆ Increase immunity.

◆ Help prevent arterial disease.

CONS

Aerobic exercise doesn't necessarily strengthen or stretch muscles. You may have to do this separately. Also, be warned that if you exercise so hard that your muscles hurt (a state called "the burn") you are then exercising anaerobically. Your muscles are complaining because of a lack of oxygen and a build-up of lactic acid. If you keep pushing yourself, you'll ache a great deal afterward.

MUSCLE STRENGTHENING

This involves working your muscles against resistance. Examples include weightlifting; exercising with weights; carrying a backpack; digging the garden; and cycling along flat ground or uphill (not downhill, though this does allow you to rest and enjoy the scenery).

PROS

Working your muscles against resistance increases their bulk. This makes them capable of greater exertion and increases their need for energy. This allows you to:

◆ "Sculpt" your body contours.

◆ Develop more power in particular muscles.

◆ Burn more fat.

CONS

However, muscle-strengthening exercise lacks many important benefits of aerobic exercise, including aerobic cardio work. Also, unless you stretch your muscles afterward, repeated strengthening exercises can make muscles shorter.

STRETCHING

This elongates your big muscles. Examples include stretching arms to catch a ball; reaching for things on high shelves; holding any stretch for at least 30 seconds; and certain yoga postures (*see page 140*).

PROS

Remember that lovely feeling from a long, luxurious early morning stretch? This is nature's way of preparing muscles, tendons, ligaments, and joints to move, support, and balance you in the day ahead. Stretching prevents active muscles from shortening, and inactive muscles, tendons, and joints from stiffening, and relieves muscle tension. Regular stretching:

◆ Increases flexibility.

◆ Benefits balance.

◆ Improves posture.

◆ Can make you feel brighter and more energetic.

◆ Relieves aching in back and shoulders by releasing muscle tension.

◆ Combats post-workout aching.

◆ Prevents muscles from shortening.

CONS

Stretching doesn't boost the blood flow or breathing rate, so it has no major influence on health beyond the benefits of the muscles and joints being stretched.

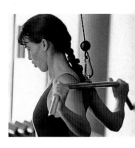

Stretching exercises improve flexibility and posture, while preventing muscles from stiffening and contracting. They are crucial before and after intensive workouts.

Weight training concentrates on strengthening individual muscle groups.

CHOOSING WHAT'S RIGHT

Deciding to take more exercise is a good idea if you are relatively inactive. The next step is choosing what to do. This isn't a final decision but something you'll do many times. You're unlikely, for example, to continue any activity for long if it bores you. You may want to add some other form of exercise because it sounds fun. Or you may dislike what you've chosen, or find it doesn't fit in with your life. One important thing to consider when choosing what to do is your personality type. Ask yourself if you're a loner, or a more sociable person who enjoys doing things with others.

BELOW: Choosing the right exercise is very important. A gentle stretch class is a good way to tone up.

BELOW RIGHT: You may prefer the excitement of a fast volleyball game.

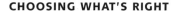

If you prefer your own company, choose something like a daily solitary walk or cycle ride, or exercising to a video. If, on the other hand, you prefer company, investigate hiking groups, a dance class, or group "spinning" (riding an exercise bike in a gym with others, and all varying your exercise intensity at the same time).

Another vital factor is what turns you on. You may need to experiment to discover what you like best, because you're clearly more likely to continue exercising if you enjoy it and find it gives you a buzz. If you enjoy change, it is sensible to try something different from time to time to stop yourself going stale. If you find yourself losing interest, switch to something else without delay. For example, just because you enjoy a Pilates class when you first begin, this doesn't mean you have to do it forever. Simply swap to something like weight training instead.

HOW MUCH, HOW LONG?

◆ On most, if not all, days of the week, everyone needs at least half an hour of either low-intensity aerobic exercise (such as walking, gardening, housework), or moderate-intensity aerobic exercise (such as brisk walking, dancing, jogging, cycling, swimming).
◆ This half-hour needn't be taken all at once, you can split it into separate shorter sessions.

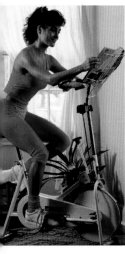

You can exercise on a bike among others at the gym, or do it at home where you can read in peace.

◆ For cardiovascular benefit, and to burn fat, include three sessions a week of exercising for 30–60 minutes with your heart-rate in the cardio range (*see page 28*).
◆ Everyone needs some stretching exercise, on most, if not all, days of the week.
◆ Do some muscle-strengthening exercise at least twice a week, and preferably every other day. Daily exercise is as important as eating or brushing your teeth, so discover the time of day that suits you best then program that time into your diary.

How does a busy person fit exercise into an already crammed day? One answer is to walk or cycle some or all the way to work. However, you'll arrive feeling hot and sweaty so unless you can shower, you might prefer to travel to work in a friend's car or via public transportation, then walk home.

Another idea is to do two things at once. For example, ride an exercise bike while catching up with the news on TV, or keep a friendship going by chatting as you speed-walk around the block, or swim 20 lengths in the pool. Some people increase their exercise levels by doing everyday activities slightly more vigorously. Suggestions include going upstairs twice as fast as normal, or swinging your arms as you walk around at home.

PREVENTING INJURIES

Get the okay from your doctor before starting a fitness program if you haven't exercised for a long time and you're overweight or hesitant, or if you have a history of high blood pressure, diabetes, or heart or other serious disease.

If you want an exercise instructor or personal trainer, choose one who is well qualified and keeps checking that you are exercising safely.

Warming up, stretching, and cooling down
Start with a warm-up, such as marching, low-impact jogging, slow stepping on to the bottom stair, or shoulder or hip circles. This warms muscles, making them more flexible and less likely to be damaged, and helps prevent stiffness. Don't take off outer clothing layers until you're warm.

Now stretch your muscle groups one by one. This helps prevent damage from sudden stretching during exercise.

Later, when you've finished exercising, gradually wind down your activity level, walk around

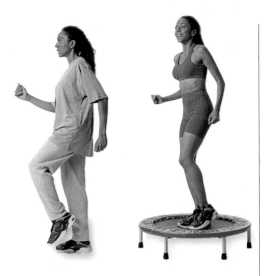

slowly for two or three minutes, then do some more stretches. Keep warm by putting on more clothes or going indoors.

Monitoring your exercise level Build your level gradually over several weeks, increasing the frequency of exercising before its intensity. Aim to get slightly breathless, so you can hear your breathing, but never exert yourself so hard you can't talk. If you overexert yourself, you won't continue for long and your muscles will ache.

Using equipment Use equipment only if you know how to do so safely.

Doing muscle-strengthening exercise Aim to do a muscle-strengthening workout every other day; this gives your muscles time to recover between workouts.

Keeping hydrated Drink frequently to replace fluid lost while exercising. For short periods of intense exercise, drink half a glass of water beforehand, then another half-glass every 20 minutes. For longer sessions, have homemade drinks containing half fruit juice, half water, with a small pinch of salt in each half pint. Avoid commercial sports drinks as they are expensive and sugary. For snacks, it is best to eat fruit and you can quickly restore energy with a banana.

Exercising and eating Some people say that exercising after a meal helps burn up excess calories. Others recommend, "After lunch, rest a while, after dinner run a mile." So what's really best? The answer depends on your situation.

Aerobic exercise makes the body burn more calories for up to 48 hours, regardless of mealtimes. (And it doesn't make you eat more — researchers say people are no hungrier on exercise days than rest days.) You can help this increase in metabolic rate to burn fat by eating no sooner than one hour after you have taken exercise.

Eating increases the circulation of blood to your stomach, intestines, and digestive organs, while exercising increases it to the muscles, lungs, and heart. If a fit, healthy woman exercises after a heavy meal, her body readily diverts blood to the muscles, lungs, and heart, though she might feel full for longer because her digestion will slow down. But if an unfit, unhealthy person exercises after a heavy meal, she may become breathless and easily fatigued, so it's better for her to exercise before eating, or at least two hours afterward.

Before taking aerobic exercise, warm up by doing some brisk marching on the spot or low-impact bouncing on a trampet.

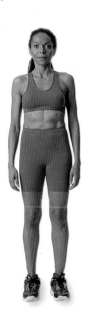

Bananas are packed with energy-giving nutrients.

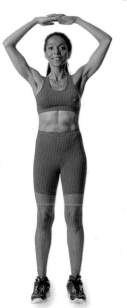

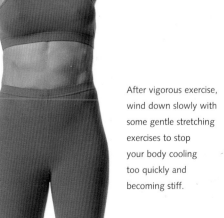

After vigorous exercise, wind down slowly with some gentle stretching exercises to stop your body cooling too quickly and becoming stiff.

RELAXING, PLAYING, AND MANAGING STRESS

Many women today live their lives as if they were high-performance racing cars. They function in top gear much of the time, make sudden changes of speed and direction, and need high-octane fuel in the form of the "stress hormone" known as adrenaline. If this seems familiar to you, bear in mind that continually pushing yourself hard encourages tension and stress. You might be able to keep going for a few days, weeks, or even months. But if you neglect your needs for too long you're bound to pay eventually. And you might even become an "adrenaline junkie," so used to getting the most out of yourself that you simply can't stop.

RIGHT: Many women have stressful jobs but need to be able to relax both their mind and body when not at work.

THE BENEFITS OF RELAXING

What you need if you are not to "crash" is frequent services. Points to include in your service check-up manual include nutritious meals, regular exercise, and enough fresh air and light. And one of the most important points for any woman, no matter how busy, is time to relax.

This relaxation needs to be of both mind and body. It's impossible to relax physically if your mind won't stop whirring. Similarly, you can't wind down mentally if your scalp, back, and shoulders feel tense, or your guts feel all twisted up.

Sometimes it's hard to rest from the demands of everyday life – but that's exactly when they start taking their toll. Stiff shoulders, an aching back, or tension headaches are often the first signs of a need to relax. The huge (but unconscious) effort involved in maintaining muscle tension depletes the body's energy. This combination of tense muscles and low energy would make even Superwoman tired, irritable, and low. It can also encourage painful and heavy periods, a less than satisfying sex life, and fertility problems.

Muscle tension can also encourage hyperventilation (*see page 13*) and many illnesses, including the irritable bowel syndrome (*see page 161*) and asthma (*see page 167*). It does this by reducing the local circulation and trapping the free flow of fluid, or charged particles (ions) or other energy, between the layers of connective tissue (fascia) that separate various muscles and organs. A lowered blood-flow to already inflamed tissue means it does not get the nutrients it needs to recover.

When you are tense, any pain – not just that from stiff muscles – is harder to manage. This is because poor circulation allows pain-provoking chemicals (such as certain prostaglandins) to build up, and because your body doesn't make endorphins – natural "feel-good" substances that help combat pain.

Unless you allow your muscles to relax, your body will become tired and you will feel you have no energy.

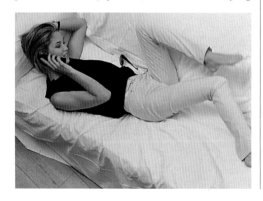

TAKING ENOUGH TIME
TO RELAX ENCOURAGES:
◆ Creativity ◆ Good circulation
◆ Rewarding relationships ◆ Optimal digestion
◆ Contentment ◆ Better sex
◆ A healthy breathing style ◆ Greater fertility
◆ Refreshing sleep ◆ Relief from pain
◆ An attractive posture ◆ Healing of many illnesses

HOW TO RELAX

There are countless ways of relaxing. What to choose depends on what's available, the practicalities involved, and personal preference. It's fascinating that what different individuals find relaxing varies so much. For example, one might love a shoulder rub yet another might loathe it. Someone with a rewarding home life may switch off from workaday concerns on their way home, while a person who dreads going home may find their shoulders stiffening. Similarly, work is relaxing for some but stressful for others.

It is important for everyone to participate in some relaxing and enjoyable activities each day. It can be educational to make a list of what you find relaxing, and how often you do it.

If you can't immediately think what helps you to wind down, use this list to jog your memory.

WAYS OF RELAXING – WHICH DO YOU DO?

◆ Sitting down with a cup of tea or coffee (as long as its caffeine doesn't hype you up).
◆ Having one or two alcoholic drinks.
◆ Watching TV.
◆ Meeting other people for a social activity.
◆ Listening to – or making – music.
◆ Having a cigarette (not really acceptable healthwise).
◆ Going to the movies.
◆ Enjoying a long, scented bath.
◆ Going to the hairdresser.
◆ Making time for a cuddle.
◆ Having sex.
◆ Being given a massage.
◆ Painting your nails.
◆ Putting on make-up.
◆ Window-shopping.
◆ Cooking and eating.
◆ Eating out.
◆ Going on vacation with family or friends, or on your own.
◆ Walking, cycling, swimming, or taking other exercise of your choosing.
◆ Gardening.
◆ Phoning a friend for a chat.
◆ Reading.
◆ Attending parties, celebrations, or festivals.

PROGRESSIVE MUSCULAR RELAXATION

Whatever your preferences, one particular aid to relaxation – progressive muscular relaxation – can come in handy when times are tough.

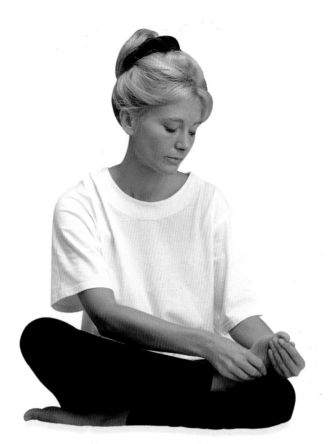

A foot massage is often a particularly enjoyable way of relaxing.

HOW TO RELAX

Choose a warm, quiet place and lie down comfortably. Make sure you are breathing "into your stomach" (*see page 11*) – check by putting a hand on your stomach and feeling it going up and down. Now you're ready to start.

1. First, firmly clench your foot muscles for three or four seconds, holding your breath as you do so, then relax your feet, let go of your breath, and breathe normally again.
2. Repeat by tightening your calf muscles, then letting go.
3. Do the same with your thighs, buttocks, pelvic floor, stomach, and chest muscles in turn.
4. Now on to your hands, forearms, upper arms, shoulders, neck, and face, one after the other.
5. Rest quietly, or sleep for a while if possible.

This exercise has stood the test of time. Its main advantage is that it helps you to learn what your muscles feel like when really relaxed.

Knowing this will help you recognize excess muscle tension and stop it early, any time, any place, before it makes trouble. Get into the habit of relaxing whenever you have a few moments to spare in a busy day.

EFFECTIVE STRESS MANAGEMENT

Now let's take a look at stress itself. Scientists define a stress (or "stressor") as any of the hundreds of things that provoke reactions in us. Repeated stresses are essential for life. However, we are unaware of many of them, and the ones we do know about, we don't perceive as overtly stressful.

But some stressors are challenging or threatening. These trigger the "fight or flight" reaction – a series of mental and physical changes that make us ready to protect ourselves by attacking, defending or running away. This sort of stress affects the hypothalamus and pituitary gland that, in turn, stimulate the adrenal glands and sympathetic nervous system. The result is raised levels of adrenaline and noradrenaline. These are both hormones (substances that have effects throughout the body) and neurotransmitters (substances enabling nerves to carry messages). They prepare the blood vessels, heart, and muscles for immediate action.

Stresses of this sort are a normal part of life and they can be exciting, invigorating, and challenging, pushing us to heights we've never dreamed of. But if they are intense, prolonged, or unrelieved, we may experience them as unpleasant. It's now that we call them stress, and feel "stressed."

RECOGNIZING STRESS IN YOUR LIFE

Signs of stress vary but can include:

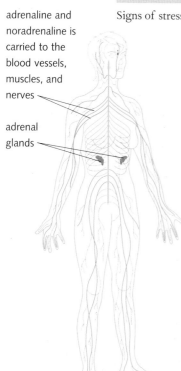

The "fight or flight" reaction to stress stimulates the adrenal glands to secrete more adrenaline into the system in order to prepare the body for action.

adrenaline and noradrenaline is carried to the blood vessels, muscles, and nerves

adrenal glands

- ◆ Muscle tension.
- ◆ Shaking or sweating.
- ◆ Anxiety.
- ◆ Depression.
- ◆ Hyperventilation.
- ◆ Fatigue.
- ◆ Lowered immunity.
- ◆ An eating disorder.
- ◆ Smoking.
- ◆ Drinking too much.
- ◆ Promiscuity.
- ◆ Lack of interest in sex.
- ◆ Working too hard.
- ◆ Being unable to work.
- ◆ Difficulty sleeping.
- ◆ Aggressive or abnormally passive behavior.

Recognizing your personal signs of stress is important, because you can then do something about it. Sometimes, though, you may realize you're stressed only when someone else points it out.

DECIDING TO DO SOMETHING ABOUT IT

Many stressed people don't realize they can help themselves. But anyone in this situation – and that's all of us sometimes – can take steps to discover and use more effective stress-management strategies than the ones they're currently using.

CHOOSING STRESS-MANAGEMENT STRATEGIES

The following long list of strategies includes ideas for preventing, banishing, or minimizing stress, as well as for learning to live with it. Read it through and tick by any item that looks interesting. Then, take your time and pretest each ticked item by imagining yourself doing it.

LIFESTYLE STRATEGIES

- ◆ Eat healthily.
- ◆ Eat regularly.
- ◆ Have more carbohydrate and less protein.
- ◆ Lower your caffeine intake.
- ◆ Take daily exercise.
- ◆ Get enough sleep.

RELAXATION STRATEGIES

- ◆ Practice relaxation techniques.
- ◆ Make time to play.
- ◆ Find a hobby.
- ◆ Be open to new interests.
- ◆ Have enough breaks.
- ◆ Arrange fun trips.
- ◆ Go on vacation.
- ◆ Spoil yourself.
- ◆ When the day is done, focus on pleasant happenings.
- ◆ Allow yourself to laugh and cry when you want to.
- ◆ Spend time on meditation and/or prayer.

ENVIRONMENTAL STRATEGIES

- ◆ Deal with unnecessary physical stressors, such as an uncomfortable chair.
- ◆ Make your surroundings more attractive.

BALANCE AND PERSPECTIVE STRATEGIES

- ◆ Have realistic expectations.
- ◆ Boost your self-esteem.
- ◆ Recognize what really matters.
- ◆ Do what you really want to do.
- ◆ Challenge "shoulds," "oughts," and "musts."
- ◆ Share responsibility.
- ◆ Let yourself make mistakes and then learn from them.

- Let others make mistakes and learn from them.
- See each stress as a challenging opportunity.
- Accept the inevitable.
- Say "no."
- Don't always be perfect.
- Discard unnecessary information.
- Dwell on positives, not negatives.
- Tolerate situations you can't change.
- Accept that you can't have everything you want.
- Separate thoughts from feelings.
- Put problems in perspective without magnifying them.
- Don't jump to conclusions.
- Remember that terrible times will pass.

SELF-MANAGEMENT STRATEGIES

- Accept yourself.
- Recognize, affirm, and develop your good points.
- Be a good, caring friend to yourself.
- Listen to the messages from your mind and body.
- Be assertive, not passive or aggressive.
- Practice problem-solving.
- Improve decision-making skills.

TIME-MANAGEMENT STRATEGIES

- Prioritize tasks.
- Set realistic deadlines.
- Do important or difficult things when fresh.
- Anticipate and plan how to deal with expected stresses.
- Make time for yourself each day.
- Don't overcrowd your diary.
- Delegate.

RELATIONSHIP STRATEGIES

- Enjoy and nurture intimate relationships.
- Deal with problems.
- Nurture friendships.
- Encourage and affirm others.
- Recognize and develop good points in others.
- Separate your feelings from those of others.

OUTSIDE HELP STRATEGIES

- Offload problems on family or friends.
- Arrange professional medical, financial, legal, or other help.

WAVE GOODBYE TO OLD STRATEGIES – SAY HELLO TO NEW ONES

When you're feeling stressed, jot down in a diary who or what the trigger is. Also, note how you behave, and what thoughts go through your mind. You will soon have a knowledge base from which you can experiment with new stress-management strategies, and move on with your life. The immediate aim is to stop your adrenaline level being uncomfortably high for too long. You'll know when it drops because your familiar signs of stress will disappear.

Saying goodbye Be kind to yourself about how you've dealt with stress until now. What you may be finding now is that what worked for you ten years ago, or even yesterday, isn't the best way of managing stress today.

Being kind to yourself also means looking at the pluses of your old strategies as well as their minuses. Otherwise, when you're experimenting with the feel of new strategies and finding them rather strange, you'll run the risk of looking back to the advantages of your old ones and not giving the new ones a proper chance. This is something that happens time and time again to most of us.

Try thinking about the plus points of one of your current stress-management strategies. For example, if you smoke to relieve stress, its plusses might be that

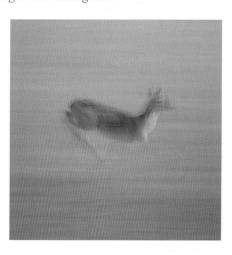

The rush of adrenaline gives this deer the signal to flee from danger. In our life we can't always flee so we may need to find ways to reduce our stress levels.

it makes you feel more clear-headed and in control. Or if you comfort-eat, the advantages might be that it makes you so sleepy you can't think about your problems. Once you've pinpointed these old plus points, try thinking about which of the new strategies you're considering will produce the same benefits. Those that do might be the very ones you most need.

When you try something new, be aware it will probably feel very odd at first. Don't worry, practice will make it more familiar – and hopefully it will eventually become second nature.

> **MOST IMPORTANT**
> Don't forget to assess the advantages and disadvantages of any new strategy so you can decide whether it really has helped. If the rewards aren't what you most need, or the downsides outweigh the rewards, try something else.

SMOKING, ALCOHOL, AND DRUGS – THE REAL QUESTIONS ANSWERED

You might think that smoking and drinking alcohol are relaxing. But chemicals from inhaled smoke raise stress-hormone levels, while alcohol depresses brain activity. This means it can switch off inhibitions and cause stress by triggering aggressive or other overexcitable behavior. It can also cause accidents by reducing judgment, concentration, and coordination. It takes the body an hour to burn up one unit (see opposite) of alcohol, which means several drinks can affect your driving ability for many hours. Too much alcohol can also make a person vomit, reduce her sex drive, and cause a hangover.

The long-term health effects of smoking can be serious. Both smoking and passive smoking (breathing someone else's smoke) encourage many illnesses, including chest infections, heart disease, several cancers (including cervical cancer), autoimmune disease, and, in a baby exposed before or after birth, premature birth, and crib death.

DRINKING TOO MUCH ENCOURAGES:

◆ Obesity (alcohol is high in calories, low in nutrients, and dampens hunger for more nutritious foods).
◆ High blood pressure (though drinking a little – 1 US alcohol unit/1–2 UK alcohol units a day – may make high blood pressure less likely).
◆ Strokes (with more than 2 US alcohol units/3 UK alcohol units a day).
◆ Liver damage.
◆ Brain damage (such as poor memory and depression).
◆ Heart disease (with more than 2 US units/3 UK units a day).
◆ Alcohol addiction (which is most likely if you have addictive traits in your personality).
◆ Cancer of the mouth, throat, stomach, liver, pancreas, colon (unless you eat plenty of food rich in folic acid), and breast (drinking 1–4 US/2–5 UK units a day increases the risk by 41 percent).
◆ Osteoporosis (because alcohol lowers the level of parathyroid hormone and weakens the muscles whose contractions boost bone-density).

DRUGS

Using and supplying "recreational drugs" such as marijuana, ecstasy, cocaine, and heroin are illegal in the USA, UK, Australia, and many other countries. However, the fact remains that increasing numbers of people take drugs for pleasure. The more often you take drugs, the more likely it is that your health will be damaged by them. Some successfully limit their intake and come to no harm, but from time to time someone has a serious health problem – or even dies – after taking drugs just once. A few become addicted to a drug, or to the danger and excitement of the drug subculture. This is more common in those who have a personality problem that encourages addictive behavior, and in those who turn to drugs as a way of managing stress. *See page 57* for some of the dangers.

The temptation is to think that alcohol makes you more sociable. However, in excess it is extremely antisocial, causing irrational behavior and unpleasant side effects, and can lead to long-term health problems.

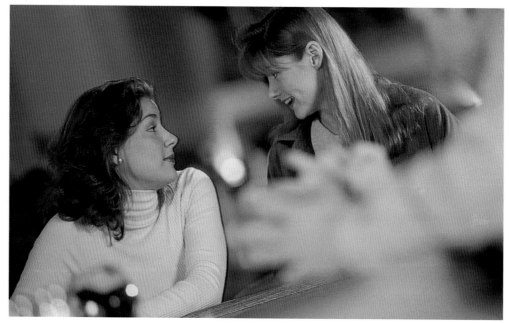

LIMITING RISKS FROM ALCOHOL

If you are pregnant, or planning to become pregnant, then first *see page 79*.

Women in the UK are advised to consume no more than 14 units of alcohol each week, with no more than two or three on any one day, and not to drink to the daily limit every day. In the US, where alcohol units are bigger, experts recommend no more than one unit a day. However, being under 18, or thin, may mean your limit should be lower.

Don't confuse your limit with that of a man. There are four reasons why women develop a higher blood-alcohol level after drinking the same amount of alcohol as men. Women are smaller. Their stomachs empty more slowly, giving alcohol more time to be absorbed. Their bodies contain proportionately more fat and less muscle, so they have less body water with which to dilute alcohol. And their livers produce less acetaldehyde dehydrogenase, the enzyme that breaks down alcohol.

In the UK, 11 percent of women and 28 percent of men now drink too much. However, the female figure is rising, and the gap between the sexes is narrowing. Young women are the most likely to exceed the limit: 22 percent of 16–24-year-olds drink over 14 units a week, compared with 16 percent of 25–44-year-olds, 13 percent of 45–64-year-olds, and 7 percent of over-65s. Working full-time makes women nearly twice as likely to drink too much alcohol as working part-time or not at all. And having a professional or managerial job increases the risk too. As for bingeing on alcohol and getting drunk, 1 in 20 of all women does this once a week, compared with one in six of those aged 16–24.

In the USA, the picture is similar. While the overall consumption of alcohol is falling, men are cutting back more than women, and bingeing on alcohol and getting drunk is an increasingly worrying problem among women in their 20s.

BREAKING A HABIT

If you smoke or drink too much, or find drugs a problem, ask: "Is this activity stress-related?" You're more likely to reduce or stop your habit if you identify your motivation.

IS IT BECAUSE YOU:

- Want to be part of the crowd?
- Want to boost your confidence?
- Enjoy the buzz it gives you?
- Want to communicate more freely?
- Want release from stress?

These are potent motivations, so you need to find creative means of meeting your needs in other ways.

If your habit developed from a need to handle stress, you must search carefully for new stress-management strategies, because stress can encourage such problems as heart disease, depression, and accidents. But get one thing straight first. The way you chose to reduce your stress was probably the best you could find in your circumstances at the time, so don't reproach yourself. Now that it has become an unwanted habit with health risks, register the fact that your habit is the problem, NOT YOU. There are several ways to do this.

WHEN GIVING UP, START WITH THIS THREE-POINT PLAN:

1. *Work out why you enjoy your habit* so you can find stress-management strategies that offer similar advantages without the danger.
2. *Identify how you usually feel before you start*. For example, feeling exhausted, frustrated, angry, or anxious might make you want a drink. Drowning painful emotions may help you cope, but only temporarily. So you need stress-management strategies that allow you to deal with difficult emotions in more lasting ways.
3. *Once you've started using new stress-management strategies, don't give up if you relapse*. If you have a drinking binge, simply write off that day and start fresh the next. Take things one day at a time.

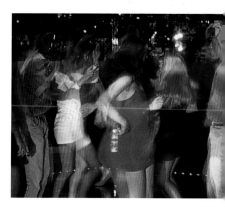

The heady atmosphere of a nightclub can lead people to drink and smoke too much and take drugs. Be aware of the danger signs and keep control of your intake.

SLEEP

A good night's sleep is worth its weight in gold, because we wake brighter, more refreshed, and better able to meet the challenges ahead. Sleep also allows our brains to process and file information and solve problems.

When we sleep we lose our normal ability to hear, see, smell, feel, and taste. However, this doesn't mean we can't do these things. Any strong enough stimulus is perceived by our sleeping selves, and affects our dreams and depth of sleep, or might even wake us. We can speak during sleep too, and lots of people do. Sleep-talk isn't consciously driven, though it may reflect something we're dreaming or worrying about. But what happens when we sleep?

Dreaming can stem from something you have done during the day, or might be the way in which your subconscious resolves issues while you are asleep. Dreaming a lot doesn't necessarily mean you have had a "disturbed" night.

DOES THE BRAIN SLEEP?

The sleeping brain certainly isn't inactive. While our conscious minds rest, our brain cells continue to produce waves of electrochemical activity that is orchestrated by neurotransmitters, substances that enable messages to travel along nerves. The rhythm and frequency of these brainwaves alternate between two patterns: one associated with REM (Rapid Eye Movement) sleep, the other with non-REM sleep. During REM sleep our eyes and

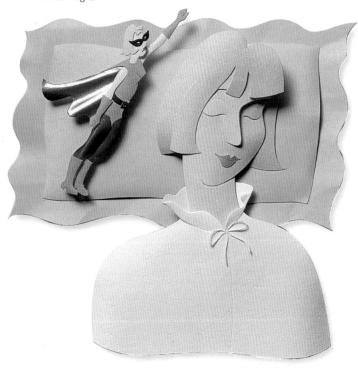

bodies move, we dream (and may speak), and we're easily aroused. Conversely, non-REM sleep is deeper and quieter.

We need a balance of both kinds of sleep to refresh both our bodies and minds. Without enough we lose mental and physical acuity. We feel tired and dull, coordination suffers, and we become slow and depressed (*see page 205*).

GETTING THE RIGHT AMOUNT OF SLEEP

You are an individual and the amount of sleep you need depends on your age, stage of life, and current activities and experiences. There is no single "right" amount for all people or at all times of any individual's life, though most of us need at least seven hours in 24, and some several hours more. So be guided by how you feel. If you're tired when you wake and don't soon feel brighter, you may need more sleep, or better quality sleep.

SIESTAS, NAPS, AND SLEEPING IN

Some people function better in the late afternoon and evening, and enjoy a longer evening, if they have an afternoon siesta. Others cope well with occasional short naps, or sleeping in weekly. The important thing is to recognize what's best for you.

DREAMING

During REM sleep the brain creates dreams as part of its information filing and retrieval processes. Dreams can be mundane or extraordinary, pleasant or exciting. Sometimes they are so frightening or shocking that we call them nightmares.

Some women dream more before a period, or when pregnant; others when stressed. Inexplicably, some people have prophetic dreams – they dream something happens before it does. We have a lot to learn yet about our slumbering selves.

ENHANCING YOUR SLEEP
Use these tips to promote a good night's sleep.

YOUR BED

◆ Check that your bed and mattress aren't too hard or soft.
◆ Make sure your pillow has the right degree of softness and support. People have strong views about their pillow(s) but it's often best to choose a firm one if you sleep on your side; a medium-firm one if you prefer to sleep on your back; and a soft one – or none at all – if you're a stomach-sleeper.
◆ Invest in good quality sheets or comforter covers.
◆ Choose blankets, a comforter, or other covers that keep you at the right temperature and are big enough to cover you and stay put.

YOUR BEDROOM

◆ Keep street light out with drapes made from heavy material, or light-excluding blinds.
◆ Heat or cool the air as necessary.
◆ Ideally have an open window or other source of fresh air.

NOISE

◆ Invest in earplugs if someone's snoring stops you sleeping – or go to another room yourself, or ask them to.
◆ Insulate windows if you live near a noisy road.

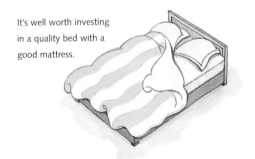

It's well worth investing in a quality bed with a good mattress.

EXERCISE

◆ Take half an hour of exercise each day, ideally five or six hours before bedtime, rather than just before.

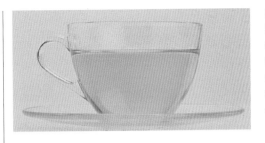

Regular tea and coffee both contain caffeine, so consider switching to herbal tea or decaffeinated coffee in the late afternoon and evening.

FOOD AND DRINK

◆ Eat a healthy diet which provides soothing nutrients, including calcium, magnesium, manganese, zinc, and vitamin B.
◆ Avoid a large, rich meal in the evening.
◆ Have your last "proper" meal early, and keep later snacks small and light.
◆ Have as a nightcap a honey-sweetened cup of chamomile, lemon balm, linden (lime) blossom, vervain, or hop tea.
◆ Remember coffee, tea, and caffeine-containing soft drinks after 4pm can interfere with sleep.
◆ The position on alcohol isn't so clear. Alcohol relaxes muscles so if you're tense, drinking in moderation in the evening may help.
◆ Some people find a hot, malted, milky nightcap very calming and comforting; others find it interferes with a good night's sleep.

RELAXATION

◆ Before bedtime, enjoy a warm bath scented with a chamomile teabag or a few drops of lavender oil.
◆ Listen to soothing music.
◆ If worry – about work or money problems, for example – stops you sleeping, consider discussing solutions with a friend or counselor.
◆ See whether reading helps you to drop off.
◆ Relax by cuddling, or having sex.

A HEALTHY SLEEP REGIME

◆ Say "no" to an evening nap, however tempting.
◆ Aim, if possible, to have a regular bedtime and rising time.
◆ Adopt a routine in the two or three hours before bedtime.
◆ Keep your bedroom for sleeping, not working, watching TV or phoning friends.

Warning: See your doctor if you've slept badly for more than two weeks, and are exhausted, depressed, desperate, or unable to drive or cope with your job or family.

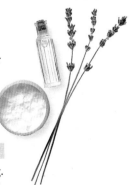

Lavender oil in the bath or dried sprigs inside your pillow will help you to relax and will encourage sleep.

RELATIONSHIPS

From the day we're conceived to the day we die we all exist in relationship to others. We all have or had a mother, father, and other relatives, and most of us have friends, colleagues, neighbors, and others we know well. We also continue to exist in people's minds long after we're gone.

But although we all have relationships, these may be active or inactive, rewarding, draining, or of no importance at all. What they are like depends partly on how much we nurture and value them.

WHY RELATING IS GOOD FOR YOU

Good relationships have many benefits. They help us feel loved and lovable, valued and valuable, happier and less stressed. All this, in turn, enhances our immunity and resistance to disease. Some relationships spur creativity. Others simply make life worth living and make unpleasant life events seem much less important.

BEING PART OF A COMMUNITY

Belonging to a family, living in a neighborhood, working with colleagues, and joining a class, club, or other social group are but a few examples of being in a community. As a member of any community you belong to a group. And sometimes a group can go places and achieve things an individual member cannot. Women's groups, for instance, have made great strides in improving community, national, and international facilities in recent decades. They have also done a lot to boost their members' self-esteem and empower them to make the most of their lives.

NURTURING YOUR RELATIONSHIPS

A relationship is most likely to thrive if it's nurtured. Having said this, everyone's heard of friends separated for 50 years who then resume their friendship as if they had been never parted.

Women tend to be much better than men at opening up to their friends. It's good to have someone with whom to share life's many ups and downs.

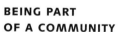

But most relationships reward both parties only if they're enjoyed, valued, and carefully and lovingly maintained, polished, and enriched.

PREVENTING DIVORCE

The twentieth century saw an explosion in divorce and separation. Some people are undoubtedly happier apart, but in parting many cause themselves and their children increased heartache. So how can an unhappy, unfaithful, or warring couple enhance their relationship and go on to grow as individuals together, instead of separately?

One excellent way of enhancing a relationship also helps each individual to grow. Ideally both members of the couple need to do it, but often it can help even if just one does so. It involves learning four proven methods that help individuals to live together, enjoy each other, and not damage each other.

THESE ARE:

- ◆ Empathic listening (*see opposite*).
- ◆ Conflict resolution (*see opposite*).
- ◆ Encouragement (*see opposite*).
- ◆ Stress management (*see page 34*).

Sounds too simple? Just try, with professional help if need be, and you may be surprised by how effective this package can be.

EMPATHIC LISTENING SKILLS

Some people seem naturally able to listen empathically. Most of us, though, have to learn by imitation, instruction, and practice. Learning the necessary skills often proves to be one of the most valuable things a person can acquire. But first, what exactly is empathy anyway?

It certainly isn't sympathy – feeling concerned or sorry for someone. Empathy means imagining what it's like in someone else's shoes, feeling what they feel. When someone listens to us in an empathic way, we feel they care, and we also feel really heard and understood. As a result we know ourselves better. And we don't feel alone. These are the three steps to empathic listening.

STEP 1

Put your own emotions aside. You can do this only if:
◆ You are aware of your obvious and underlying emotions.
◆ The time and situation are right.

STEP 2

Identify the other person's main emotions. For this you need to:
◆ Seek every clue, with each of your senses, including the sixth. Listen to what they say and how they say it. Watch their body language. Note any hints from their dress, the colors they wear, their hair and bearing. And sense how being with them makes you feel, as your body and your mind may be picking up on their emotions.

STEP 3

Tell them what emotions you think they're feeling, bearing in mind these guidelines:
◆ Remember that the primary difficult emotions – the ones that cause trouble if unrecognized and mismanaged – are fear, anger, sadness, and despair. These come in many guises and have many names, so put on your detective's hat.
◆ Say what you think their main emotion is by suggesting – "It seems to me you're feeling sad" or, "It sounds like you're angry about …"
◆ If you are wrong, they won't mind. They will soon put you right if they can, and if they can't, the search will start them thinking.

CONFLICT RESOLUTION

Conflict is natural and to be expected at some time in any relationship. These six steps will help you to resolve it:

1. Decide who needs hearing first.
2. Agree that whoever listens first will try to listen empathically.
3. Say how you feel only when it's your turn to be heard. Then concentrate on expressing your main emotions, using "I feel …" statements, not "You make me feel …" statements.
4. Continue to take turns listening and speaking until each of you feels heard and understood, even if your conflict isn't yet resolved. Recognizing how someone feels doesn't mean you agree with their explanation of why they feel that way. You are simply hearing how they feel, and how they interpret what's going on. And that's important.
5. Together, brainstorm solutions and ways of moving toward resolution.
6. Acknowledge the peace that comes from working toward resolution.

ENCOURAGEMENT

This is different from praise. It involves noticing what the other is attempting to do, describing this in some detail, and then using empathic listening skills to recognize and name the positive emotions their activity gives them.

Take as an example a young child showing you a painting. You might say something like, "I can see a nest in that tree, some bright yellow flowers in the garden, and a girl on the swing with such a big smile that she must be having a lovely time. I expect you're really pleased with your picture." If possible, try to encourage those around you several times each day.

Each generation has something to learn from the others, and some children find it easier to talk to their grandparents about their worries than to confide in their parents.

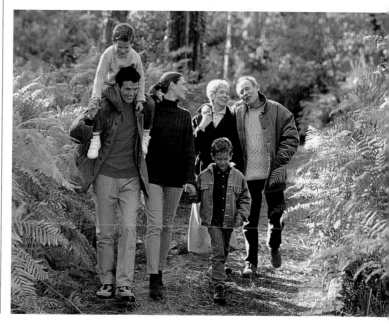

There is a strong relationship between sex and health. Good sex makes you feel good, and when you feel good you enjoy sex more.

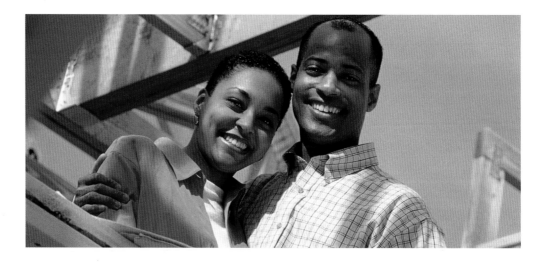

GETTING PHYSICAL

Sex is probably an important part of your relationship with a partner, and a good sex life can certainly enhance your feeling of wellbeing. But sometimes, other influences interfere with the desire for sex.

LIBIDO, PLEASURE, AND ORGASM

Our sex drive, or libido, is a natural pleasure that's ours by right. It is also changeable. Sometimes, for example, we experience more delight and have more rewarding or frequent orgasms than others.

Many things can influence our sex lives. Some are external issues such as comfort, privacy, and the needs of young children. But most women say the biggest influence is the way they feel emotionally. Feeling happy, loved, and lovable – content with life in general, and our partner in particular – helps make sex enjoyable. But it is not necessarily a requirement for enjoyable sex (*see right*).

Good health is a positive encouragement for sex, whereas feeling ill, exhausted, anxious, or depressed dampens desire, partly because we can't forget such problems. The stress of feeling unwell affects our sex drive by changing the levels of hormones such as adrenaline (which is also a neurotransmitter), cortisone, estrogen, and testosterone. Food and drink, exercise, and exposure to daylight also affect these substances.

A healthy diet provides the nutrients we need if we are to express and enjoy our sexuality; iron, zinc, vitamins B, C, and E, essential fatty acids, and plant hormones are particularly important. Exercise makes us fit for sexual activity and also increases the levels of endorphins (natural "feel-good" substances). And ultraviolet light boosts both endorphins and estrogen.

SEX – WITH WHOM AND HOW OFTEN?

Only you know the answers to these questions. They will be determined by a great many things, including your upbringing, education, experience, friendships, personality, morals, beliefs, and opportunities.

A person's choice of partner and subsequent sex life is a source of neverending fascination, perhaps never more so than now when so many women are struggling to discover how best to live their lives and form lasting and rewarding sexual relationships.

EXPRESSING YOURSELF THROUGH SEX

Being unaware of suppressed feelings such as anger, fear, sadness, or despair can sabotage desire. However, it's possible to use sex as a way of bringing these emotions to the surface. If, for example, you avoid sex or find it unrewarding, try some detective work. Use empathic listening skills (*see page 41*) on yourself to see if you can pinpoint unrecognized emotions such as anger – which might masquerade as boredom, frustration, irritation, or being cross. Recognizing and naming emotions is the first step to owning and accepting them. Once you accept them, you're free to use them constructively to improve life for you and your partner, rather than allow them to remain uncomfortable or dangerous.

Sex can be experienced and enjoyed when you feel all kinds of things other than "loving" or "nice". Sex in these situations can be a way of expressing such emotions while at the same time transforming them into positive, constructive energy. Many great writers', musicians', and artists' work has been fueled by anger or despair. And the art of great sex is no different.

PROS AND CONS OF DIFFERENT CONTRACEPTIVE METHODS

Worldwide, the three commonest contraceptive methods are condoms, the Pill, and natural family planning (which includes the sympto-thermal method, see below, and the tendency of breastfeeding to suppress ovulation). Others include diaphragms, caps, coils, hormone-releasing coils, hormone implants and injections, and female condoms. In developed countries condoms and the Pill are the most popular.

Male condom A thin cover for the penis.

PROS

◆ Man is responsible.
◆ Available over the counter.
◆ No side effects.
◆ Used as needed.
◆ Prevents disease transmission.

CONS

◆ Lessens his sensations.
◆ Changes her sensations.
◆ Easily forgotten, broken, or dislodged.
◆ A woman may have to insist on a man using a condom.

Female condom A thin bag which lines the vagina and vulva.

PROS

◆ Woman in control.
◆ Available over the counter.
◆ No side effects.
◆ Used as needed.
◆ Prevents infection.

CONS

◆ Reduces sensation for both.
◆ Feels unpleasant.
◆ Expensive.

The Pill A combination of estrogen and progestogen (synthetic progesterone), or progestogen only. This prevents ovulation, fertilization, or the implantation of the fertilized egg.

PROS

◆ Convenient.
◆ Some women feel healthier.
◆ Not related to the sex act.
◆ Doesn't interrupt sex.
◆ Eases some period problems.
◆ Lowers ovarian cancer risk.

CONS

◆ Easily forgotten.
◆ Some women feel less healthy.
◆ Must be taken every day at the same time (possibly with one week a month off).
◆ Can have hormone-induced side effects, such as nausea, tender breasts, and headache.
◆ Makes blood clots more likely.
◆ Raises breast cancer risk.

◆ Offers no protection against disease transmission.

Natural family planning This includes: detecting your fertile days and avoiding sex on these days. One way is to detect changes in vaginal mucus, the cervix, and body temperature (the "sympto-thermal" method). Another is to measure urine hormones with an electronic monitor.

PROS

◆ No side effects.

CONS

◆ A condom – or abstinence – becomes necessary on fertile days, which is when many women feel most like sex.

Another method is the lactational amenorrhea method (LAM). Breastfeeding frequently and regularly, without a pacifier or limitation of sucking time, can suppress ovulation for over a year. (Used with the sympto-thermal method.)

PROS

◆ No side effects.
◆ Longer break from periods.

CONS

◆ Disrupted breastfeeding triggers ovulation, making method unreliable.

Withdrawal The man ejaculates outside the vagina.

PROS

◆ No medical side effects.

CONS

◆ Some loss of pleasure for both.
◆ Extremely unreliable.

Diaphragm or cap These cover the cervix.

PROS

◆ Side effects rare.
◆ Used as needed.

CONS

◆ Must insert and remove each time.
◆ Involves pre-planning.
◆ Interrupts sex unless inserted beforehand.
◆ Reduces her sensations.

◆ Must be used with a spermicide.
◆ It must be fitted for size by a doctor.
◆ Its size must be reassessed after weight loss and childbirth.

Coil This plastic or copper device in the womb prevents implantation of a fertilized egg.

PROS

◆ Generally no change in sensations for her or him.
◆ Once inserted can be forgotten.

CONS

◆ Can cause period problems and backache.
◆ Increases risk of pelvic infection.
◆ Must be removed by a doctor to enable pregnancy.
◆ Man may be aware of strings.

Hormone-releasing coil This coil releases progestogen to prevent pregnancy.

PROS

◆ As for coil.
◆ Effect continues for five years.
◆ No side effects because the coil releases the equivalent of only two progestogen-only pills a week.

CONS

◆ As for coil.
◆ Hormone-induced side effects (*see above*).

Hormone implant Progestogen implants are inserted beneath the skin.

PROS

◆ Lasts five years

CONS

◆ Must be inserted and removed by a doctor.
◆ Removal sometimes difficult.
◆ Hormone-induced side effects (*see above*).

Hormone injection Progestogen is injected into muscle.

PROS

◆ Lasts two to three months.

CONS

◆ Hormone-induced side effects (*see above*), including heavy bleeding.

What you choose will depend on your age, stage of life, health, partner, previous contraceptive experience, and how serious you are about not wanting to get pregnant. These issues are discussed later.

FULFILLING YOUR POTENTIAL

Each of us is a unique individual, even if we have an identical twin. We have different experiences from conception onward, and even though some experiences are shared, we each have a different vantage point and that, in turn, helps shape who we are. Given that each person is unique, it is clearly good sense to make being truly ourselves the most useful and rewarding experience it can be. No one else can do this for us, and we can't live life for anyone else either.

KNOW YOURSELF

Recognizing and valuing your uniqueness and specialness is the basis of having self-esteem. We have this gift of life, it's a once-only existence (on this earth) and we owe it to ourselves to "love" ourselves. This means accepting, knowing, and caring for ourselves, and making the most of our abilities and potential for loving. Of course, recognizing the uniqueness and value of others is vitally important too. The old adage "love your neighbor as yourself" makes good sense, because if you don't love yourself, you can't truly love anyone else, and vice versa.

Part of knowing yourself is recognizing the influences that shape you. Among them are your body rhythms, the daily and monthly variations in mind and body that result partly from changing hormone levels. Other influences include upbringing and education, as well as feelings and behaviors – both of which are shaped by your genes, personality and experiences. Your daydreams and hopes and aspirations can also play their part.

Two interesting ideas about the personality and brain could help you know yourself better. The first is the discovery that the right and left sides of the brain each govern particular types of thoughts and abilities. For a right-handed person, the left side governs rational intellectual activities, while the right is responsible for creativity and daydreams. Some people seem more influenced by their left brain, others by their right.

You owe it to yourself to discover where your strengths lie and to work toward fulfilling the potential within yourself.

The second idea is the psychoanalytic concept that each individual's personality has both a "masculine" part (the animus) and a "feminine" one (the anima). The "masculine" part craves action; it is goal-oriented (or "product-centered") and tends to live for the future. The "feminine" is the nurturing and accepting part; it tends to enjoy the actual process of doing something, and enables us to be aware of the present moment. You can help yourself live your life more fully by accepting the existence of both your "masculine" and your "feminine" sides, and encouraging one or the other when necessary.

FINDING THE BALANCE

Many children while growing up come to believe they are either bright or stupid. Those who don't do well at academic subjects are often guided toward other areas of the curriculum instead. And those who do do well academically frequently spend little or no time on artistic, creative, or more practical subjects. This judgmental splitting of gifts and abilities into good or bad, present or absent, sometimes leads to a girl's real potential remaining locked up for years.

Yet many teachers and parents persist in labeling children according to what they currently do well, and what currently interests them. Perhaps this is just human nature. But wouldn't it be better if, rather than a mother saying, for example, "Polly is our artist, and Sophie is the academic," she were to say, "At the moment Polly loves her painting, and Sophie is more into books"? Anything rather than exclude the possibility that Polly may turn out to be able academically, as well as with her paintbrush, and that Sophie may become a budding jazz saxophonist, as well as having a first-rate academic mind.

Think about the labels you've grown up with, and whether they've held you back or, perhaps, helped you. Remember you can always discard them or add others. Or you can refuse to be labeled and instead leave the way open for all sorts of interesting twists and turns ahead and, hopefully, some wonderful surprises.

PLANNING YOUR LIFE

Although some planning is a good idea, letting life take its own route from time to time can be exciting and challenging. After all, life changes so much that it's hard to make concrete plans. So as with many things, the best solution may be a good balance – in this case a combination of taking control and at the same time being open to new ideas and opportunities. That way you can dare do something different from time to time. And you'll rarely be bored.

REORGANIZING YOUR LIFE

There will be times when your life doesn't go the way you want, and you'll need to make adjustments, big or small. But you don't have to wait until things have become uncomfortable to make a start. It makes sense to stop, think, and take stock every six months or so. This will help you to redirect your life before you get too stuck.

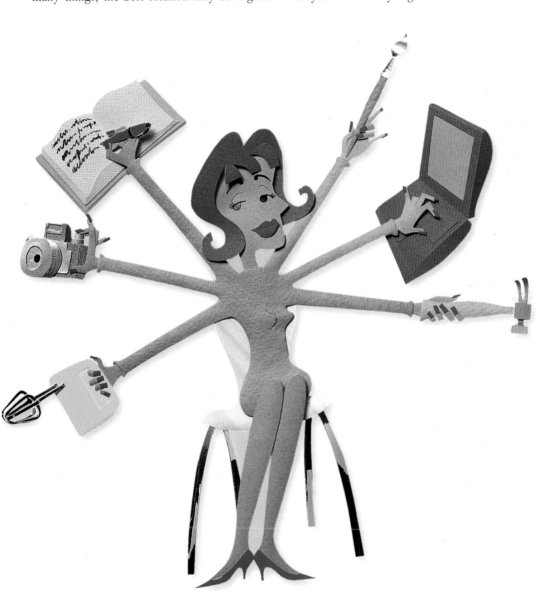

Everybody has a range of different talents, so don't feel you should be pigeonholed into one area of expertise. Life has a habit of surprising us, so be prepared to be flexible and change your plan if presented with an enticing opportunity.

LOOKING GOOD

We can't all look like models, but whatever our body style or size, we can maximize our looks with a healthy diet, regular exercise, good grooming, and with clothes and personal adornment that suit and please us. Most people evaluate new acquaintances almost entirely on looks, because the way others look is so revealing. This is fine if the way you look is what you want to portray. If not, you need to swing into action.

First, analyze your appearance – with a friend if it helps. Focus, for example, on your clothes.

ASK WHETHER THEY LOOK:

- Comfortable.
- Well put together.
- Just pulled on.
- Fashionable.
- Like those of a fashion victim.
- As if they are chosen in colors that really suit you.
- Dramatic.
- As if you are seeking attention.
- Shabby.
- "Loud" in color.
- Serviceable.
- Cheap.
- Well worn.
- Dull.
- Well cared for.
- Dowdy.
- Expensive.
- Quirky.

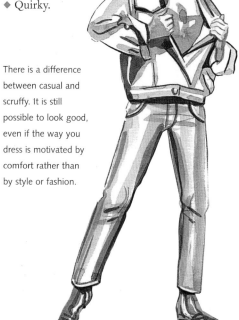

There is a difference between casual and scruffy. It is still possible to look good, even if the way you dress is motivated by comfort rather than by style or fashion.

SECOND, CHECK ON YOUR HEALTH AND WELLBEING:

- Are you unwell? Looks can be sapped by, for example, eating poorly, or having anemia, chronic fatigue, or a thyroid condition.
- Are you stressed or depressed? These states could affect your looks without you realizing.
- Are you angry or sad? Many of us act out emotions in the ways we present ourselves.

CHANGING YOUR APPEARANCE

Before-and-after photos of women who have changed their looks are endlessly fascinating. They are the equivalent of "rags-to-riches" novels. Everyone has the power to change their appearance dramatically if they wish. So if you don't think your looks suit you, try experimenting:

DOING YOUR OWN "MAKEOVER":

- Cut, color, or restyle your hair.
- Use more or less make-up – or use it differently.
- Change your shape with exercise and healthy eating.
- Learn which clothes look best.
- Choose different glasses frames, or invest in contact lenses.
- Adjust your usual expression.
- Improve your posture.

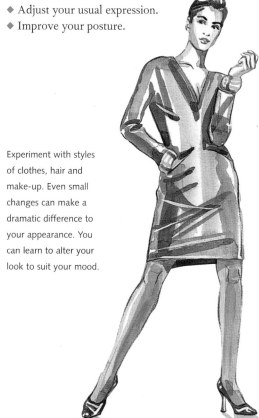

Experiment with styles of clothes, hair and make-up. Even small changes can make a dramatic difference to your appearance. You can learn to alter your look to suit your mood.

NATURAL ALTERNATIVES TO PLASTIC SURGERY

Plastic surgeons instruct patients extremely carefully about skin care after surgery, especially facial surgery. Patients must be non-smokers, eat a skin-friendly diet (rich in beta carotene, vitamins C and E, flavonoids, minerals such as selenium and silicon, and plant hormones) and avoid excess UV light. In the long term these tips are probably as beneficial as the knife, or, indeed, more so. And you can do them at home.

Facial exercises involve daily sessions of moving the muscles that tighten the jaw-line, firm the cheeks and smooth the fine lines above the mouth. Iron out frown lines by easing them flat with your fingers. Note how this relaxed state feels, and learn to maintain the feeling afterward.

Healthy eating, exercise, and weight loss (if necessary) are also good for toning thighs, stomach, and bottom, and (if you are overweight) lightening heavy breasts.

PLANNING YOUR WORKING LIFE

The nature of work is changing rapidly. No longer do we stay in the same jobs forever. We can now expect to learn many skills and do several different sorts of job over our lifetime. Even the most specialized worker will find that developing new areas of expertise helps link areas of knowledge and make their existing skills more useful.

When choosing a career, remember that if it involves lengthy training it's usually easier, both practically and financially, to get it under your belt when you are young. Conversely, initiatives offering equal access to college, and to distant learning schemes, mean you can embark on many sorts of formal education at any age.

Whatever you do, and whatever your age, aim to choose something you enjoy. Being fulfilled and interested at work helps make life sing. Some employers use psychometric tests to try to ensure a good fit between employee and job. These assess personality, attitudes, aptitudes, and leadership and problem-solving skills. Careers advisors also offer these privately.

WORKPLACE HAZARDS FOR WOMEN

Any job can be hazardous, not just those involving obvious physical danger, such as working on the factory floor or with chemicals. Employers have a duty to make working conditions safe. But you should also use your common sense to make your work safer, or stop doing it if necessary.

Some of the most neglected workers are those in sedentary jobs. Sitting down all day, perhaps working at a keyboard, can promote backache, varicose veins, hemorrhoids, and repetitive strain injury. If you have a sedentary job, get up and walk around for five minutes every half-hour or so. And make sure you fit in your half-hour of aerobic exercise each day.

If you work outside much of the day you run the risk of your skin aging prematurely, and of developing skin cancer from the harmful effects of too much UV light on your skin. Shading your skin with a wide-brimmed sunhat, never letting it burn, and keeping out of the sun for the two or three hours around noon probably give the best protection. Using factor 15 sunscreen is sensible too, though the long-term benefits are unproven.

During pregnancy it's best to avoid work that necessitates standing up most of the time, or carrying heavy weights, as both these increase the risk of having a miscarriage.

Some occupations are particularly stressful. These include management and certain professions such as teaching and dentistry. Because most jobs are potentially stressful, it pays to know your signs of stress (*see page 34*) so you can alleviate the triggers or use more effective stress-management strategies when necessary.

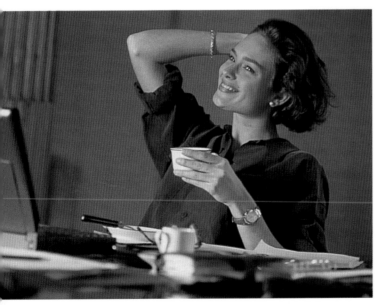

Some elements of your working life are within your control. Posture, diet, taking breaks, drinking plenty of water, and lighting and stress levels are all crucial factors in workplace comfort.

SOUL AND SPIRIT

Not so long ago, many people in most countries shared a religious faith, or a set of common beliefs. These gave meaning to life, reinforced ancient truths through vivid stories, and laid down a moral code that promoted harmony.

Nowadays things are different. Young people worldwide are more likely to travel and settle elsewhere, and adults often have to uproot themselves to get work. This means that communities almost everywhere are less stable, which makes it harder for individuals to develop the relationships and structures that encourage a shared faith. This helps explain why, over the last three or four decades, there has been such a marked growth in new age beliefs, therapies, and teachings.

SPIRITUAL SUSTENANCE AND CHALLENGE

"New age" ideas have bubbled up from many sources, including psychology, Eastern religions and practices, philosophy, mysticism, folk beliefs, and traditional healing methods. They are not connected in any formal way, yet have many common strands. For example, there is often a focus on such concepts as knowing yourself; loving yourself and each other; living authentically, in the moment, and in harmony with the environment; and realizing that everyone, and everything, on the planet is interdependent in some way.

These ideas are often presented in a very user-friendly fashion. But none of them is new. They represent various facets of ancient wisdom in attractive modern packaging. And they echo similar teachings from the major world religions: Judaism, Christianity, Islam, Hinduism, and Buddhism. The first three religions incorporate the concept of a creator God, an idea that has stood the test of time over several millennia. Christians also believe that Jesus was the son of God who died in order that we could have life after death. And Christians also believe that the Holy Spirit, the "breath of life," is a part of God. Hindus believe that there are many gods, each aiding the understanding of a particular part of the human psyche. They also talk of Brahman, the divine "soul" within the universe from which we all come and to which we all return.

However, the belief in "a higher power" that is a force for good is not confined to religious people. Many others believe in this without calling it "God". The fact is that most human beings, young and old, have a yearning for something greater than their own power and understanding to fill them and provide meaning. Buddhists have a fundamentally different belief. They assert that it is possible to attain perfect peace – nirvana – by our own efforts. Instead of taking sides, and affiliating ourselves either with a religion or the new age, it might be better simply to listen openly and learn from each other. There is no reason at all why new-age ideas shouldn't enrich people with a religious faith, or why new agers shouldn't explore the richness of religious teachings and, perhaps, their need for the divine. In this way, we can all develop a better understanding of why we are here and how we can best live our lives. Such tolerance of others and their beliefs keeps us humble and ever open to the possibility that others may hold some keys to the essential truths about life and death.

WHERE TO LOOK AND WHAT TO LOOK FOR

If you feel attracted to a particular faith or religion, don't be put off from trying to find out as much as possible about it. Constantly search and open yourself to listening and learning – it's never too late to meet your need for spiritual sustenance.

SPIRITUAL LIFE AND HEALTH

Having an active spiritual life doesn't prevent or cure all ills. However, it has provable links with health. Church attendance, for example, seems to benefit mental and physical health. Researchers in the USA report that churchgoers are less likely to divorce, commit suicide, and have drug or alcohol problems. They experience less heart disease; recover faster from burns and hip fractures; and are less likely to have high blood pressure, or need hospital admission.

◆ A 1987 review published in *Social Science Medicine* said that 22 out of 27 studies found that the more often a person went to church, the better was his or her health.

◆ A 1992 review in the *American Journal of Psychiatry* found that over 90 percent of studies into religious commitment and health showed that having a relationship with God and participating in religious ceremonies benefits mental health.

The reason for this is probably the teachings the religions give. They encourage us to enrich our spiritual lives with activities that emphasize the values that really matter. Such activities contribute to spiritual wellbeing which, in turn, can benefit physical health. But you don't have to be a churchgoer to benefit from a spiritual life.

Any one of us – religious, new-ager, both, or neither – can nurture our spiritual life by doing certain things each day.

Here are some examples:

◆ Meditating (*see page 142*).
◆ Living simply, without greed or excess.
◆ Seeking help from a spiritual teacher when our spirits are low or we feel hopeless.
◆ Celebrating the belief that each of us is more than just a mind and a body.
◆ Recognizing, feeling sorry for, and making amends for wrongdoing.
◆ Praying to and worshiping God or a "higher good". Making time for such activities will link you in spirit with millions of others around the world who are following a similar path. It is also very likely to lift your spirits and make you feel better emotionally. A fulfilling spiritual life can also refresh and strengthen your inner resolve and make you better able to cope with everyday activities and challenges.

This has repercussions for physical health. There is good evidence that feeling brighter boosts immunity, reduces the risk of heart attacks and other arterial disease, aids pain-management, and speeds recovery from illness. Meditation, for example, has been widely researched and shown to be beneficial to health (*see page 142*). Many people find that spiritual practices can help them to cope with emotional ill health too. If you're anxious or depressed, for example, spiritual practices can offer hope. And however unpleasant or hard an experience may be, and however rough and angry it may make you feel, many of those who come through difficult times say it is possible – eventually – to learn from adversity, and make good come from it.

Last but not least, spiritual teachers encourage the use of gifts and skills to help others feel noticed, cared for, and loved. This, in turn, enhances their emotional and physical health, and helps their own spiritual growth.

SUCH SKILLS AND GIFTS INCLUDE:

◆ Teaching.
◆ Encouraging.
◆ Helping others.
◆ Practicing discernment over family and community decisions.
◆ Giving.
◆ Being compassionate.
◆ Leading.

You'll be surprised how much inner peace and joy you'll experience as you exercise the great privilege of using your gifts and skills to do this work for the benefit of others.

Taking a few moments every day to sit quietly and comfortably and focus your thoughts inward will refresh you and strengthen your inner resolve.

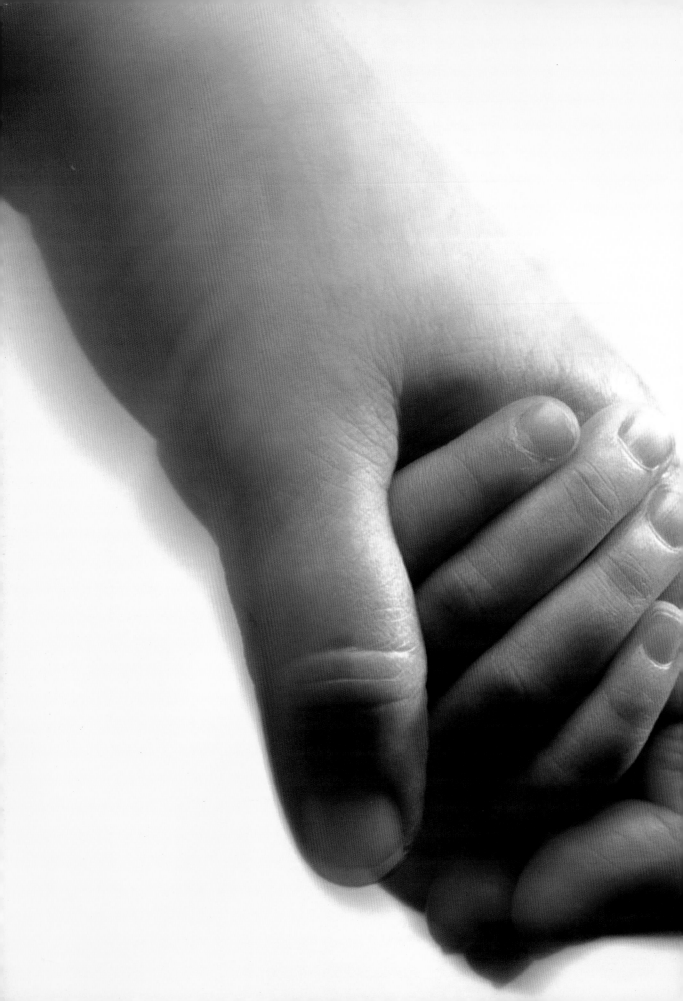

PART 2

Health in a Lifetime

SPECIFIC MEASURES FOR EACH AGE OR STAGE TO BALANCE LIFESTYLE, MAINTAIN HEALTH, AND PREVENT ILLNESS

CHILD TO WOMAN

Many years lie between the first signs of impending womanhood and becoming a physically mature young woman — which is just as well, because so much has to happen. On a physical level, you become able to reproduce, and your body gets into the habit of preparing each month for the possibility of pregnancy. On an emotional level, your relationships with the opposite sex and, perhaps, others too, start to change.

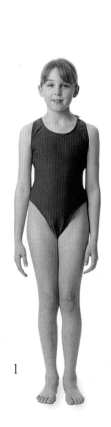
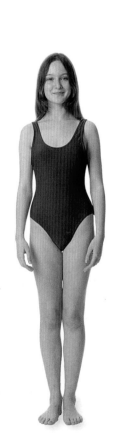
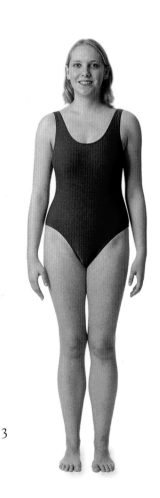
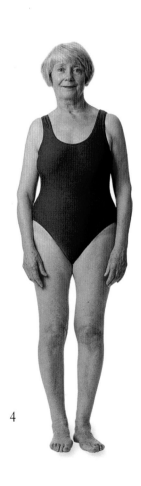

1   2   3   4

The challenging journey from child to woman is easier if you know what to expect from each stage.

1. At around ten years old many girls go through a growth spurt and other signs of maturity start to appear.

2. Teenage girls must learn to deal with periods and with the emotional turmoil that often goes with adolescence.

3. The childbearing years can be a woman's most challenging time when she may find herself devoting most of her energies to others.

4. Beyond the menopause women are free from of the burdens of the reproductive cycle yet can remain comfortably aware of their sexuality and self.

CHANGES IN YOUR BODY

You'll probably start to grow faster for a few years from around the age of ten-and-a-half years. Your reproductive system will probably begin maturing from around 10 to 12 too, though quite a few girls notice the first signs when a bit younger or older. First you'll see some breast-swelling and then some pubic and underarm hair. And you'll gradually develop curves. This is because your newly high

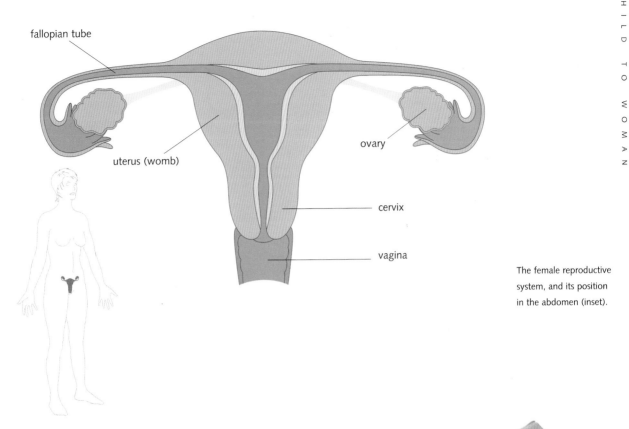

fallopian tube

uterus (womb)

ovary

cervix

vagina

The female reproductive system, and its position in the abdomen (inset).

level of a hormone called estrogen encourages fat to be laid down in your breasts, hips, and thighs.

PERIODS AND OVULATION

The first period marks an important stage on your journey from childhood to womanhood. It's also a pretty amazing and startling event, and in some parts of the world one that's actively celebrated.

Around 9 in 10 girls have their first period ("monthly" bleed from the womb) between the ages of 11 and 15 – the average age being 13. But some begin at 9 or younger, and others later. If your periods haven't started by the time you're 16, it may be wise to see your doctor. Periods generally begin when a girl weighs 42–52kg (92–114lb) and when 17 percent of this weight is made of fat. In the average girl periods come every 28 days, but a range of 20–35 days is perfectly normal.

For the first few months you probably won't release an egg from one of your ovaries (ovulate). So for a while you won't get any of the cramp-like aching some older girls get when their periods start.

If you can't talk with either of your parents about periods and growing up, ask a female relative, or your biology teacher. Some girls are shocked by their first period because they simply didn't expect it.

When you have a period you'll need to use sanitary protection. Most girls start with pads and leave tampons until they're older. Choose pads that are thin, highly absorbent and large enough to protect your underwear. A waterproof back and sticky wings make life easy. Take fresh pads to school in a wash-bag. And ask a friend who's already started having periods what to do with used ones (or ask a teacher).

CHANGING EMOTIONS AND BEHAVIOR

The teens are a time for recognizing, coming to terms with, and enjoying your developing sexuality. This is also a time for learning to relate to others in a more adult way. However, there'll still always be a childlike part inside you. Being able to recognize the difference between your "child" and "adult" sides helps you avoid slipping unknowingly back into childish behavior, and explains why someone behaves in a patronizing way toward you.

Choose the sanitary protection you feel most comfortable with. Most teenagers use sanitary napkins at first.

53

HEALTH

As you become a teenager, you start sharing the responsibility for protecting your health. A healthy lifestyle will help you feel well and boost your energy. It's also very important for your future wellbeing, as what you do now lays the foundations for the rest of your life.

FRESH AIR
Aim to get some fresh air every day if possible.

FRESH AIR IS:

◆ Brimming with oxygen.
◆ Lacking in the high levels of carbon dioxide found in crowded, poorly ventilated places.
◆ Free from vehicle-exhaust gases, smoke, and other pollutants.

Fill your lungs with fresh air by going for walks. If it's winter and the daylight hours are short, walk to and from school – or at least some of the way – as far from busy roads as possible.

SKIN CARE
Homemade skin-care products are often just as good as expensive commercially produced ones. So what do you need to keep your skin looking good? If you're prone to pimples, *see page 148*. But if your skin is clear, you need only two things:

◆ A moisturizer to prevent your skin from becoming too dry, especially in cold, dry, windy, or sunny weather. Creams and oils act as moisturizers by trapping a layer of the skin's natural moisture. Sweet almond oil is a pleasant one to use (add the oil from two capsules of vitamin E to a small bottle of almond oil to help preserve it, and store in a cool, dark place, such as the refrigerator). Another is a simple cold cream from the drugstore. You can make this smell wonderful by stirring in a few drops of lavender, neroli (bitter orange) or – though this is expensive – rose oil.

◆ Something to remove your make-up each night. Cleansing milks or creams are now more popular than soap and water. To get rid of stubborn eye make-up, use some sweet almond oil applied with a cotton ball.

LIGHT
It's all too easy when you're studying to get relatively little bright daylight on your eyes and skin. Yet you need light to keep well. Make a point of going outside for half an hour or so during the daylight hours each day, even on a cloudy day.

YOUR HOME ENVIRONMENT
If you're doing lots of homework, make sure you are sitting comfortably; otherwise you risk hunching over your books and getting an aching back and shoulders. Another tip for your back when carrying school books is to spread the load by wearing a backpack or to use a shoulder bag and sling the strap right over your head.

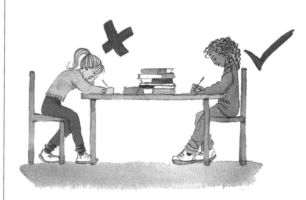

Sit squarely on your chair and keep your back straight. If you slouch you are more likely to get a backache.

Choose a bag that distributes the load evenly, rather than a shoulder bag that puts weight on just one shoulder.

HEALTHY EATING

The nutrients you get from eating healthy, well-balanced meals and snacks are vitally important for your development and growth. For example:

◆ Flavonoids, plant hormones, and a good balance of essential fats (*see page 25*) are necessary for well-balanced sex hormones, and for healthy skin and hair.

◆ Minerals such as calcium, magnesium, and boron build strong resilient bones. Resist any temptation to drink lots of coffee, or carbonated soft drinks such as cola, root beer, and ginger ale, as these can take calcium from your bones. One or two cans a day shouldn't be a problem.

Teenage girls are particularly likely to be short of iron, calcium, and riboflavin (vitamin B2), so make sure that you are eating enough foods rich in these nutrients (*see page 25*), especially if you are slimming or are a vegetarian or vegan. Slimming isn't wise. It's better to take half-an-hour's daily aerobic exercise, eat normal amounts of a healthy diet, and watch your body slim naturally as you grow.

EXERCISE

All types of exercise – aerobic, stretching, and strengthening – are beneficial at your age (*see page 28*). Weightbearing exercise (the sort that transmits weight to the feet) is especially good for developing bones. Examples include walking, dancing, and tennis. Transmitting your weight to your feet even though they aren't on the ground, such as with cycling and rowing, counts too.

RELAXATION AND PLAY

Learn to balance your life so you make enough time to relax and enjoy yourself, even when you're busy during the week with a full school day, family life, and homework. Try to vary your leisure activities and avoid the trap of lounging in front of the TV too much.

One suggestion for when you're studying for exams is to divide your day into thirds – studying during any two, and relaxing during the other.

STRESS MANAGEMENT

Teenagers can get just as stressed as adults. Indeed, stress may sometimes feel so overpowering that it's hard to know how to handle it. Adults get lots of advice about stress management but there's no reason why you shouldn't benefit from the information built up by stress counselors and others over the last 20 years. Turn to *page 34* to discover your signs of stress and find fresh ideas for handling them; then next time you feel fed up, try some new stress-management strategies.

SLEEP

Like most young people, you may sometimes want to go to bed late and then sleep in until late in the morning, if you can. That's fine if your commitments allow it and your parents agree. But take care that your sleeping pattern doesn't mean you never see your family, or prevents you from getting enough fresh air and daylight.

FAR LEFT: Carbonated drinks fill you with bubbles and may contain sugar that can rot your teeth.

Even at the height of studying, make time for some exercise and fun each day.

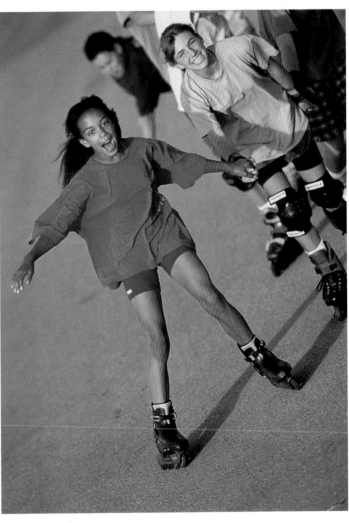

WORK

Relaxation, play, stress management, and exercise have all been mentioned – but what about work? Schoolwork, homework, domestic work, garden work, community work, babysitting – there's work in every part of life. And there are many ways in which work can affect how you feel.

Many young people's parents have seen and probably lived through a huge amount of change in the workplace, with lay-offs, unemployment, downsizing, being passed over for promotion, and so on. Careers are hardly ever for life nowadays, as they were for your grandparents' generation. And you may have heard that jobs are getting harder for young people to find.

But never have there been so many opportunities for education or training as today so to put things into perspective, let's go through some of the positives of the workplace.

PAID WORK CAN:

◆ Give you a good standard of living.
◆ Make life run smoothly.
◆ Be interesting.
◆ Civilize a society.
◆ Benefit others as well as yourself.
◆ Allow you to learn new things.
◆ Provide company.
◆ Give you a sense of purpose.
◆ Let you join with others to work toward a common goal.
◆ Encourage skills.
◆ Keep you in shape.
◆ Build community spirit.

Try to make some connections between working and keeping healthy by ticking any of the above that are true for you and your work. Next, think of any other positive aspects of what you think of as "work". This is worth doing, because by identifying what you find positive about working, you'll be pinpointing some of the benefits to your physical and mental health. "Keeps you in shape" is one obvious example, but "Provides company" promotes health too, because it can prevent loneliness and encourages interaction and friendships.

There can, of course, be a darker side to work too. Continued overwork can damage your health, and working without taking due care or safety precautions is plain stupid.

Take the subject of too much work first. It's interesting that employees have official regulations to protect them from being overworked (though they may still do so from choice, or because they fear they'll lose their jobs). Child actors, for example, can work only within strictly supervised limits. But schoolchildren have only their parents and themselves to monitor how much homework and other work they do. So it's vitally important to learn to pace yourself, to have adequate breaks, and to balance work and play. This is especially true if you're doing a job before or after school.

But what about the other side of the coin; young people who don't work hard enough? If you fall into this group, think long and hard about what people are trying to tell you – and what you're trying to tell them. A clearer understanding of this may change your perspective.

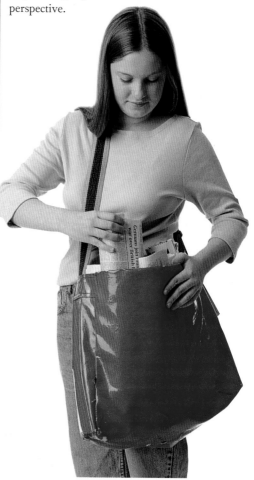

A part-time job provides welcome finance, boosts your self-esteem, and provides a sense of purpose.

YOUR APPROACH TO LIFE

The lifestyle choices that you make at this stage will have a big impact on your health, both physically and emotionally.

One of the many good things about being a young person is that you have a great deal of choice open to you. Depending on your age, stage, and situation you can decide what subjects to concentrate on studying. You can monitor how much work you do at home, and how and when you relax. You can make the arrangements for your social life. And depending on where you live, you'll be able to take yourself to meetings with friends and to other social events on foot, by bike or public transportation, or maybe by car.

All this means you probably have a lot more control over your lifestyle than you did when you were a child. It also means you have to take more responsibility for making choices or, perhaps more important, noticing when something you've decided on isn't going well, so you can try something else instead.

Having choices is like having rights of any kind – it brings responsibilities. And this taking on of choices and responsibilities is a major part of becoming an adult.

Having fun, and making serious life choices often go hand in hand.

DECIDING ABOUT DRUGS

Some decisions are more challenging than others. One example is drugs.

The standard advice given to all young people is "Don't do drugs." But nevertheless a fairly hefty proportion of teenagers ignores this. It has to be said that most come to no harm, and that many of those who are harmed have pre-existing problems. Either through desperation and bravado, or as a way of managing their stress, they use drugs too much, too often or without thinking about safety. A very few sink into the underworld of addiction and require a lot of professional and other help to pull out of it.

But, and this is a very big but, some apparently perfectly normal young people – those who have caring parents and are getting on okay at school and with their friends – are unexpectedly severely and permanently damaged by drugs.

Occasionally a young person who takes a single tablet, thinking it'll give them a high, ends up dead. You can't tell beforehand if you are going to be affected in this way. And you have no way of knowing what is really in a tablet or capsule unless you take it to a laboratory to be analyzed. But who's going to do that?

So clearly it's safest not to do drugs at all, ever. And if you feel emotionally unstable or upset this advice could be absolutely vital.

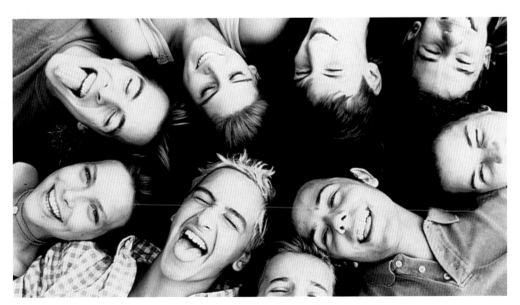

YOUR RELATIONSHIPS

Everyone knows relationships affect health. Good ones make you happy, make depression less likely and boost immunity. Conversely, bad ones are stressful, and can lead to stress-related disorders (*see pages 32 and 34*).

Your relationship with your parents is particularly important. There's no such thing as "typical" teenager–parent relationships. Teenage girls are as different from each other as are people in any other age group, and the same goes for parents.

Don't shut your parents out of your life. Talk over your problems with them and consider what they have to say.

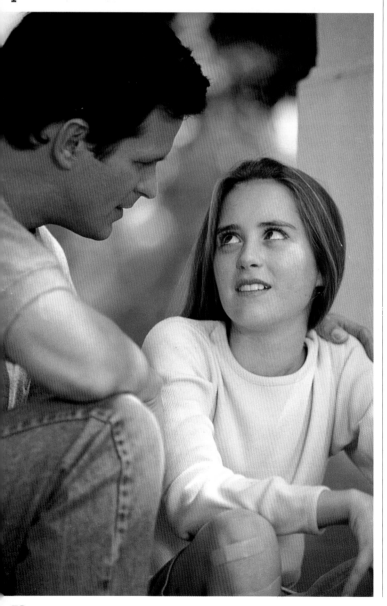

YOU AND YOUR PARENTS

One characteristic applies to most teenagers though, in spite of all their differences. Teenagers of both sexes frequently need extra parenting to help them on their way to independence. Indeed, some psychologists call this time "the second childhood." If insufficient good parenting (from parents or others) is available, certain challenging emotions and problems may be forced underground until some time later in life when someone else provides it.

Parenting skills include empathic listening, encouragement and conflict resolution (*see page 41*), and teaching teenagers how to solve problems.

GOOD COMMUNICATION

The fascinating thing is that a large part of good parenting is simply good communication. If neither your parents nor anyone else communicates well with you, demonstrating their skills in depth and with patience, you may have to resort to learning and practicing them yourself. Then who knows what might happen? Your parents might even learn from you how to communicate more effectively.

It is worth knowing that having a teenage girl around can raise feelings and issues for parents that existed for them when they were teenagers and which remain unresolved. So they may have personal issues to work on too.

Learning communication skills will help you manage stress better now and in the future. This should mean you're less likely to experiment with second-class and potentially dangerous stress-management strategies such as smoking, drinking too much alcohol, drug-taking or sleeping around, eating too much or too little.

One parenting skill not yet mentioned is the ability to set boundaries and make sure they're adhered to. Growing up is uncomfortable when discipline is too lax. It feels boundariless, frightening, and unsafe. And if a teen can't deal with the resulting fear, anger, or other difficult emotions, these may go underground, into the unconscious mind. Here they can trigger unsafe, "acting out" behaviors, such as hanging out with the wrong crowd, showing off by driving too fast, having fights and tantrums, getting pregnant "by mistake,"

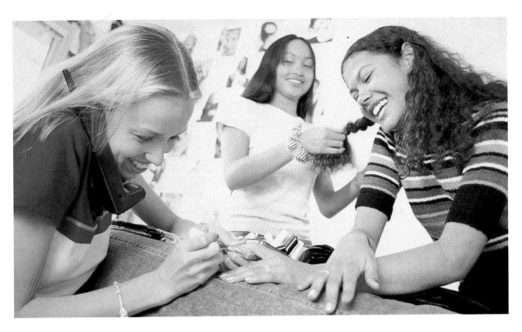

The friendships you form when you are young often last your whole life, because you share so many significant experiences.

developing an eating disorder, staying out late, or not getting homework done.

One final responsibility we have when we're young is to treat our parents with respect and consideration. Almost all parents love their children and try to do their best. And it's good to acknowledge this with good humor and affection.

RELATIONSHIPS WITH FRIENDS AND THE OPPOSITE SEX

Just as your relationship with your parents influences how you feel – and therefore your health – so too do your friendships. These help you grow and develop emotionally. Remember a time when a friend made you feel delighted, sad, angry, frustrated, excited, hopeful, hopeless, or happy? Experiencing these emotions gives you the chance to learn how to deal with them. And developing empathic listening skills, to use both with yourself and with your friends, is the key, along with conflict resolution skills to relating well to others throughout your life (*see page 41*).

You'll probably find that the way you deal with difficult emotional situations changes from time to time simply because some methods you try don't work well – neither resolving your feelings, nor mending things between you and others.

This is good, because all your life you'll have repeated experiences of challenging emotional situations between yourself and others. If now, as a young person, you can learn a range of effective ways of dealing with them, you'll be better equipped when you're an independent adult.

Relationships tend to be very intense at this time of life. It's a time when we feel very strongly about our parents, friends, and, of course, boys. Friends who are boys aren't just good friends like our girlfriends are. Once hormones are up and running, girls and boys are almost always aware of each other's sexuality. But that certainly doesn't mean you have to like or even want each other. Most ordinary heterosexual and so-called platonic friendships have sexual overtones too, even if both of you acknowledge that things will go no further between you.

Being friends with boys can be excellent practice for your future relationship with a partner. One reason why so many adult partnerships fail is because those involved haven't learned how to be friends as well as lovers. When the first flush of being in love subsides, they have nothing left.

This takes us back to the importance of learning to deal with emotional issues in friendships. In any relationship there are bound to be different points of view that can lead to disagreements and upsets. When conflict happens in a pair-bonded relationship, you both have to be able to deal with it, and move on together. Otherwise it may be tempting to split. And this isn't always for the best.

Unfortunately, but hardly surprisingly, the problems involved in separation and divorce can cause illness in either partner. As for children of divorced parents, it has been shown that they're more likely to suffer from stress-related problems, achieve less at school and at work, and to experience broken marriages themselves.

VIRGINITY, SEX, AND CONTRACEPTION

Staying a virgin until marriage was once widely considered the counsel of perfection, even though not everyone did it. Then in the 1960s increasing numbers of young people rode roughshod over this long-held moral code by going for sex without commitment – the hippy ethos of "free love".

Ever since, many adults have dithered over what to teach young people about sex before marriage. Often their only message is about "safe sex," which means using condoms or the Pill so you don't get pregnant, and using a condom to lower your risk of sexually transmitted infection.

If you have no clear moral guidelines, you'll have to choose for yourself from several options:

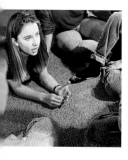

Don't let peer pressure influence your thinking about sex. Make sure that your views are your own.

THESE INCLUDE:

◆ Stay a virgin until you marry or settle down with your partner.
◆ Wait until you're in a "committed," loving relationship.
◆ Sleep with a number of different partners.
Today's pressures mean many teenage girls and boys find it difficult to stay virgins. But just because you have casual sex doesn't mean you're actually ready for sex and for the responsibilities to each other that go with it.

Many teenagers feel at heart that casual relationships of this sort debase sex. Indeed, casual, uncommitted sex is very rarely emotionally and spiritually enriching. Casual sexual partners are also less likely to use reliable contraception. And if you are unprotected or poorly protected by contraception, you run the risk of sexually transmitted infections and unwanted pregnancy.

SEXUALLY TRANSMITTED DISEASES

Infections aren't always easy to recognize. Yet if untreated they can cause pelvic inflammatory disease (*see page 188*) and infertility (*see page 195*). Some researchers recommend a test for one particular infection, chlamydia (*see page 183*) every six months for sexually active adolescent girls.

PREGNANCY

When teenage girls get pregnant by mistake they are faced with some agonizing choices. If a girl chooses to continue with the pregnancy she is burdened with baby care, her baby is more likely to grow up without the close involvement of its natural father, and society partly foots the bill. Having said that, some girls manage very well, especially if they have parents who are prepared to help.

The alternatives to having your baby and caring for it yourself are:
◆ Having an abortion (termination of pregnancy), which may leave some sadness and guilt forever, and denies the baby its life.
◆ Continuing with the pregnancy and having the baby adopted – which is a terrible wrench, but allows the baby's life to continue.

CONTRACEPTION

The only really reliable way of preventing pregnancy and infection is to abstain from sex altogether. If you don't, use reliable contraception such as the Pill (*see page 43* for its pros and cons, and *page 71* for starting).

Your partner should use a condom also to help protect you both from infection. Don't just rely on a condom alone for contraception, though, because it could well slip off or break.

In the UK, if you have unprotected sex (for example, because you miss a Pill – *see page 71*) then emergency contraception from a doctor, taken within 72 hours, usually prevents an unwanted pregnancy.

AGE OF CONSENT

There are legal as well as moral and other personal reasons for deciding when to start having sex. However, the minimum legal age at which a girl can agree to sex varies from country to country and, in the USA and Australia, from state to state.

Country	Minimum legal age for sex
England, Wales, and Scotland	16
Northern Ireland	17
USA	Varies from 14 in Hawaii and Pennsylvania to 18 in Arkansas and Virginia
Australia	Varies from 13 (in wedlock) in Western Australia to 16

YOUR INDIVIDUALITY

Part of being a teenager is discovering who you are. One day you'll look in the mirror and see yourself as if for the first time, just as you might look at someone new. But who you are isn't just about looks. The most important thing is what makes your mind tick.

Each generation hands down a moral code to its young. In most societies this code changes only slightly from one generation to another. Most of us, for example, know that we shouldn't kill or hurt others, or steal, and many of us have been taught to tolerate other people's beliefs and accept their differences.

Your parents and teachers will have handed you a moral code. However, it may not always be easy to stick to it, and sometimes you'll stray from it.

If this happens to you, and you let down yourself, your family and friends, or your school, it's good to do something about it.

AIM TO:

◆ Recognize what you've done wrong.
◆ Say sorry.
◆ Make up for it, if possible.
◆ Accept any punishment gracefully.

Everyone does wrong sometimes — it's part of being human. But we can learn from our mistakes, get help, if necessary, to avoid them in future, and end up making good come from them.

FULFILLING YOUR POTENTIAL

Accepting that you can move on like this and continually redefine your behavior if necessary is an important part of realizing that you have some control over your life. It helps define who you are — someone who recognizes right from wrong. And it allows you to be true to yourself and to fulfill your potential.

Another way of fulfilling your potential is by putting something back into the various systems that have helped you get this far — your family, your school, and your community. Learning to recognize and, where practical, help meet the needs of those around you is a vitally important part of living in any community. It also helps you to be happy with yourself and to create a sense of achievement that you have helped to do something worthwhile.

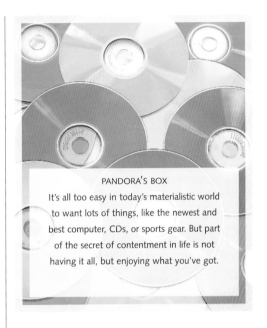

PANDORA'S BOX
It's all too easy in today's materialistic world to want lots of things, like the newest and best computer, CDs, or sports gear. But part of the secret of contentment in life is not having it all, but enjoying what you've got.

SOUL AND SPIRIT

The teens are a time when many of us become particularly interested in big questions, such as "Why are we here?" and "How did life on earth begin?" Thinking about possible answers and discussing them with friends, family, and teachers helps your spiritual side develop. Considering the possibility that there is more to life than just body and mind — that each human being has another dimension formed by her soul and spirit — is exciting and worth exploring. And realizing there may be something beyond ourselves, a higher power for good, can give purpose to our lives.

Get involved in your local community. Doing voluntary work is a good way to find out more about yourself while also benefiting other people.

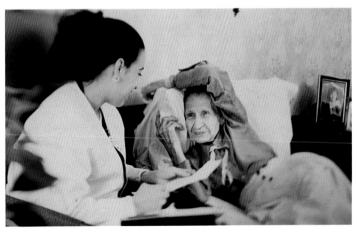

YOUNG WOMAN

As a young woman in your 20s or early 30s you have a lot of choices to make. This is a time for choosing where to live and what work to do. It's a time for seeking a partner to give you the pleasure of pair-bonding, sex, and, perhaps, children. And it's a time for firming up on what sort of person you want to be in terms of your behavior, your beliefs, and the way you handle your emotions.

Making choices can be exciting but it also takes energy. Given that you'll probably want to live life to the full, you'll find yourself playing hard and working hard. And it's now that you need to be especially sure that you're looking after your health.

Making time to be with friends and to share your current challenges, difficulties, and achievements, as well as your hopes and plans for the future, helps to bring a sense of balance to a busy lifestyle.

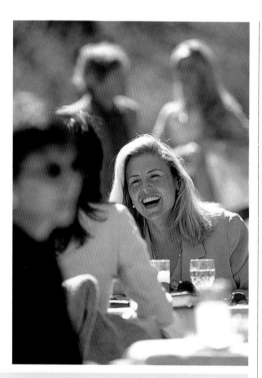

LOOKING AFTER YOURSELF

Most young women have family and friends to take an interest in their health and wellbeing. Employers, too, have a duty to care for their employees' health. However, during the transition from being a teenager living at home with your parents, to being a mature, independent woman, you'll gradually need to take over most of the responsibility for your health yourself.

THIS INCLUDES:

◆ Eating well and getting enough exercise and exposure to natural light.
◆ Using appropriate contraception if you are sexually active, unless you want to get pregnant.
◆ Learning to treat common ailments, using natural remedies and therapies when possible.
◆ Deciding when to see a doctor or other practitioner, and making it happen.
◆ Working out acceptable and effective stress-management strategies.
◆ Asking for help from family, friends, or, perhaps, a counselor or psychotherapist, if you get overstressed or depressed.
◆ Seeing your dentist regularly.

BALANCING WORK, RELAXATION, AND PLAY

Try to balance your duties at work with your responsibilities and leisure pursuits at home. You can assess this balance in three ways.

YOUR ENERGY LEVEL

When tired or exhausted, either rest more or do something to restore your mental and physical energy, or both. Eat a healthy diet with plenty of foods rich in vitamin B *(see page 25)*. And however little you may feel like it at first, consider whether you need more exercise: even if your work is physically onerous, you may not be getting a good balance of aerobic, strengthening, and stretching exercises.

First, consider how you feel. If you are over-stressed, you may need to make some changes to your life or to the way you cope with stress. Second, jot down the things that give you pleasure, and work out how often you do them. If this isn't nearly often enough, try reapportioning your time. Third, if you have too much leisure time, think about signing up for a course to learn something new, or working as a volunteer in the community.

HEALTHY EATING

If you are the one doing the shopping and food preparation, you may want to experiment with new ideas, buy take-out foods and super-market ready-meals, or cook familiar family recipes. Whatever you do, you need a well-balanced, nutrient-laden diet (*see page 24*). Several things are particularly important.

YOUR SPECIAL NEEDS

Strong bones Minerals such as calcium, magnesium, and boron make bones dense, hard, and resilient. The density of minerals in your bones is still building up to its lifetime peak. Most young women reach this "peak bone density" in their early 30s. This density needs to be as high as possible if you are to avoid having fragile, easily fractured bones (osteoporosis) later in life.

Encourage your bones to lay down minerals by eating plenty of mineral-rich foods. Good sources include dairy foods, root vegetables, green leafy vegetables, fish, meat, nuts, seeds, and bread and other foods made from cereal grains. Be warned, though, that eating too much animal protein (such as meat, fish, and eggs), and not enough vegetables and fruit, encourages minerals to leach out from bones. Having too many carbonated soft drinks has the same effect, too.

Balanced hormone levels Your body needs a good balance of progesterone and estrogens to prevent period problems, premenstrual syndrome (*see page 186*), polycystic ovary syndrome (*see page 193*), and other causes of lowered fertility.

One way of encouraging this is by eating foods rich in plant hormones (*see page 25*). These are similar in structure (though not identical) to your own hormones. Researchers believe that plant hor-mones, like your own, can latch on to the hormone receptors that cover each body cell. Latching on to receptors enables hormones to act by triggering certain cellular activities. Plant estrogens are less powerful triggers than your own estrogen. But if your estrogen level is low – which means some estrogen receptors are empty – then plant estro-gens can latch on to empty receptors and thereby switch on certain estrogen-controlled cellular activities. This helps prevent health problems due to a low estrogen level. Similarly, if your own estrogen level is too high, then by latching on to estrogen receptors and so taking the place of your own estrogen, plant hormones can prevent prob-lems resulting from too much of your own.

Reliable eating habits When busy studying, working, or socializing, you may not have much time to think about food. And if you're existing on a shoestring at college, you may want to spend

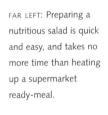
FAR LEFT: Preparing a nutritious salad is quick and easy, and takes no more time than heating up a supermarket ready-meal.

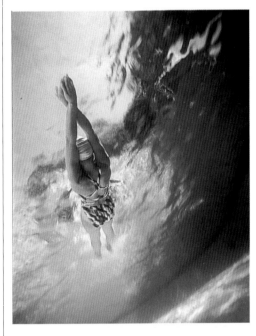
Swimming exercises your whole body without putting unnecessary strain on your joints.

your money on other things, like travel, CDs, or clothes. However, try not to neglect your diet and skip meals, as this could make you tired and irri-table and lead to bingeing. Bingeing regularly over the months or years encourages the polycystic ovary syndrome, with disrupted periods, hairiness, and lowered fertility.

Effective stress management Some young women manage stress by eating too much or not eating enough. At worst this leads to obesity (*see page 165*), or to bulimia or anorexia nervosa (*see page 206*). Remember that however hopeless you feel, you can – with help if necessary – always find other ways of managing stress.

HEALTH AT HOME AND AT WORK

This is a time of life when regular exercise is never more necessary, yet sometimes it's hard to make it happen and fit into your day.

Exercise is most practical and likely to happen if it suits your lifestyle. It's best if it takes place naturally, without having to be planned for, but it's better to plan for it than not to do it at all. Remember you don't have to do your daily half-hour of aerobic exercise all at once. You can take it in ten-minute chunks, spaced throughout the day if you prefer. Here are some ideas.

EXERCISE FOR WORKING WOMEN:

◆ If you commute by train, walk to the station instead of taking the car.
◆ If you go by bus, walk to the bus stop instead of getting a ride, and consider walking on to the next bus stop instead.
◆ Walk upstairs at work instead of taking the elevator or escalator. Or if you work high up in a skyscraper, walk the last few flights.
◆ Avoid sitting down during your lunch break, go for a walk instead.

EXERCISE FOR MOMS AT HOME:

◆ Take a brisk half-hour walk with your baby in the stroller or baby carriage.
◆ Run upstairs at home.
◆ Use an exercise video.
◆ Go to a gym or pool with a playpen so your baby can sleep safely or, with luck, watch contentedly while you exercise.
◆ Go to a gym or a pool with another mom and take turns caring for each other's baby while the other swims.
◆ Consider attending an exercise class with a nursery.
◆ Throw away the TV remote control.

LIGHT

It's wise to encourage the peak bone mineral density (BMD, *see page 179*) that you reach in your late 20s or early 30s to be as high as possible. Vitamin D will help your bones take up calcium and, while you can absorb this vitamin from your diet, the best way of getting it is from the action of bright daylight on your skin. Research has found that just two hours a week of sunlight on your bare face, arms and legs between 11a.m. and 3p.m. in the summer allows you to make and store enough vitamin D to meet your needs throughout the coming winter. However, too much sun can burn your skin, make it age prematurely, and encourage skin cancer. So always take care not to overexpose yourself (*see page 17*).

YOUR HOME ENVIRONMENT

When you choose where you want to live, it's worth putting health considerations somewhere near the top of your list. For example:
◆ If you live in a town or city, it might be wise (especially if you have asthma) to live somewhere with fresher air, such as several stories up, or on a hilltop, or to move to the suburbs or beyond.
◆ Choose somewhere dry. If necessary, pay a surveyor to measure moisture levels, then take steps to make your home damp-proof.
◆ Avoid the stress of poor soundproofing. A noisy neighbor can stop you sleeping and generally make your life hell.
◆ Have gas appliances checked annually for safety and to ensure there are no carbon monoxide emissions.

Take a brisk walk in the park with your baby. You will benefit from the exercise and you will both enjoy the fresh air, whatever the weather.

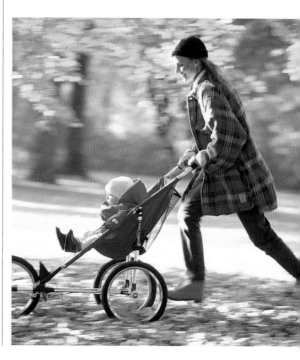

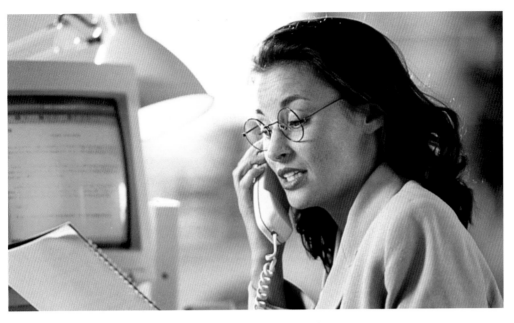

Have a five-minute break from your desk every hour, if possible. Take your lunch break and go for a quick walk before eating something light but nutritious.

HEALTH AT WORK

As a young woman out in the world of work, studying at college or working as a full-time mom looking after your children, you have a duty to look after your health. You owe this to yourself, to those who love and rely on you, and to your employers or college staff. Being young doesn't make you immune to the pressures of poor working conditions. But it could mean you don't know how to do anything about them.

Two of the commonest health concerns for young women are fatigue and period problems.

Fatigue Feeling tired generally results from burning the candle at both ends – working hard and playing hard. This is fine sometimes but it isn't if you lose out on sleep and rest.

As a student, for example, you may find that if you party until the early hours on Friday and Saturday nights, then sleep until noon, your energy level the next day is fine. But if you continue partying through to Sunday night, you might miss classes on Monday morning because you can't get out of bed.

Some ambitious young women determined to get ahead in their careers find themselves working very long hours. But if working late for days on end means you return to work jaded and not feeling at your best, this is clearly unproductive for you and your employer.

As for young mothers, they may have broken nights and early mornings, and these, together with staying up late to get some uninterrupted time, may make them exhausted.

Period problems The hormones produced by the pituitary gland in the brain are largely responsible for the timing and length of your periods, as well as for how heavy they are. The levels of these hormones are strongly influenced by various lifestyle factors, including the food you eat, your body weight, the amount of exercise you take, the exposure your eyes get to bright daylight, your emotional state, and your stress level.

Working too hard can lead to period problems if it means you spend too little time attending to your basic needs in these areas. You may, for example, suffer from period pain, heavy periods, irregular periods, or your periods may even stop completely if you do not look after yourself.

Take your sports clothes to work with you and go straight to the gym, pool, or squash court on your way home.

YOU MAY HAVE PERIOD PROBLEMS IF YOU:

◆ Eat a diet that doesn't provide you with enough nutrients.
◆ Lose too much weight.
◆ Take too much or too little exercise.
◆ Go outside in bright daylight too infrequently.
◆ Are shocked, or feel emotionally disturbed for long.
◆ Feel overstressed for a long period of time.

So if, as a young woman at work, you become overtired, or develop period problems, look to your lifestyle first. Making simple adjustments to the way you live your life could work wonders.

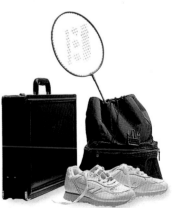

STRESS

Being overstressed can show in many ways (*see pages 32 and 34*). Two in particular – eating disorders and drinking too much – are becoming more common in young women.

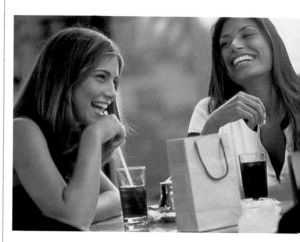

EATING DISORDERS

These often begin as a reaction to uncomfortable feelings that we haven't yet acquired the "emotional intelligence" to deal with differently. Having an eating disorder (*see pages 206 and 165*) acts as a reasonably effective defense against the pain of unacceptably difficult emotions. This is because the concentration on eating in a disordered way takes your mind off what's really going on inside. And it gives the impression that you – rather than your feelings – are in control.

You might, for example, smother frustration or grief by gorging on cookies even though you aren't physically hungry. You might deny yourself food to control guilt. You might make yourself vomit to forget despair. Or you might eat – or not eat – to display rage in a way that isn't actually murderous or suicidal.

EATING DISORDERS INCLUDE:

◆ Anorexia nervosa – losing weight by starving, despite feeling hungry.
◆ Bulimia – binge-eating then vomiting or purging.
◆ Compulsive eating, leading to obesity.
The trouble is that an eating disorder is neither an effective stress-management strategy, nor a good defense against emotional pain.

AN EATING DISORDER:

◆ Relieves stress only temporarily.
◆ Makes you feel uneasy.
◆ Hurts you physically.
◆ Doesn't effectively communicate your underlying feelings to others.
◆ Provides no avenue for negotiation.

If you have an eating disorder, you deserve better. So try this two-pronged approach:
◆ Learn to recognize and name your emotions using empathic listening skills (*see page 41*), if necessary with the help of a trusted friend, a counselor, or other expert. Naming emotions throws light on them so you can see what you're dealing with. And talking about them often shrinks their power.
◆ Work out other ways of managing stress (*see page 35*).

DRINKING A LOT OF ALCOHOL

More and more young women are drinking more than the recommended limit of one US unit or two UK units a day (*see also page 37*).

WARNING SIGNS OF DRINKING TOO MUCH INCLUDE:

◆ Needing alcohol every day.
◆ Having an alcohol-related problem, such as drink-driving.
◆ Turning down other activities so you can drink.
◆ Having to have more alcohol than before to produce the same effect.
◆ Feeling irritated if questioned about drinking.
Drinking too much over many months or years raises the risk of breast and certain other cancers, liver and pancreas damage, memory loss and, with more than three units a day, high blood pressure, heart disease, and strokes.

So sort out your drinking problem fast. Keep a drink diary. Confine drinking to a particular part of the day. Increase your number of alcohol-free days. And accept help from your doctor or an agency offering advice, counseling, and support.

YOUR APPEARANCE

How you look reflects the time and care you put into your appearance. This, in turn, mirrors how good you feel about yourself. And feeling and looking good are important parts of staying well.

Over the last few decades the media has devoted an enormous amount of coverage to beauty and image. You have only to look at magazine racks to see the wide variety of titles appealing particularly to women in their 20s and 30s. Page after page debates fashions, shows before-and-after photos of women who've had makeovers, and discusses the pros and cons of various cosmetics, creams, lotions and potions to beautify the face, body, hair, and nails.

So what are you to make of them? Do you really want to become a fashion victim by slavishly following the latest styles? Is the advice focused carefully enough on you and your lifestyle, skin, hair, and body shape? Or is reading women's magazines more a way of relaxing, and doing what women down the ages have always enjoyed — watching other women, seeing how they care for and adorn themselves, and getting a few tips for themselves into the bargain?

Once you see all this information for what it really is — passive, relaxing entertainment — you can then begin to do some realistic thinking about your own appearance.

To make the most of what you've got and to feel good about yourself, you need to do some careful assessments. Focus one by one on your shape and size; hairstyle, color, and condition; skin type and coloring; and wardrobe. Think too, if you use them, about your make-up, skin-care products, and perfume. To give yourself a helping hand, you could buy one of the excellent practical guidebooks on improving your individual style. Or you could enlist the help of a good friend, or even pay to see an image consultant. Doing it this way means you concentrate on your own needs and opinions, instead of those of other women in a magazine photo or article.

CHOOSING CLOTHES

Many women agree that the best use of their money and wardrobe space is to build up a capsule wardrobe containing a few good quality items, such as a couple of well-fitting jackets, some

trousers, skirts, and dresses in neutral colors such as beige, black, or navy. Keep them well maintained, and introduce changes with tops and accessories such as scarves and jewelry. Casual clothing, being cheaper, gives more flexibility for experimentation.

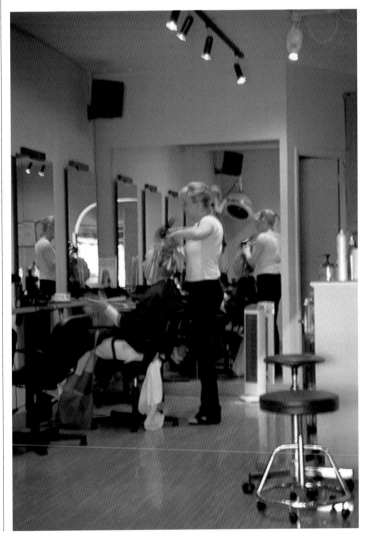

BELOW: Discuss with your hairdresser which hairstyle will best suit your face and hair.

ABOVE: Your hands are as visible as your face so keep them well cared for and keep your nails clean and manicured.

ALTERNATIVES TO PLASTIC SURGERY

The two plastic surgery operations most favored by young women are breast reduction and breast augmentation. The back pages of many women's magazines are full of advertisements for private clinics offering plastic surgery. Many of these clinics are staffed by young surgeons who've had no special-ist plastic-surgery training, and are therefore under-trained to provide an expert service.

Part of the service offered by experienced plastic surgeons in-cludes a realistic assessment of a woman's need for the proposed surgery, her psychological state, the likely outcome, and the risks involved. But some of the clinics that advertise to the public neglect this area. The result can be disappointment, wasted money, and unexpected and some-times disastrous side effects.

And some inexperienced or time-pressed "counselors" in these clinics fail to offer the women who consult them a down-to-earth outline of any alternative ways of dealing with their dissatisfaction.

Take large breasts. A woman's breast-size fluctuates throughout her life according to her weight, her natural estrogen level, whether she's on the Pill or other hormonal contraception, whether she's pregnant or breastfeeding, and whether she's pre- or postmenopausal.

It's often possible to shrink large breasts nat-urally and safely by eating a healthy diet rich in plant estrogens; taking a daily half-hour of aerobic and muscle-strengthening exercise – including strengthening exercises for the pectoral muscles in the upper chest; keeping your Body Mass Index (BMI) between 20 and 25 (*see page 27*); and asking for a progestogen-only Pill instead of one that contains estrogen.

◆ The combination of a healthy diet and aerobic and muscle-strengthening exercise will help shed excess fat from the breasts.

◆ Doing muscle-strengthening pectoral exercise will help keep your breasts in good shape as they slim down.

◆ The plant estrogens, being weaker than the your own natural estrogens, may prevent your estrogens from encouraging fat to be deposited in your breasts.

◆ A progestogen-only Pill won't have the breast-enlarging effect of one that contains estrogens.

◆ Drinking bottled water means you'll avoid exposure to any recycled estrogens present in piped water.

As for small breasts, it's well worth doing pectoral muscle exercises and learning to maintain a really good posture, both of which make the most of small breasts. Try putting on a few pounds if you're underweight. Eat foods that are rich in plant estrogens, as this could make up for any lack of estrogen (though most women with small breasts don't lack estrogen). If you use contraception, talk to your doctor, because you might like to go on an estrogen-containing Pill for its enhancing effects on breast size.

Drink plenty of bottled water to help keep your skin clear.

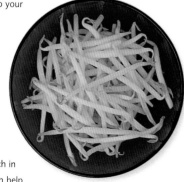

Choosing a diet rich in plant estrogens can help reduce breast size.

YOU AND MEN

Most young women are all too aware of the opposite sex, and most want at some stage to find someone with whom to have an intimate and sexual relationship, share their life and, perhaps, have their children. Indeed, the 20s is the time when many women choose their partner, although increasing numbers of women in Western countries are now putting their career first in their 20s, and delaying partner selection until their 30s.

But what has this got to do with your health? The answer is, a great deal. Any activity that takes so much time and mental space is bound to impact strongly on your physical and mental wellbeing. To help ensure that this impact is positive and life enhancing, rather than negative and energy sapping, here are a few tips.

BE FRIENDS

Try to base close relationships with men on friendship as much as sexual attraction. Friendship is also very important as a sexual attraction develops into something stronger, and it remains vital when two people commit themselves to living together. Friends like being together. They enjoy doing things – though not necessarily everything – together. And they like having separate sides to their lives so that they can meet others, learn fresh things on their own, and bring back new ideas – "seed-corn" – to enrich their relationships with each other.

BE REALISTIC

If you're in a close relationship, don't expect your man to meet all of your needs. No one can do that. This unrealistic expectation is an important reason behind the failure of so many marriages and long-term live-in relationships. And it results in the emotional pain surrounding separation and divorce that is responsible for so much mental and physical illness in later life.

Instead, realize that when things go wrong in life they often affect both of you at the same time. So neither is best able to support the other. This means you may each need to look to a good friend, close relative or professional counselor for extra help and support. Expecting or even insisting that your man should meet your every need can be doomed to failure in such situations, and could easily send you from man to man in search of the non-existent perfect partner.

BE A GOOD LISTENER

Learning to listen in an empathic way (*see page 41*) to yourself and your man means you'll be able to accept yourself and him as individuals, rather than using him as a mirror in which to see yourself. In this way you each retain your own viewpoints, emotions, needs, desires, and dreams.

Friendship is vitally important within our family, with our girlfriends, with our colleagues, and with our one-to-one partner.

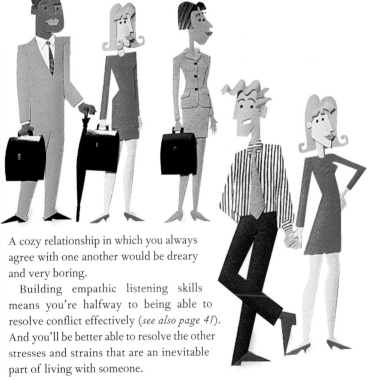

A cozy relationship in which you always agree with one another would be dreary and very boring.

Building empathic listening skills means you're halfway to being able to resolve conflict effectively (*see also page 41*). And you'll be better able to resolve the other stresses and strains that are an inevitable part of living with someone.

PERIODS AND OVULATION

Many young women today find their life disrupted by difficult periods. It can be difficult to separate the emotional and physical influences of any aspect of health, but sometimes it's almost impossible when it comes to period problems. However, what can help is to look at your feelings as well as your physical health.

This is partly because the way you feel at an emotional level alters the levels of neurotransmitters in your brain. These influence the hypothalamus. And this, in turn, affects the output of the gonadotrophic hormones from the pituitary gland that stimulate your ovaries and so influence ovulation and periods.

Each month, in the first half of your menstrual cycle, your brain's pituitary gland releases a gonadotrophin called follicle-stimulating hormone. This stimulates the development of between 10 and 20 egg follicles in your ovaries. Each of these follicles contains an immature egg, and all produce estrogen, but only one egg develops to maturity. Once this leaves the ovary, your pituitary gland releases another gonadotrophin – luteinizing hormone. This triggers the follicle left behind in the ovary by the departed egg to become a "yellow body" (corpus luteum) that releases progesterone and estrogen.

You now see why strong or longstanding emotions can exert changes in your ovaries. For example, feeling anxious when overstressed can prevent the hypothalamus from telling the pituitary to release follicle-stimulating hormone and luteinizing hormone. This, in turn, lowers the levels of estrogen and progesterone, and can prevent ovulation (and therefore pregnancy too). Even if you don't ovulate, you can still bleed each month, but your periods will be irregular and you can't get pregnant.

Warning: Don't kid yourself, though, that feeling anxious is an efficient contraceptive, because it most certainly is not.

EXERCISE AND DIET

Your emotions aren't the only things that can affect periods and ovulation. Intensive exercise can also have an effect on the hormones controlling both these aspects of your physiology. If you train too hard, your periods may stop. This is because your body responds to the stress of training by producing hormones that act on the hypothalamus to stop the pituitary gland from releasing the gonadotrophins that control ovarian function.

Your body weight and eating pattern can also affect your ovaries. If your weight falls too low, your periods will stop. If it's too high for your height because of binge eating, you may develop an imbalance of the gonadotrophins produced by the pituitary gland. The result is the development of multiple small cysts on your ovaries (*polycystic ovaries, see page 193*), the cessation of ovulation, and scanty, irregular periods.

The daily length of exposure of your eyes to bright light is yet another thing that affects the pituitary gland. Too little light means your hypothalamus is understimulated. This makes your brain's pineal gland produce too little of another hormone called melatonin. This makes you less likely to ovulate, which can make your periods irregular.

Both exposure to light and healthy vigorous exercise contribute to a well-functioning menstrual cycle.

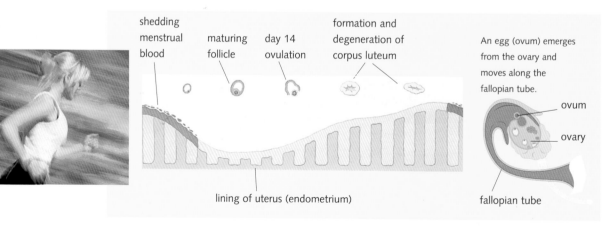

shedding menstrual blood

maturing follicle

day 14 ovulation

formation and degeneration of corpus luteum

An egg (ovum) emerges from the ovary and moves along the fallopian tube.

ovum

ovary

lining of uterus (endometrium)

fallopian tube

SEX AND CONTRACEPTION

Nowadays sex is mainly for fun, not babies. Most probably you, like lots of young women, want to have a baby when the time is right. So in the meantime you'll need contraception that interferes with sex as little as possible and protects you from pregnancy until you're ready to start a family. Most young women choose the Pill, but it's wise to insist on a condom as well (to protect you both from infection) unless you were both previously virgins, or you have been faithful to each other for many months.

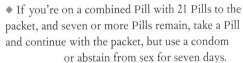

THE PILL

If you're about to start the Pill, several things are worth knowing.

THESE ARE:

◆ A medical check is essential.
◆ You need a Pill to suit your age, stage of life, and medical history. The estrogen content of combined oral contraceptive pills ("COCs," containing estrogen and progestogen) varies from 20–50 micrograms; the lower-estrogen ones have a reduced risk of producing estrogen-related side effects, but allow a very slightly higher chance of pregnancy. Progestogen-only pills ("POPs") contain no estrogen.
◆ Many monthly packs contain only 21 pills, so you have seven Pill-free days between packs. "Everyday" packs contain 28 Pills: 21 active and seven inactive ones.
◆ With some types of Pill you have no periods for months at a time.
◆ You may have scanty periods and irregular bleeding, especially early on.
◆ You'll need urgent attention for symptoms that may result from a blood clot. These are pain or swelling in your leg, chest pain, breathlessness, coughing up blood-stained sputum, a severe headache, or weakness in one side of your body.
Pill failure Oral contraception can fail if you forget a Pill by more than 12 hours (three for an "everyday" combined, or progestogen-only Pill), or if you start a packet late, have severe diarrhea or vomiting, or take antibiotics.

◆ If you're on a combined Pill with 21 Pills to the packet, and seven or more Pills remain, take a Pill and continue with the packet, but use a condom or abstain from sex for seven days. Have your usual seven Pill-free days before the next packet.
◆ But if six or fewer Pills remain, take a Pill, use a condom or abstain from sex for seven days, and when you finish the packet, start the next right away. You may not have a period until after the next packet, but that doesn't matter.
◆ If you're on an everyday Pill, and six or fewer active Pills remain, take a Pill at once, use a condom or abstain from sex for seven days, continue with the active Pills, miss the inactive ones, then start the next packet.
◆ If you take a progestogen-only Pill more than three hours late, use a condom or abstain from sex for seven days.
◆ In the UK, if you had sex during your normal Pill-free week and start your next packet late, consider emergency contraception (from your doctor). Emergency contraception within 72 hours of unprotected sex (the "morning-after" Pill) usually prevents pregnancy.

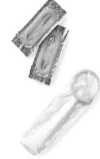

The Pill alone won't protect you from sexually transmitted infection – only condoms or a long-term, faithful relationship can do that.

Take contraceptive advice from a professional who will be able to talk you through your needs.

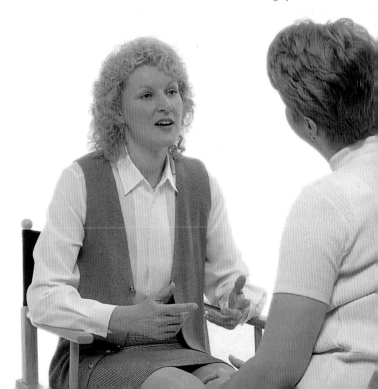

PREVENTING SEXUALLY TRANSMITTED DISEASES

Sexually transmitted diseases (*see also page 183*) are a growing problem because both casual sex and repeated short-lived faithful relationships readily spread infection like wildfire.

The only sure way of protecting yourself is to have sex only with one lifelong partner, and for him never to have had – or have – sex with anyone else. The next best bet is for you both to remain faithful. However, it's possible for a man or a woman to be infected without knowing before entering a new sexual relationship.

◆ Soreness – this can accompany thrush, trichomonal infection, and herpes virus infection.
◆ Genital blisters or ulcers – these are important signs of a herpes virus infection, and can make urination painful.
◆ Discomfort during sex – can accompany any sexually transmitted infection.
◆ Painful urination – can result from herpes blisters, gonococcal infection, or soreness of the vulva following scratching of the skin with any itchy infection.

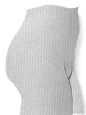

Look after your sexual health. You have a duty to your male partner to say if you have an infection.

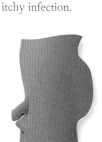

Be aware that infections can sometimes be "silent," and that a man may not reveal his sexual history.

If you know there's a problem, you can use a condom (which gives good, though not complete, protection), and – if you're infected – stop your partner from performing oral sex on you until the infection has been successfully treated.

But sometimes an infection is "silent," with no recognizable symptoms or telltale signs. So it's wise for new sexual partners to use a condom for some months unless they are both sure they are infection-free.

EARLY SIGNS OF INFECTION INCLUDE:

◆ An abnormal vaginal discharge (*see page 192*).
◆ Low abdominal pain – can mean the infection has spread beyond the vagina into the womb or pelvis, causing pelvic inflammatory disease (*see page 188*). This can result from any one of several sexually transmitted infections.
◆ Bleeding between periods or after sex – the bleeding can also result from pelvic inflammatory disease.
◆ Fever – can be a symptom of pelvic inflammatory disease.
◆ Genital itching – common with thrush and herpes-virus infection.

FAR RIGHT: A condom offers some protection against infections.

IF YOUR PARTNER HAS AN INFECTION, HIS SYMPTOMS MAY INCLUDE:

◆ A discharge from the penis.
◆ Pain on passing urine.
◆ A rash or other skin change on his genitals.
If you or your man suspect an infection, refrain from sex without a condom – and from oral sex, and see a doctor for diagnosis and treatment.

HEALTH SCREENING

Worthwhile screening tests for this period in your sexual life include:
◆ A chlamydia test – every six months to a year, unless you are having sex only with one faithful boyfriend.
◆ A Pap (cervical) smear every year in the USA (every three to five years in the UK) for sexually active women over 20. This involves a doctor or nurse putting an instrument called a speculum into your vagina, then gently removing some cells from your cervix. These are examined in a laboratory for any signs of abnormality that could one day, if not treated, progress to cervical cancer.

HAVING CHILDREN –
IF, WHEN, AND WITH WHOM?

Down the ages most young women have wanted to have babies at some stage in their lives. And today's young woman is no exception. The question, for many, is When? Almost completely reliable contraception has meant that for the first time ever women can now choose if and when to get pregnant. This, of course, means we can also choose how many children we want.

You might think this is good news. And in many ways it is. Apart from freedom from unwanted pregnancy, and the choice of family size, using reliable contraception means you're not repeatedly pregnant throughout your reproductive life, like millions of women throughout history. But while the freedom to choose is an enormous advance, it also presents some dilemmas.

One is that you have to make a choice, whereas before there was really reliable contraception, conception was much more unpredictable. Making a choice means weighing up the pros and cons of if and when to get pregnant. That can be hard. So in this sense things were perhaps easier before the arrival of reliable contraception.

Another dilemma is that once you've decided to try for a baby, you might not necessarily conceive when you want to, or even – for some women – at all. So you move from thinking that you have the choice to realizing with increasing certainty as your period comes each month that you're going to find it difficult or even impossible to have a baby (*see page 195*).

SINGLE PARENTHOOD

For some young women the problem isn't deciding whether or when to have a baby. They know they want one – perhaps even as soon as possible – but they haven't yet found a partner with whom they want to start a family. This, of course, isn't a modern problem. What's fascinating today is that more and more young women are getting pregnant outside committed relationships and opting to start motherhood as single parents, sometimes not even letting the fathers know. This too isn't new, but with welfare programs, nurseries, and the option for mothers of young children to work, it's sometimes easier financially than it used to be.

Having said all this, the vast majority of young women who willingly get pregnant already live with the fathers of their children in committed relationships. Increasing numbers of babies, however, are being born outside marriage, though some unmarried parents go on to legalize their relationships later.

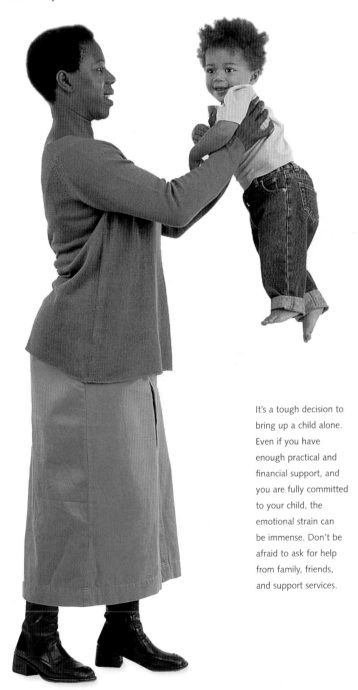

It's a tough decision to bring up a child alone. Even if you have enough practical and financial support, and you are fully committed to your child, the emotional strain can be immense. Don't be afraid to ask for help from family, friends, and support services.

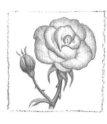

PREGNANCY AND BIRTH

The whole process of reproduction – from sexual attraction to partner selection, intercourse, conception, pregnancy, birth, and breastfeeding – may be something all mammals do, but it is still a complete and utter miracle. It's also of central importance to most women's lives. For you are likely to find that your sexuality and ability to attract and want a partner occupy a large part of your thoughts. And conceiving, bearing, and nurturing a baby will change the course of your life forever.

This section looks at how you will know you're pregnant, follows the changes in you and your baby during pregnancy, then discusses what happens during labor and the birth itself. It also shows how you can care for your baby and yourself during pregnancy and birth.

FERTILITY

Your fertility will peak in your 20s, but your biological clock means that from your late 20s onward you'll become less and less likely to conceive. This is because your egg supply is limited. At birth you had around a million eggs. By the time you started periods, the number had already fallen to 250,000. Since then, you've lost hundreds in each menstrual cycle. When only 25,000 or so are left (probably when you are around the age of 37) they'll be lost twice as fast. And the fewer your eggs and the older they are, the lower your fertility. Indeed, the average woman's reproductive ability begins to fall from her mid-30s onward.

A new test developed in the UK (the G-test, which involves an ultrasound scan, a pituitary gland-stimulating drug, and three blood tests) reveals how well a woman's ovaries are working and whether she can afford to wait to get pregnant or not. A man's fertility also falls with the passing years.

BOOSTING FERTILITY NATURALLY

Aim to have sex when you're most fertile. Whatever their cycle length, women almost always ovulate 14 days before their periods start. So with a 28-day cycle, for example, you'll probably ovulate on day 14 (counting the first day of your period as day one), so you'll be most fertile on days 10–15 (and particularly on days 13–15).

For conception to occur, an egg must be fertilized within 24–36 hours. Sperms usually live up to 72 hours, so the best time for sex is from 72 hours before, to 36 hours after, ovulation.

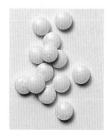

Women trying to become pregnant are now advised to take folic acid supplements.

SEX AND FERTILITY

FREQUENCY OF SEX

To try and become pregnant, have unprotected sex once each day in the week before you are due to ovulate. If your partner (or you) can bring you to orgasm, so much the better. Stay lying down with a pillow under your hips for 15 minutes after sex.

SMOKING AND DRINKING

Stop smoking and limit your alcohol intake to make early miscarriage less likely.

YOUR FOOD

Eat a healthy diet with plenty of foods rich in vitamins B, C, and E, folic acid, selenium, and zinc to nourish your eggs. And start taking folic acid supplements now (*see page 78*).

FOODS THAT UPSET YOU

Avoid foods to which you are sensitive as they could reduce your fertility.

STRESS

Learn to manage stress effectively (*see page 34*) because stress hormones can prevent ovulation.

KNOWING YOU'RE PREGNANT

Some women have a sixth sense about being pregnant. They know they've conceived even before there are any obvious signs, and before a test could reveal pregnancy hormones. A few women seem to know right from conception. But many suspect that something has happened only when their periods are late or they experience morning sickness. And a very few go right through pregnancy without realizing they are pregnant. But what signs are likely?

A missed period is usually the first sign, though some women experience a little monthly bleeding at around the time they would have had periods, for the first one, two, or three months. In addition, you may notice other changes.

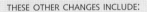

THESE OTHER CHANGES INCLUDE:

◆ Uncharacteristic fatigue.
◆ Nausea from about two weeks after your missed period.
◆ Increasingly full and, perhaps, tender breasts.
◆ More frequent urination.
◆ Food cravings. These are often for salty or unusual foods, such as pickles or sardines; a few women even find themselves attracted to coal or earth.
◆ Unusual hunger.
◆ An aversion to coffee, tea, or alcohol.
◆ A metallic taste from certain foods.

If you want to confirm your pregnancy, buy a test kit from the drugstore. Use this any time after the day that your period would have been due. Alternatively, ask your doctor to arrange a pregnancy test for you.

Working out your "due date" Using a calendar, take the first day of your last period, go forward nine calendar months, then forward one more week.

Your response to being pregnant The way you feel will depend partly on whether you're pleased or shocked to find yourself pregnant. If you've been planning this baby, then discovering you're pregnant is probably going to be a huge thrill. Indeed, many women find they think of little else. The change in how you feel from being an "ordinary" non-pregnant woman to one who is expecting a baby is much greater than you might have imagined.

Whatever you happen to be doing, you will probably find that your mind keeps returning to the baby inside you. Indeed, many women focus almost totally on their pregnancy and tend not to look beyond the birth to the practicalities of life with a baby.

In contrast, many fathers-to-be are often very interested in what life is going to be like when the baby is born.

You and your partner Now is an excellent time for you both to practice your skills of empathic listening and encouragement (*see page 41*). Once your baby is born, life will change a lot. And using these skills will help you to recognize and validate each other's emotional reactions to this change.

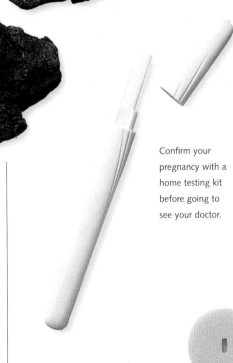

Left: Cravings for unusual foods – or perhaps even coal and earth – are not unusual in early pregnancy.

Confirm your pregnancy with a home testing kit before going to see your doctor.

Once the pregnancy is confirmed, you will find your baby occupies your thoughts for much of the day.

YOU AND YOUR GROWING BABY

Your baby's life begins well before your pregnancy starts to show. After the first four weeks, the organs, limbs, and face begin to form, the heart starts beating, and the nervous system begins to develop.

The average woman is pregnant for nine calendar months, which is 280 days, or 10 four-week months. You and your doctor can work out when your baby is due and this date can be confirmed by a scan, if necessary.

However, only seven babies in 100 arrive on the "expected date of delivery". A perfectly normal pregnancy can last anywhere between 37 and 42 weeks. Some babies are born prematurely, before this time, and some, if there's no obstetric intervention, after this time.

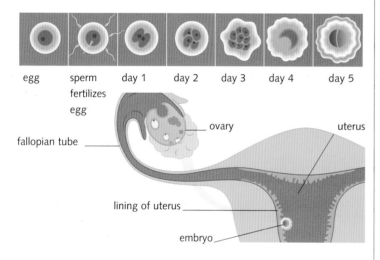

egg | sperm fertilizes egg | day 1 | day 2 | day 3 | day 4 | day 5

fallopian tube · ovary · uterus · lining of uterus · embryo

As the weeks go by, this is what you may notice, and this is how your baby will grow and develop.

MONTH ONE (1–4 WEEKS)

Your baby's life begins – and you become pregnant – when your partner's sperm fertilizes your egg. This event, known as conception, normally occurs in one of the fallopian tubes (the passage-ways running from near each ovary to the inside of the womb). The microscopically small newly fertilized egg makes an epic six-day journey through the fallopian tube to the womb. By the time this tiny scrap of life arrives safely there, the original single cell (carrying genetic material from both of you) has become an embryo, a ball of dividing cells the size of a sugar grain. This embryo then nestles into the womb lining.

During this time you'll miss your period (or bleed only a little), and may experience some of the other early signs of pregnancy.

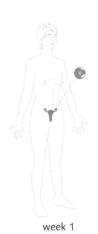

week 1

MONTH TWO (5–8 WEEKS)

Your baby grows to 2.5cm (1in) long. The organs, arms, legs, and face start developing, the heart begins beating, and the nervous system is nearly fully developed.

You'll probably find the early signs of pregnancy now become more obvious. In addition, your skin may be dry or flaky. You may notice pimples for the first time in years. And you could sometimes feel faint, especially if you stand for some time in a hot, relatively airless place.

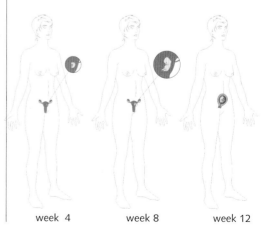

fetus · placenta · umbilical cord

In the third month the baby's face becomes more defined. Also, morning sickness might lessen.

MONTH THREE (9–12 WEEKS)

Your baby grows to 6.5cm (2½in) and is now called a fetus. The skeleton and external genitals begin to appear. The arms have already grown long enough for your baby to be able to touch its face; the fingers and toes are developing; and the legs start to kick, though you won't feel them for some time. The face looks more like a face, though the lower jaw isn't fully developed. The eyelids gradually cover the eyes, then remain shut until month seven. And hair begins to grow.

If you've been feeling sick, you'll probably find this lessens now. You may notice some weight gain. And you'll feel warmer than usual.

week 4 · week 8 · week 12

MONTH FOUR (13–16 WEEKS)

Your baby grows to 16cm (nearly 7in). The kidneys and other organs are working, finger and toenails now start to grow, and the eyebrows and lashes appear.

You may find you feel very well and much less tired, and you may notice some swelling of your lower abdomen.

MONTH FIVE (17–20 WEEKS)

Your baby grows to 25.5cm (10in) and scalp hair begins to appear. The fingers have short nails, and the cartilage (gristle) of the skeleton is being hardened by minerals such as calcium and magnesium. When awake, your baby may suck a thumb (or finger or fingers), and move his or her arms or legs.

You may look "blooming". You'll probably feel very well, with thicker, shinier hair and a glowing complexion. You may dream more than usual, though your memory may not be as sharp as before. You might feel your baby moving and kicking from about 18 weeks.

MONTH SIX (21–24 WEEKS)

Your baby grows to 33cm (13in) and, because the brain cells are maturing fast, may react to stimuli such as noise or warm bath water by moving around – and perhaps even turning somersaults – in the fluid in your womb.

You'll probably feel fine, and be aware sometimes of your baby's movement. Your expanding womb pressing on your diaphragm may mean you breathe harder during exercise.

MONTH SEVEN (25–28 WEEKS)

The average baby now weighs almost 1kg (2lb), about the weight of a large bag of sugar, and can open its eyes and maybe hiccup too.

A baby girl's ovaries now contain about 7 million eggs, though by birth this number will have fallen to around a million (*see page 74*). A baby boy's scrotum has developed by now too.

You'll have a "bump" and may sometimes notice your womb tightening with "trial" or "Braxton Hicks" contractions. These are similar to the contractions during an orgasm, or at the beginning of a period or labor itself. If you put your hand on your abdomen during one of these contractions you'll feel your womb hardening as it tightens.

MONTH EIGHT (29–32 WEEKS)

Your baby probably now weighs about 1.5kg (over 3lb) and can swallow.

Your energy levels will probably fluctuate, and you'll sometimes feel very tired and have backache. Almost every pregnant woman looks pregnant now.

MONTH NINE (33–36 WEEKS)

Your baby may weigh as much as 2.5kg (over 5lb) and be starting to settle into the final birth position.

You could find that the weight of the baby, amniotic fluid, womb, placenta, and extra fat is becoming much more burdensome now.

MONTH TEN (37–40 WEEKS)

Your baby grows more. The average birth-weight is 3.5–4kg (7½–9lb).

You may need extra rest, but could also be surprised by a surge of energy.

After nine months your baby will be fully formed and will gradually settle into his or her birth position, and the head will be engaged ready for delivery.

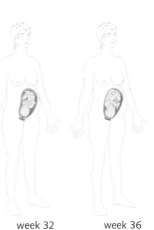

baby

umbilical cord

placenta

The stages of the developing fetus inside your ever-expanding bump. You might feel your baby move from about 18 weeks. By the end of your pregnancy you can feel quite cumbersome.

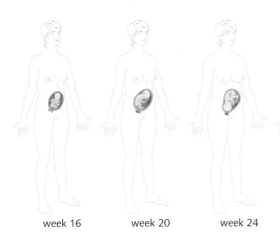
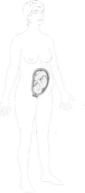
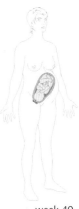

week 16   week 20   week 24   week 28   week 32   week 36   week 40

YOUR DIET IN PREGNANCY

The food you eat now has to nourish you and your baby. If you don't eat enough, or if you eat a poor-quality diet, your baby may not grow and develop as well as possible. You also increase your risk of going into labor prematurely, which may be bad for the baby.

Research suggests that if a pregnant woman eats badly, her baby has a higher risk of developing certain illnesses as an adult. These include high blood pressure, diabetes, heart disease, and strokes. This sounds scary, so what exactly should you be eating?

Good nutrition in pregnancy isn't rocket science. The food you need is basically what you get from an ordinary healthy diet (*see page 24*). But several nutrients are particularly important, so here are some practical tips.

Orange juice and other vitamin C-rich drinks and foods help you to absorb iron.

Green vegetables will boost your vitamin levels and help prevent constipation.

JUNK FOOD?

Eating a little "junk" food (food so highly processed that it has lost most of its original nutrients) is all right *if you eat only a little and, most important, eat enough nutritious foods as well.*

So don't fill up with white bread, cookies, cake, candy, and sugar only to find you don't want anything else. Instead, eat wholegrain foods (such as wholewheat bread and brown rice); vegetables, salads and fruit; dairy foods; vegetable oil; fish, meat, and eggs; seeds and nuts (though not too many, and not if you are allergic to them). Only then should you have a small amount of junk food if you still want it.

THREE ESPECIALLY IMPORTANT NUTRIENTS

Researchers say the nutrients most likely to be lacking in a woman's diet in pregnancy are folic acid, calcium, and iron.

◆ *Folic acid* is a B vitamin. It is named after the Latin *folium*, meaning "leaf," because it is found in particularly large amounts in leaves, though it is also found in some other foods (*see page 25*). Having too little during very early pregnancy could, at worst, mean your baby develops a spinal defect called spina bifida. Experts now advise every woman to take folic acid supplements from the time she starts trying for a baby until the end of the 12th week of pregnancy, or throughout pregnancy. Take 400 micrograms a day (unless your doctor recommends more).

◆ *Iron* is a mineral present in many foods (se*e page 25*). Help your body to absorb iron by drinking orange juice or eating other vitamin C-rich foods with meals, but avoiding tea and coffee until an hour after a meal.

◆ *Calcium* is another mineral present in many foods (*see page 25*). Eating canned fish such as sardines and salmon, complete with their soft bones, will help increase your intake, as will homemade chicken soup made from boiled chicken-bone stock enlivened with a tablespoon of vinegar (to help release calcium).

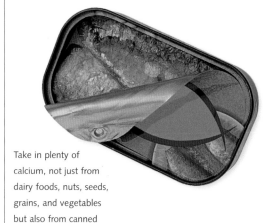

Take in plenty of calcium, not just from dairy foods, nuts, seeds, grains, and vegetables but also from canned fish such as salmon and sardines.

EATING FOR TWO?

During the first six months of pregnancy, you won't need any more food than the time before you were pregnant, which is good news if you continue to be plagued by nausea. Even after six months you need only around 200 extra calories a day. One reason this extra requirement is so small is that most women become less physically active in later pregnancy, because of the weight and bulk that they are carrying.

WHAT TO AVOID

For some years pregnant women have been advised to avoid liver because its vitamin A content was considered too high for safety. However, a little liver is almost certainly perfectly safe. There are only a few foods that are really worth taking care to avoid because they might, at worst, harm your baby.

FOODS WORTH AVOIDING:

◆ Those foods containing raw egg (such as mayonnaise), because of the risk of infection with *Salmonella*.
◆ Those that might cause infection with *Listeria*, including pâté; soft, mold-ripened cheeses such as Brie and Camembert; feta cheese; blue-veined cheese; soft ice cream; unpasteurized milk; precooked poultry; cooked chilled food – unless thoroughly reheated; preprepared salads – unless washed thoroughly; and undercooked meat.

◆ Those that might cause infection with *Toxoplasma*, including raw or undercooked meat; and unwashed salads, vegetables, and fruit. (Further precautions against *Toxoplasma* infection include avoiding being with a sick cat; disinfecting your cat's litter box each day; and wearing rubber gloves when handling cat litter, raw meat, or soil.)

SUPPLEMENTS

Apart from taking folic acid (*see opposite page*), you might consider a multivitamin and multimineral supplement especially formulated for pregnant women. Adding a supplement of certain poly-unsaturated fatty acids (docosahexanoic, arachidonic, and gamma-linolenic acids) ensures that

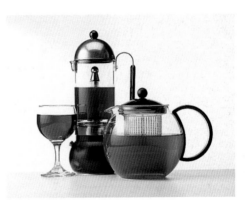

RIGHT: Cut down your caffeine intake. Also the very latest research suggests it's ideally best to say no to any alcohol.

BELOW LEFT: Avoid raw eggs and soft, mold-ripened cheeses, because of possible infection with *Listeria* and *Salmonella*.

your baby's developing brain and eyes receive enough of these important nutrients. If, against all advice, you continue to smoke, take a twice-daily supplement of vitamin C to replace the 25mg of the vitamin that will be destroyed by each cigarette.

DRINKS

In the USA, pregnant women are advised not to drink any alcohol. The advice in the UK is that small amounts are safe, but recent research suggests it may well be better to avoid any at all. Getting drunk is very irresponsible.

You can carry on drinking a moderate amount of tea and coffee, but it's probably best not to drink a lot of either. A "moderate amount" provides 320–360mg of caffeine a day. (A 6fl oz cup of average-strength brewed coffee contains 80–90mg, a cup of instant coffee 60mg, and a cup of tea 40mg.) It's worth noting that a can of cola provides 40mg of caffeine, though you can buy decaffeinated varieties.

OVERCOMING COMMON PROBLEMS

Try sips of water, ginger cookies, or dry bread to relieve nausea before you get out of bed.

Most women suffer only a few, if any, medical complaints during their pregnancy. And some women say they've never felt better.

NAUSEA

Pregnancy nausea is related to high levels of placental hormone called chorionic gonadotrophin. Thankfully it usually improves by 12 weeks.

To counteract nausea, sip water and eat a little dry bread or a ginger cookie. Have small, frequent meals, and try chewing fresh ginger root, or drinking ginger, peppermint, or lemon balm tea. Avoid fatty foods, and anything bitter, such as coffee, lettuce, or brussels sprouts. Ask your doctor's advice about taking supplements of vitamins B6 and C. Avoid traveling and getting overtired. Acupressure sometimes helps: lightly press point PC6 (three finger-widths above the crease on the front of the wrist, between the two tendons in the center of the forearm) for two minutes, or wear an acupressure wristband (sold for seasickness). A cup of chamomile tea every two hours may help. Herbal remedies made from tamarind can be useful, but consult a medical herbalist for safe, personalized advice.

When you rest make sure your back is supported and your legs are raised.

FATIGUE

Eat a healthy diet, don't work too hard, manage stress effectively (*see page 34*), and put your feet up whenever possible.

HEARTBURN

Don't eat or drink too much; avoid rich meals; don't eat any fruit after a meal; eat slowly and relax at mealtimes; drink fluids only between meals; and avoid alcohol. Leave several hours between eating and bedtime. Have an extra pillow, or prop up the head of the bed. And ask your doctor or pharmacist to recommend an antacid, or a "rafting agent" such as an alginate.

CRAMP

Take daily exercise. Eat a healthy diet containing magnesium-rich foods (*see page 25*). Have a warm bath before bedtime and keep warm in bed. One unexpected remedy recommended by a surprising number of people is a cork or a magnet beneath the mattress! A firm massage can relieve cramp, as can stretching the muscle.

VARICOSE VEINS

Get a daily half-hour of exercise. Avoid standing, keep legs uncrossed when sitting, rest more and, when you do, put your legs up. Support tights may help. Eat a healthy diet with plenty of foods rich in vitamin C and flavonoids. (*See pages 25 and 173.*)

HEMORRHOIDS AND CONSTIPATION

For hemorrhoids, drink more water, eat more fiber-rich foods (*see page 25*) and take regular exercise (*see page 175*). The advice is the same for constipation. If you are taking iron tablets, ask for an alternative that doesn't encourage constipation. Don't take laxatives without consulting your doctor. (*See also page 162.*)

BACKACHE

Exercise regularly and check your posture. Stretching often relieves muscle tension, as does massage. When sleeping on your side, put a pillow between your knees, or bend your upper leg at hip and knee, push it slightly forward, and rest it on a pillow. When sleeping on your back, put a pillow or two beneath your knees. If necessary, consult an osteopath or chiropractor. (*See also page 198.*)

CARPAL TUNNEL SYNDROME

Nerve pressure from fluid retention can lead to tingling and numbness in the thumb and first three fingers, symptoms known as the carpal tunnel syndrome. (*See also page 201.*)

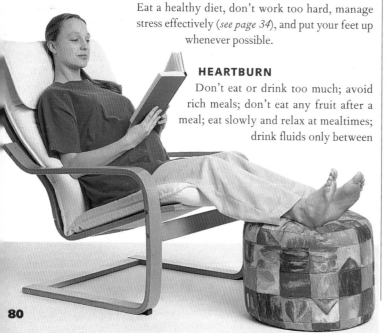

ITCHING

Put two tablespoons of baking soda in your bath water – but don't soak for too long. Afterward, apply some moisturizing cream mixed with a few drops of lavender oil. See your doctor if itching lasts more than a few days, or if you look sallow. Persistent itching can result from a liver problem that resolves after delivery, but doctors must monitor such a pregnancy closely and may need to induce labor early.

THRUSH AND BACTERIAL VAGINOSIS

Itching and a vaginal discharge due to *Candida* infection (thrush) are common. You can treat the infection with antifungal cream and suppositories bought over the counter (*see also page 192*). Another infection, bacterial vaginosis, is easily mistaken for thrush. This can trigger preterm labor, so if thrush treatment doesn't work, consult your doctor. Bacterial vaginosis is treated with antibiotics.

URINE LEAKS

Doing pelvic floor exercises several times a day (*see page 136*) helps prevent any urine from leaking. Don't let your bladder overfill, and avoid movements that trigger leaks.

BLEEDING AND MISCARRIAGE

One pregnant woman in ten bleeds a little in early pregnancy, but continued bleeding and stomachache are usually signs of miscarriage.

If you bleed heavily, or feel faint, call an ambulance, or your maternity unit. You may have a low-lying placenta (placenta previa) and need an emergency cesarean. If you are bleeding lightly, call your doctor. If a scan shows your baby is alive, there is a nine-in-ten chance that all will be well. Your doctor will check your blood group. If you are Rhesus-negative, you'll need an injection of antibodies (anti-D immunoglobulin) to prevent trouble next time you are pregnant.

It's unlikely that anything you do will influence your baby's chance of survival. However, don't have penetrative sex, or an orgasm, until a day or two after the bleeding stops, and don't use tampons. Don't lift heavy weights or stand for long, and have a few days off physically onerous work. Two in five miscarriages are unexplained, but there are known possibilities.

THESE INCLUDE:

◆ A damaged or abnormal baby.
◆ An immune problem, such as antiphospholipid syndrome, in which antibodies create small blood clots in the placenta. Treatment is with aspirin (and, perhaps, heparin to help prevent clots).
◆ Pre-eclampsia (high blood pressure and, possibly, protein in the urine, and ankle swelling).
◆ Too little folic acid.
◆ Infection.
◆ Diabetes.
◆ Being overweight.
◆ Excessive alcohol or smoking.
◆ Environmental hazards (such as pesticide or radiation exposure).
◆ A hormone imbalance (for example, with polycystic ovaries, *see page 193*). Four out of five repeated miscarriages are associated with polycystic ovaries.
◆ A misshapen womb.
◆ A weak cervix.
◆ Fatigue and stress may play a part.
Many of these factors also encourage preterm birth, or the need to induce labor.

As long as you feel well you should continue to take gentle exercise.

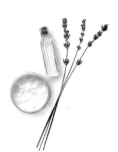

Add baking soda to the bath to relieve itching. Afterward apply some moisturizing cream mixed with a few drops of lavender oil.

Relaxation and breathing exercises can help reduce the stress and fatigue that may encourage a miscarriage.

CARING FOR YOUR UNBORN BABY

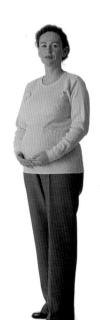

Pregnancy is an excellent time to focus on your own health as well as that of your baby. Everything you do affects your baby, and while babies are remarkably resilient, there's a lot you can do to maximize wellbeing for both of you. This way you have the best chance of feeling healthy during pregnancy and afterward – which is good for your baby. And the baby has the best chance of growing and developing normally, staying in the womb for the full term of pregnancy, and being born in good health.

We've already looked at what you should be eating and at the supplements recommended for pregnancy (*see page 78*). But there's a lot more that's well worth doing too.

teacher or coach know you're pregnant before you begin an exercise class. Avoid any high-impact exercise that jerks or bounces the baby, or anything that makes you more than very slightly breathless. And avoid risky sports.

Warning: See a doctor urgently if you bleed; have any pain or leg swelling; or become dizzy, breathless, or nauseated. And seek help at once if your waters break, or your baby stops moving.

DAYLIGHT EXPOSURE

Bright daylight on your skin each day is the best way of obtaining vitamin D. This enables your baby to start laying down calcium and other minerals in its bones during the fifth month of pregnancy.

Keeping yourself healthy is the best way to protect your unborn baby.

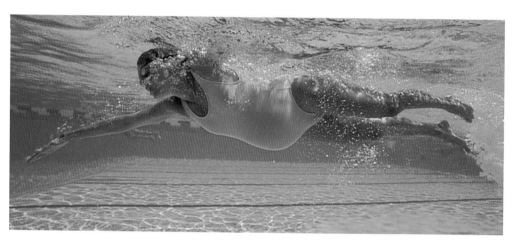

Swimming is excellent exercise, because the water supports your body and takes the weight off your joints.

Yoga offers gentle exercise with meditation and relaxation, but if you are new to it, take things very gently.

EXERCISE

Keeping active to some extent is good, however big you become. Exercise helps keep blood vessels, including those in the placenta, in good condition. While you need to lay down extra fat, exercise helps prevent you laying down too much (which would increase the risk of miscarriage). And it can help guard against high blood pressure, and pregnancy diabetes, both of which can be hazardous for an unborn baby. However, choose what you do wisely. If you've ever miscarried or had back trouble, or if you're unfit, check with your doctor before you start. Also, let your

NO SMOKING

If you're a smoker, giving up is one of the best things that you can possibly do for your baby. Smoke contains nicotine and a large number of other toxic chemicals that reduce a baby's blood supply by encouraging the placenta to become prematurely old.

This means the baby is likely to be born smaller than he or she would otherwise have been, which, in turn, raises the risk of breathing difficulties and several other problems after birth. Research suggests that it may also increase the risk of high blood pressure, diabetes, and heart disease in adult life.

If you want to stop smoking because of pregnancy or just for general better health, there's plenty of high quality "quit-smoking" information and support in the community.

MAKING A BIRTH PLAN

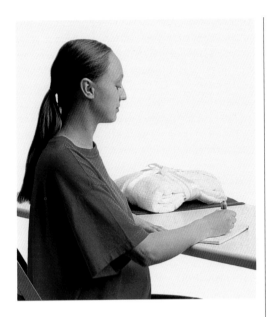

In an ideal world, every pregnant woman would know her midwife and obstetrician before she went into labor. Things aren't always like that, though, and there's a chance you'll find unfamiliar faces around you when giving birth. This is one reason why making a birth plan can be a good move. Another excellent reason is that it gives you the chance to think about the type of birthing experience you want, and to make some preparations.

Of course, things won't necessarily turn out as you want or hope, because labor and childbirth sometimes aren't straightforward, and you may need more help than you envisaged. But you can take account of unforeseen events that could alter your birth plan simply by saying that you are prepared to be flexible if necessary.

Suggestions for a birth plan include: involving a companion of your choice (such as your husband, partner, mother, sister, or friend); having any medical interventions and their possible side effects explained fully before you accept; trying to avoid any interventions unless really necessary; and wanting a peaceful atmosphere during labor, perhaps with dim lights and your choice of music.

The purpose of a birth plan is to help you guide your birth attendants, not bully them. Most midwives, obstetric nurses, and obstetricians are familiar with birth plans, and find it useful to know what each woman wants.

PREPARING FOR THE BIRTH

Practicalities Toward the end of pregnancy, make sure you've got everything you'll need to make you comfortable from a practical point of view during labor and afterward. Suggestions include: dressing gown and slippers; front-opening nightgown (for breastfeeding); a sweater or cardigan; box of kleenexes; sanitary napkins, and underwear to keep them in place; reading matter; bath things and other toiletries; a hairband or scrunchy; money for the telephone and hospital shop; massage oil; a water "spritzer" for your face; and your address book and writing gear. Leave your cell phone at home – you won't be allowed to use it because cell phones can interfere with medical electrical equipment.

Write a birth plan but be prepared to change it. Until you go into labor you don't really know how your body is going to react or what medical requirements might arise.

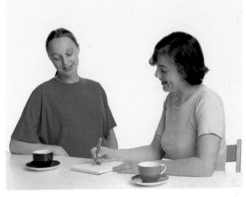

Discuss your concerns with your midwife. Make sure she knows what sort of delivery you would ideally like.

Two unusual tips Two things are said to help prepare a woman to give birth more easily. And while there's no scientific evidence that they work, you may like to follow folklore and try them.

One is to massage and gently stretch the area around the opening of your vagina for a few minutes every day toward the end of pregnancy. This is believed to help the vagina stretch more easily as the baby comes out.

The other is to drink raspberry leaf tea (a daily cup from three to six months of pregnancy, then three cups a day until you go into labor, then a cup each hour in labor if allowed). This helps the muscles of the womb to work effectively during labor. To make this tea, pour 600ml (1 pint) of boiling water over 25g (1oz) of dried raspberry leaves. Cover and leave for ten minutes, then strain. You can keep it in the refrigerator for up to two days.

GIVING BIRTH

Birth is one of life's great miracles. Your baby will come when he or she is ready, but if you feel the time is right you may be able to encourage the birth. One way is to have frequent intercourse (prostaglandins in semen can encourage labor if the baby is ready to arrive). Another way is to stimulate your nipples and have an orgasm each day (both of which can encourage labor by raising your oxytocin level).

YOUR POSITION DURING LABOR AND BIRTH

Contractions will be most effective if you remain upright and active when you're not sleeping or resting. They may also be less painful, especially if you keep changing your position to whatever feels most comfortable. For example, try leaning forward during a contraction and supporting some of your weight by holding on to something in front of you. You could do this while standing, or when kneeling with your knees bent either at right angles or completely.

Being on all fours and rocking your pelvis up and down may relieve backache. Lowering yourself on to your elbows may help even more.

If your baby is being monitored, ask for a machine with a cord long enough to let you get out of bed and remain relatively mobile.

Kneeling on the labor bed or the (clean and covered) floor may help you cope with contractions and, perhaps, help the baby on its way.

Alternatively, try a semi-squatting position, with a helper supporting you under your armpits from behind. There are three advantages to kneeling or semi-squatting. First, gravity helps the baby's descent. Second, you can make each contraction easier to bear and more effective by adjusting your position – for example, you can lean forward or backward, or move your pelvis from side to side. Last, remaining upright can make birth safer, and make you less likely to tear or need an episiotomy. It can also shorten labor.

OTHER THINGS YOU CAN DO TO EASE LABOR

Ask your companion to massage you in whatever way feels most helpful. Small, light, stroking movements with the fingers over the base of the spine are often remarkably effective. Make yourself comfortable by keeping warm, laying a cold washcloth on your forehead, or putting a hot or cold pack on your lower back, or spritzing your face with cold water. The breathing and other relaxation exercises you learned in antenatal classes should come in useful now. Your companion can act as your coach to remind you what to do and, if necessary, encourage you to keep going.

You may be offered pain relief in the form of a mask delivering a mixture of gas (nitrous oxide) and air; a TENS (transcutaneous electrical nerve stimulation) machine; demerol; or an epidural infusion.

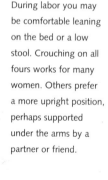

During labor you may be comfortable leaning on the bed or a low stool. Crouching on all fours works for many women. Others prefer a more upright position, perhaps supported under the arms by a partner or friend.

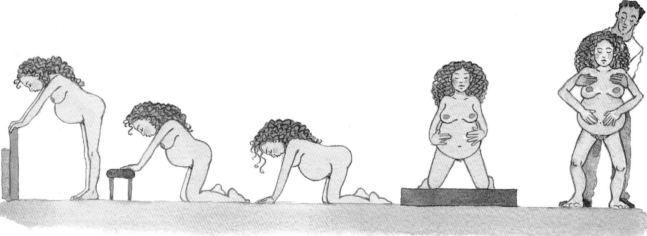

YOUR NEWBORN BABY

So here is your baby that you've been protecting and nurturing inside you for so long. Some women experience a strange feeling of recognition. Although this is the first time they've seen their baby's face (except, perhaps, on ultrasound scans), they somehow "know" their baby already.

Feel free to keep your baby with you if you can. The pediatrician will make sure all is well, and the nurses will do tasks such as labeling and weighing. A baby's birth-weight varies according to the length of pregnancy, the health and nutrition of the mother in pregnancy, and his or her own health, inherited build, and racial extraction. But the average full-term newborn girl weighs 140g (5oz) less than the average full-term newborn boy. Once the weighing is done, you'll be able to have as long a cuddle as you like.

If you need medical care, ask if your baby can stay in a crib by your bed and, if necessary, be lifted into your arms whenever you ask. If the baby needs special care, ask whether you can have a room near the special care unit, or whether the baby is well enough to be looked after in an incubator by your bed and perhaps "kangaroo style" next to your chest for some of the time.

Babies are very vulnerable to getting too hot or cold, becoming dehydrated or starving hungry, or being uncomfortably wet or soiled. Indeed, you may be surprised by just how much time it takes to care for just one small scrap of humanity! They also need plenty of focused attention and "TLC" (tender, loving care) if they're to grow and develop as well as possible. They love being looked at. They thrive on being held, stroked, massaged and otherwise caressed or groomed. And they love being talked to or sung to.

You'll find as the weeks go by that you and your baby will begin to gaze into each other's eyes. If you smile or talk, the baby will become still and attentive. When you've finished, he or she may coo, gurgle or even, after a few weeks, smile, while you watch attentively. This "dance of love" is then repeated all over again. This is the beginning of a shared pattern of communication that will one day develop into speech.

If your baby has to be in an incubator, ask what you can do to help. You may be able to help clean your baby, or change a wet or soiled diaper. You may be able to give feed milk down a tube. And you can provide breast milk (*see page 87*) to be given by tube or cup.

But more than this, you can look at your baby; talk and croon; stroke or hold (though for a very tiny preterm baby this might not be possible) – and just be there. Many babies in incubators soon learn to recognize the presence of their parents and somehow make it obvious that they like it.

Many women say that nothing can prepare you for the overwhelming rush of emotions you feel as a newborn baby wraps his or her tiny fingers around yours.

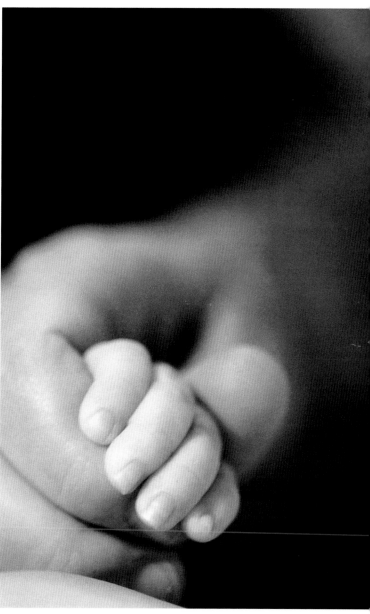

MOTHERHOOD – THE FIRST YEAR

Everything changes when a woman becomes a mother. For the rest of her life she will be in a relationship with her child – this person whom she and the father have created together and whom she has nurtured so intimately.

Being a mother can bring enormous pleasures and rewards. But it also throws up many challenges, some of them surprising. And, inevitably, it can sometimes be difficult. All this offers you the chance to grow in emotional and spiritual awareness. And it provides you and your partner with an entry ticket to the worldwide club of parenthood. Being so closely involved in the life, health, happiness, and potential of a child can raise you to a different plane of being, one where you know in your heart what is important and what isn't. It also means that when you look at another person, you see them more easily as someone else's child – and therefore as a precious and unique human being.

THE WAY YOU FEEL

Some women fall in love with their babies, and feel elated from the moment they meet face to face. Others are indifferent. And a few have somewhat negative emotions. What happens depends on your expectations of motherhood and babies, whether the baby was wanted, the birth, your health and that of your baby, and the support you get. So be gentle with yourself as you negotiate the early days, weeks, and even months of being a mom. You'll learn on the job and there's no need to feel you should be an instant expert.

A few days after the birth you may feel low, tearful, and emotional. This state is often called "the baby blues" and usually passes shortly. The cause is probably a combination of changing hormone levels, a lack of sleep, a fall in your cholesterol level (*see page 89*), and a reaction to the exertion, excitement, and, perhaps, shock of labor and of giving birth. (*See also pages 89, 181, and 202.*)

Babies soon grow up, so take time just to hold them and enjoy them.

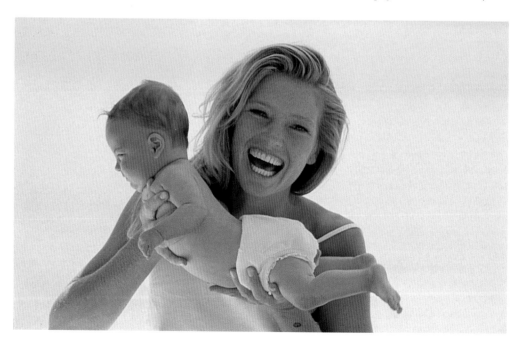

YOU AND YOUR PARTNER

The focus of the health professionals is usually on the mother and baby, with the result that the father can feel rather left out. Yet his life has irrevocably changed too. This is his baby. And he is now responsible, with you, for the care, guidance, and protection of a young human being for many years to come.

Try to make time to recognize and name your partner's feelings, and to encourage and affirm him in his new role (*see page 41*). This will help him take pleasure and pride in his child, and adjust to the new relationships in his family.

YOUR PELVIC FLOOR

As soon as you are ready, start doing pelvic floor exercises (*see page 136*). These encourage your vagina, bladder neck, cervix, vulva, and anus to return to normal more quickly.

CHOOSING HOW TO FEED YOUR BABY

The way nature intends you to feed your baby is by breastfeeding. Your milk is better than that of a cow, goat, or any other animal (however much that animal's milk is modified), because human milk is specifically designed to suit the needs of a human baby, whereas the milk of other animals is designed to suit their own young.

Breast is best so it's hardly surprising that so many women choose to breastfeed their babies.

THE HEALTH BENEFITS OF BREASTFEEDING FOR BABIES

◆ Less illness and hospitalization.
◆ Fewer infections.
◆ Fewer allergies.
◆ Less celiac disease (digestive and other symptoms from a sensitivity to gluten in cereal).
◆ Less pyloric stenosis (vomiting due to a tight stomach outlet).
◆ Less meconium ileus (a type of bowel blockage).
◆ Less appendicitis.
◆ Less ulcerative colitis and Crohn's disease (inflammatory bowel diseases).
◆ Less acrodermatitis enteropathica (a scaly skin disease).
◆ Less dental decay.
◆ Less diabetes.
◆ Less cancer.
◆ Fewer unexplained crib deaths (sudden infant death syndrome).
◆ Better jaw and mouth development.
◆ Optimal brain development.

These are all proven benefits. Researchers also suspect that people who were breastfed as babies are less prone to juvenile rheumatoid arthritis, schizophrenia, multiple sclerosis, and heart disease.

Arguably, breastfeeding is also a much more intimate and pleasurable experience for babies than is bottle-feeding.

THE HEALTH BENEFITS OF BREAST-FEEDING FOR MOTHERS

Breastfeeding is good news for you too. It provides useful contraception if you also use the sympto-thermal method (*see page 43*). And ovarian, womb, and premenopausal breast cancer, and post-menopausal osteoporosis appear to be less likely in women who've breastfed.

Many women also find breastfeeding more convenient, satisfying, enjoyable, fulfilling, and empowering than bottle-feeding, and believe it makes their relationship with their baby more intimate.

FINDING THE SECRETS OF SUCCESS

Almost every breastfeeding woman experiences some difficulties; the secret of success is learning how to overcome them. For example, if you're embarrassed in front of others, learn the knack of feeding discreetly. If you want to go out alone, learn how to express milk to leave for your baby. To pull through these challenges and overcome common problems, such as sore nipples, you'll need good information and support (*see pages 218 and 219*). Many women think they have insufficient milk, for example, but with the right help over 95 percent learn how to provide all the milk their babies need.

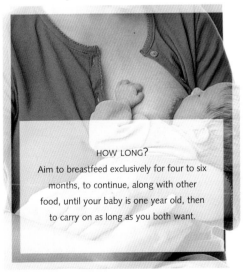

HOW LONG?
Aim to breastfeed exclusively for four to six months, to continue, along with other food, until your baby is one year old, then to carry on as long as you both want.

HEALTH NEEDS DURING YOUR BABY'S FIRST YEAR

You'll enjoy this time more if you look after yourself so you feel in good shape and well as you take on your new role as a mother.

Food and drink During the months you breastfeed you need to eat more than usual (an extra 400–600 calories a day). You also need a highly nutritious diet to replace the nutrients that go into your milk. Making milk also uses up a lot of fluid, so try not to let yourself get thirsty. Many women keep drinks by them as they breastfeed. As for alcohol, it's best to drink only in moderation; babies tend to take less milk if it tastes of alcohol, and some are fussy afterward.

Exercise Start doing postpartum exercises (recommended by the doctor or hospital) when your doctor gives you the all clear. Exercise will tone your stomach muscles and make you feel good. Build your stamina and strength slowly, and, when the time is right, see how you can fit a daily half-hour of aerobic exercise into your everyday life. Ideas include walking briskly with your baby in a baby carriage or stroller, or swimming or joining an exercise class (leaving the baby either safely nearby, in a nursery, or with a sitter).

Daylight and fresh air Get some direct daylight on your skin each day to help keep your bones strong. This is especially important if you're dark-skinned or live in northerly latitudes where the sun's rays are weaker.

Be a non-smoker If you and your partner are non-smokers, both your baby and you will be healthier. If you stopped smoking before or during pregnancy, don't restart now but continue to use alternative pleasures or stress-relieving strategies.

Your figure As long as you look after your breasts, breastfeeding itself won't make them droopy. Wear a well-fitting bra by day and do the same at night too, because your breasts are heavier than usual then.

Relaxation and play Make time each day to relax, recuperate, and restore your energy. Mothers need play just as much as their babies do! Problems can arise if the ways you used to relax before your baby are hard to fit in now that you're a mom. If this happens, do some creative thinking to find new ways of getting enough fun and pleasure.

Sleep It's a fact of life that babies wake up at night. They aren't being undisciplined or naughty, just doing what they need to do to nourish their rapidly growing bodies. It's also a fact of life that mothers need sleep. So you will need to find ways of catching up with lost sleep. You might, for example, go to bed earlier, or catnap or have a siesta during the day.

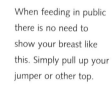

When feeding in public there is no need to show your breast like this. Simply pull up your jumper or other top.

SEX AND RELATIONSHIPS

Some women are comfortable with 'full' sex around six weeks after childbirth, others find it uncomfortable for some weeks or months.

But what's most important for you and your partner is to listen to, hug, and give each other some of the "tlc" (tender, loving care) you both need. As parents of a new baby you need extra attention and support – in other words, parenting, which is partly why psychologists call this time the third childhood (*see also page 58*).

But when sometimes you find you can't meet each other's needs, don't be surprised, and don't take it out on one another.

Instead, meet the challenge of your joint vulnerability with humor and respect, and by discussing other ways of meeting your needs. For example, you might like an evening out with friends, or a session at the hair salon. You can take the baby to either. And your partner may want time with a friend to talk about his new life to take his mind off it.

YOU AND YOUR RELATIONSHIP
WITH YOUR BABY

The most important thing is that your baby needs to know that he or she is loved. The baby will learn this from your normal, everyday interest in him or her. It won't be long before your baby starts gazing at you, following you with wide eyes, smiling, cooing, and gurgling. Then you'll soon notice what psychologists call "the dance of love". First, your baby will keep still as he or she watches you and listens to you. Then your baby will respond by cooing, gurgling, smiling, and looking intently at you, while you, in turn, gaze at him or her and listen intently. And then you'll probably both repeat this "dance," perhaps several times.

The love and interaction your baby experiences as he or she grows will provide a wonderful foundation for growing up with a loving nature and a healthy sense of self-esteem.

A ROLLERCOASTER OF EMOTIONS

One woman in two feels temporarily low when her baby is a few days old. And some mothers of young babies find that their emotions are all over the place for many months. They may, for example, seem to feel more deeply about everything that happens. However, some time in the first year one woman in ten feels mentally and physically unwell, and finds that her emotions are flattened by postpartum depression. A few become so ill that they need hospital treatment.

How to manage if you're depressed (*see also page 202*). Check you are eating well. You need plenty of nutrients so breastfeeding doesn't drain your body. Eating enough fatty foods counteracts the steep fall in your body's cholesterol level. This is expected after childbirth, but experts think that in some women it hinders the body's use of serotonin (a neurotransmitter) and encourages a state of depression.

You need some exercise. Even in the earliest days it's best not to sit or lie down all the time unless you must. It's very wise to go outside and get some daylight and fresh air every day. Somehow you'll need to catch up on some of the sleep you're losing. And you deserve some fun things, just for you, like having a good friend visit.

It's also important to have the practical and emotional support you need, including someone close – such as your partner, sister, parent, or friend – who can listen to you over and over again, if necessary, and pick up on how you're feeling. Childbirth can be a shock to the system, as can life with a young baby. This is especially true if it's your first time. Any difficult feelings about the loss of independence and the social contacts of your former life are much better acknowledged than suppressed. Don't delay in seeking expert help if you continue to feel low or become really depressed.

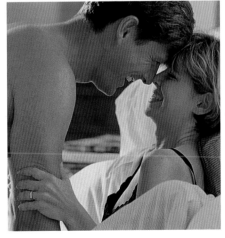

Sex can be just as good as before the birth. But take time to adjust and don't expect too much of yourself at first.

YOU AND YOUR PRESCHOOL CHILD

From the time your baby starts walking, to the beginning of full-time school, you'll be spending a great deal of time together, whether or not you work. During this time, your child needs plenty of one-to-one, focused attention. Children who have enough of this attention learn that they matter, and this, in turn, gives them the confidence to learn and to communicate.

But your needs are important too. You also need focused attention. If you don't get enough from others, it's perfectly possible to give it to yourself.

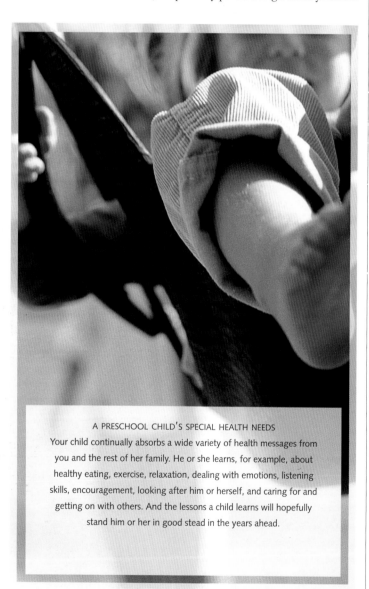

A PRESCHOOL CHILD'S SPECIAL HEALTH NEEDS
Your child continually absorbs a wide variety of health messages from you and the rest of her family. He or she learns, for example, about healthy eating, exercise, relaxation, dealing with emotions, listening skills, encouragement, looking after him or herself, and caring for and getting on with others. And the lessons a child learns will hopefully stand him or her in good stead in the years ahead.

YOUR RELATIONSHIP WITH YOUR CHILD

Accept your child's personality as an intrinsic and potentially valuable part of him or her, and you are teaching a hugely useful lesson. It's also important to separate your child's behavior from his or her personality. Human beings can generally change only their behavior, not their personalities. As the years pass, you'll guide and mold your child's behavior. And experiencing this sort of parenting, together with your loving attention, will make your child into a well-balanced individual able to take a place in the community and use his or her personality for everyone's benefit.

Role modeling You are your child's main example both of women and of mothers. All others will be compared with you forever. And what you do will be considered the norm for a good many years to come. If you are happy with what you're doing, fine. If not, now is the time to change your behavior. You might like to consider going to one of the excellent parenting courses that include learning and listening skills – topics such as developing a more creative parenting style.

YOUR HEALTH NEEDS

Quite a few women with young, preschool children start off with very good intentions of looking after their own health, but find that time is against them. Daily exercise is usually the first thing to go. Going outside each day is the next. Yet staying in shape and well is good not just for you, but for your family too. So do some creative time-management – with help if necessary – to decide on your priorities.

Another potential challenge is your diet. Some women begin to put on weight now, partly because of a lack of exercise, partly because they cook and eat "nursery food," and partly because they polish off their children's leftovers.

Daily exercise is good for you and good for your child. It is also a way of meeting other mothers and forming new friendships.

YOU AND YOUR OLDER CHILD

Being a mom is a privilege. It can also be a considerable challenge and can open windows to opportunities you never dreamed were there. For these reasons many women find that bringing up their children stretches and shapes them in unexpected and far-reaching ways. Many say it's the single most important influence in making them mature.

YOUR GROWING RELATIONSHIP

Whatever happens, you'll always be your child's mother. That's undeniable. It's also a given that your mothering style will affect your child for ever. However, after much research, psychologists affirm that mothers need be only "good enough". They don't have to be perfect for their children to grow up well balanced and ready for adult life.

As you live alongside your learning and growing child, remember that while motherhood is one of your roles, you have many others too. For example, you're probably also a lover and friend to your partner; a daughter to your mother; a sister to your siblings; a friend to your friends; and an employee or boss at work. As a whole person with many roles, you'll find that polishing and maintaining each one of them can enhance your relationship with your child.

Focusing on your child as an individual, with his or her own feelings, beliefs, and views, enhances this relationship too. Help yourself do this by honing your skills in the areas of empathic listening, encouragement, and conflict resolution. Parenting courses and some parenting books can be useful sources of creative suggestions.

YOUR HEALTH NEEDS

It's an excellent idea to make time for regular – perhaps six-monthly – assessments of your health and wellbeing while you have children this age. A mother's needs are sometimes squeezed out of the family's schedule because she's pushed for time. Yet both you and your family will feel better if your needs are met.

A SCHOOL-AGE, PRETEEN CHILD'S
SPECIAL HEALTH NEEDS
Your son or daughter absorbs health messages from many sources. You are the most important source; others include his or her friends and teachers, and the media. It is well worth discussing the pros and cons of some of these messages as they occur, so your child gradually learns he or she has a choice of behaviors when it comes to influencing health.
Your children need you to take an intense (though not excessive) interest in their ideas, hopes and fears, friends, work, and play. Having an enthusiastic cheerleader and a trustworthy, loving, skilled confidante is vitally important to the mental and emotional wellbeing of a child of this age, and to his or her self-confidence.

FOR A PERSONAL ASSESSMENT, WRITE DOWN THESE TEN HEADINGS:

- ◆ Food and drink.
- ◆ Weight and shape.
- ◆ Fitness, strength, and suppleness.
- ◆ Skin, hair, and nail care.
- ◆ Daylight-exposure.
- ◆ Fresh air.
- ◆ Relaxation and play.
- ◆ Relationships and sex.
- ◆ Emotional state.
- ◆ Soul and spirit.

Then, under each one, list any concerns or unmet needs. Next, write by each one what to do about it, and how. Lastly, put your plan into action, perhaps with the help of your partner.

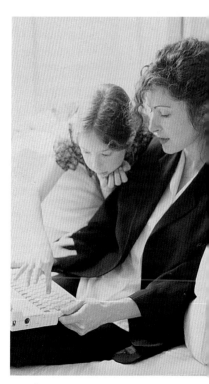

As your child's own personality develops, provide room for self-discovery but be there to offer support when needed.

ALL MOTHERS

As you put parenting into practice, you'll use the knowledge and skills you've been learning, albeit unwittingly, ever since you were born. Even bad experiences are helpful, because it's by making mistakes that you learn to put them right. Also, it's by facing your fears that you learn to move on and to "feel the fear and do it anyway". And it's by enduring difficult times that you become acquainted with painful emotions (such as rage, despair, sadness, jealousy), recognize how these color your mind and behavior, and come to accept them as potentially enriching sources for your emotional, spiritual, and creative development.

Remember that you don't need to get things right the first time. Some women believe they can be perfect moms if they only try hard enough. They then beat up on themselves when they don't achieve their goals. Such women set themselves up for failure, which is bad news for them and for their children. Their problem is an addiction to perfection, or "hubris" – the false belief they can achieve anything by striving hard enough.

Mothers encourage and empower their children if they teach by example how to learn and grow from life, whatever challenges may occur. Their acceptance of their own fallibility allows their children to accept that they, too, are human. Sometimes they will take a wrong turn, and have to get where they want by a different path.

All this is vitally important, because understanding that difficult emotions and mistakes are an expected part of human behavior, but that they can be acknowledged, and used constructively, provides you and your children with a very real sense of security.

YOU AND YOUR PARTNER

Crises in a couple's relationship are most likely to arise during the first year after a baby is born, and/or around seven years after they start living together as a couple. The key to pulling through is to see such adversities as opportunities to work on enriching your lives together. Couple-relationships are never perfect. The challenges of everyday life may sometimes come between you, and it's then that you may need assistance as you experiment with new ways of relating (*see pages 40–41*).

DO OLDER MOTHERS HAVE SPECIAL NEEDS?

Older mothers may benefit from greater maturity and worldly wisdom but, like mothers of any age, they sometimes get tired. And some women who have their first babies in their 30s or 40s seem to get more tired than younger mothers. If this happens, don't push yourself, but take time to work out how to restore a sense of balance and ease to your life. This may mean asking for help, so never be too proud to do so. Older mothers may also find that adjusting to having a child takes longer after so many baby-free years. This feeling is only natural, so be patient with yourself (*see page 105*).

YOUR HOME ENVIRONMENT

Home should be a place where everyone can be themselves. And that means you too. You need a place where you can relax, entertain friends, pamper yourself with some personal grooming, do exercises, and look after your health. However, you may need to think constructively about solitude, space, amenities, and, perhaps, the time-sharing of facilities, so your home works well for you.

Being an older mom can have several benefits – such as having older children to share the pleasures and tasks of baby care.

THE WORK/HOME DILEMMA

Women have always worked, whether they are mothers or not. Working is a vital part of staying mentally, emotionally, and physically healthy. But what exactly do we think of as work?

Over the centuries women's work has encompassed all manner of activities. These have included growing crops; tending animals; manufacturing things; painting; embroidering; healing; preaching; teaching; cooking; midwifery; accounting; housekeeping (in other people's homes or their own); and last but not least, bearing and bringing up children.

And that's what makes the "work/home dilemma" a misnomer, because the term implies that you aren't working if you're at home, or you stop being a wife and mother if you're at work. This is obviously wrong. Being at home doesn't even necessarily mean you aren't earning. And it certainly doesn't mean you aren't being useful! Bringing up children is one of the most useful things to do. Running a welcoming and comfortable home is also a vital task in any society. And the list goes on: servicing other people's needs is useful; doing voluntary community work is useful; and so is making money for your family, enriching your partner's life, and creating a place of comfort, welcome, and beauty.

The really important questions are not whether to stay at home or go out to work, but how to be useful and fulfilled, to make ends meet financially, and to ensure that your children receive what they need in the way of mothering.

Avoid the trap of feeling dissatisfied and not achieving your full potential with this four-point management plan.

YOUR MANAGEMENT PLAN

◆ List your achievements, abilities, and gifts.
◆ Add your goals for the future in each of these categories.
◆ Work out several ways of arriving at each goal and choose what seems the best.
◆ Put these strategies into practice.
A few people today enlist the help of a new breed of helper, called a coach, to guide them as they try to fulfill their potential. However, you and your partner, friend or some other trusted person can coach each other simply by using a mix of empathic listening and encouragement (*see page 41*), and common sense. The most important thing is to take an intense, focused interest in each other and to listen as well as speak.

SOUL AND SPIRIT

The vast majority of the world's population believes there's more to life than just people and the mundane practicalities of everyday existence; something beyond what is readily apparent to our five senses, and even to our sixth sense. Parenthood is a prime time for exploring your spiritual beliefs and taking them further. Along with the challenges and difficulties, there are opportunities for growth. It can also be a time for developing spiritually, opening your heart to a way of living and relating with others that transcends petty conflict and material ambition, and of learning to listen to the wisdom of your inner voice.

Whatever you decide – whether you want to be a full-time mother, or work full-time or part-time – you can always change your mind.

In addition to the practicalities of having a young baby, you need to be sure that you are fulfilled spiritually.

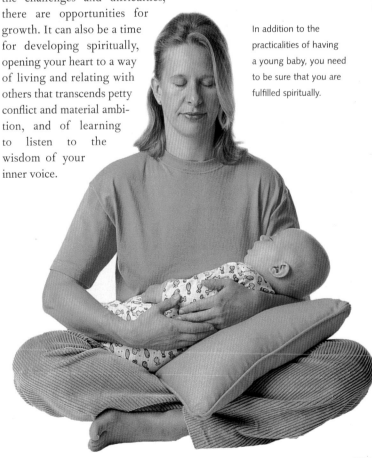

93

MATURE WOMAN

Being mature means being well developed — and reaching full maturity means being well developed in body, mind, and spirit. When you are fully mature, your body is grown. You are emotionally intelligent and able to use your intellect. And you have an active spiritual life. Whatever your age, you can continue developing emotionally, mentally, and spiritually.

Maturity certainly doesn't mean you have to come to a standstill. It simply means you are able to make the most of your capabilities and know how to adjust to changing circumstances. You can then empower others to do the same.

The age of reaching full physical maturity varies. Many women become reproductively mature in their teens and reach their peak reproductive ability in their 20s, and peak muscular prowess often occurs in their 20s or 30s. However, the age of attaining emotional, intellectual, and spiritual maturity is hugely variable.

Indeed, many women say it takes them until their late 30s to feel really mature.

When your children are grown up you have the chance to put yourself first more of the time and to do things that give you pleasure and satisfaction.

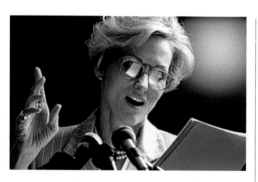

LOOKING AFTER YOURSELF AT THIS STAGE OF LIFE

A mature woman may be able to look after herself, but she doesn't necessarily have to be self-sufficient. Knowing when to ask for and accept help is a vitally important part of looking after yourself. And just because you can care for yourself doesn't mean you won't thoroughly enjoy having someone else meet some of your needs from time to time.

As a mature woman, at the prime of your life, you may have many responsibilities. But one of your main ones should be your personal health and wellbeing, because servicing yourself effectively and lovingly can bring rewards to you and your nearest and dearest for decades to come.

In order to look after yourself best, first try to identify your needs. To help you do this, let's look at some of your many possible roles.

BALANCING YOUR ROLES

Being a grown woman is rather like being a talented member of a repertory company. One moment you're acting the lead in an intense Shakespeare tragedy, the next you're in a light-hearted farce. Yet you also take your turn at prompting, managing the lighting, and taking money at the door. A mature woman today expects to have a rewarding one-to-one relationship, manage a family, have a good social life, have creative outlets, and, perhaps, work outside the home and put something back into the community. She may also care for an elderly or ailing relative, a friend or a neighbor.

Given that you have all these roles, take time to look at your life and assess whether its different sides are well balanced. Too much "doing" and not enough sitting and watching, for example, can sap energy. Too great a focus on your intellect and not enough on your feelings can allow emotional pressure to build up. And too much work might mean you don't have enough time to play.

MAXIMIZING HEALTH AND ENERGY

There'll be some times when you feel better than others. Your energy will ebb and flow according to your body rhythms and health, as well as with the season, the amount of work you do, and other external factors. Throughout these changing times try to eat well; get enough exercise, fresh air, and bright light; and relax, play, and sleep enough to restore your mind and body. Also, keep a close eye on your stress-management strategies and try new ones if necessary.

Here are a few points you might find helpful:

Your food The shape and size of a mature woman's body often reflects her self-esteem as well as the way she's cared for it over the years. So if, for example, you've put on too much weight, and become uncomfortably obese rather than comfortably curvy, ask yourself three questions:

◆ "Am I feeding myself properly?" (You may need a better diet, more exercise, and more determination to care for yourself.)

◆ "Do I have enough freedom?" (If life is cramping your style, squeezing energy from you, and not meeting your needs, then getting fat – which makes your body take up more space – could represent a need to make changes so you can break free.)

◆ "Am I trying to say something I can't put into words?" (Your body may try in many ways, including getting fat, to make you understand that you need more care and attention.)

If you are unhappily overweight, there are three things you must do. Take the time and effort to feed yourself good, nutritious food. Take steps, with help if necessary, to boost your self-esteem (*see page 44*). And don't allow unacknowledged feelings to mar your enjoyment of your body. Instead, use empathic listening skills (*see page 41*) to hear your innermost feelings, name them, and use them constructively.

Exercise Time is most women's main sticking point when it comes to exercise. So get out your diary and allocate spaces for a personal fitness program.

Light You continue to need at least 15 minutes of direct daylight each day (*see page 17*). Bone minerals are constantly being laid down and removed. But bone density decreases from a woman's mid-30s onward. And for five to ten years before the menopause women begin to lose bone even faster. So it's vital not to neglect daylight as your prime source of the vitamin D that helps calcium to strengthen bones.

Relaxation and play Even fully grown women need to relax and play. Indeed, it's fully grown women in particular who need to do this if they are to counterbalance the stresses and challenges of everyday life. This isn't an indulgence but simply sound common sense.

Managing stress Check whether your stress-management strategies are working well, without harming you. If you find, for example, that you've begun to deal with stress by drinking too much, eating too much or too little, smoking, being a "shopaholic" or workaholic, or having affairs, get help to ditch these potentially dangerous strategies, and strengthen your repertoire of effective, life-enhancing ones instead (*see page 35*).

Health screening

Several medical tests may be valuable.

WORTHWHILE SCREENING TESTS FOR THIS TIME OF LIFE INCLUDE:

◆ A Pap (cervical) smear – every year in the USA and every three to five years in the UK (*see page 72*).

◆ An eye test for glaucoma (raised pressure in the eye that is symptom-free until it damages the eyesight) – every two years over the age of 40, or, if you're short-sighted, or have diabetes or glaucoma in your family, from age 35.

◆ A blood-pressure check and cholesterol measurement – every two years or so may be advisable, particularly if there's heart disease in your family.

◆ An ultrasound scan of your ovaries and a mammogram – every few years may be advisable, particularly if there's ovarian or breast cancer in your family.

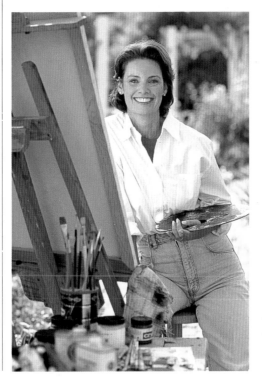

Now is a good time to try something different, to meet new friends, and to develop fresh interests.

95

YOUR HOME

Maslow's hierarchy of needs model. Maslow suggested that there are five sets of goals which may be called basic needs. He arranged these into a series of levels according to their importance. As those at the bottom of the pyramid are met, the next level becomes the priority, and so on to the top.

The psychologist Abraham Maslow described a hierarchy of human needs:

Ultimate needs
Self-esteem needs
Belonging and love needs
Safety needs
Physiological needs

A parent's basic needs, as shown at the bottom of this pyramid, are for air, food, and water, because without these we can't live. But on the very next level come "safety needs". And one of these is shelter. (Others are security, order, stability, and freedom from such things as chaos and anxiety.)

The shelter of a home is such a basic need that the idea of anyone being homeless – be they a runaway kid, a political refugee, or the victim of a natural disaster – is extremely unsettling to us all. And, of course, being homeless isn't something that happens only to others. Perhaps you've already experienced it. Perhaps you are threatened with having to leave your home now because you can't pay the mortgage or rent. Or perhaps you want to leave your partner but have nowhere to go.

It's easy to take home for granted. But when times are tough, acknowledging the security of a roof over your head is an important part of holding on to the hope that life will be good again. Some people even make a prayer of thanksgiving for their home a part of their daily routine.

DOES YOUR HOME ENCOURAGE WELLBEING?

As a householder it's worth making periodic checks to make sure your home continues to be a healthy place to live. For example, a home that doesn't keep you warm and dry encourages arthritis, asthma, bronchitis, and stress-related illness. And some homes, while warm, have poor ventilation and high levels of moisture, which encourages the fungal spores and house dust mites that can trigger eczema and asthma.

COMMON SENSE AND FENG SHUI

Feng shui (pronounced "fung shway") is a collection of ideas and advice from the East about the effects of where you live and work on your health, wellbeing, and likely success in life. It's been built up over the centuries and is now fashionable – and taken very seriously – in certain Western circles.

Many of the suggestions – such as siting a home or workplace so as to take advantage of the environment and not putting the front door directly in front of a staircase or the toilet right next to the kitchen – are based on sound common sense and hygiene. Certain others – such as putting mirrors in particular places and using colors creatively – can enhance the feel of a home and might make living in it more enjoyable and energizing. If the concept appeals to you, you could try incorporating some of the ideas and practices of feng shui to help you to reorganize your home, eliminate clutter, and make it a more pleasant place to be in. If, however, the idea that various parts of your home represent certain aspects of your life, such as wealth and health, seems too superstitious, don't pursue it.

BENEFITING FROM NATURE

Many women derive pleasure from the natural world around them. Mountains, hills, forests, fields, rivers, and the ocean, for example, can inspire awe, wonder, and delight. The night sky is full of fascination, while the sky by day provides an ever changing vision of color and cloud formation. And many of the animals with whom we share this planet can be a source of relaxation and delight as we admire them, care for them, or interact with them. The pleasure and happiness we derive from contact with the natural world is a potent aid to health, partly as they raise our level of "feel-good" chemicals called endorphins.

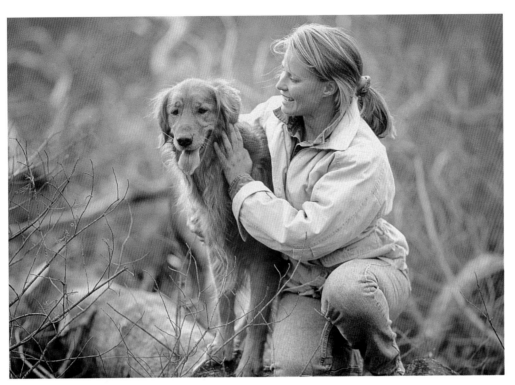

Keeping a pet is a proven way to beat stress. In addition, a dog makes you go out in the fresh air for long walks, which do you both good.

Having a pet Studies show that caring for a pet can benefit health in several ways. The presence of a pet counteracts any loneliness and gives some people a reason for living. Stroking an animal reduces stress-hormone production, lowers the levels of cholesterol and fats in the blood, and also reduces blood pressure. And having to exercise a dog means you get more exercise too.

Fitting your garden to your needs If you have a garden (if not, see below), you can mold it – for example, by changing the shape of the paths, seating areas and flowerbeds – to make it more pleasing and comfortable. If you don't know what to do, ask for help. And if you can't afford to pay someone, offer your skills in return or teach yourself from a book.

Growing healing herbs Animals often seek out certain plants to eat when they are unwell – cats, for example, choose long grass when they feel sick.

Using herbs to treat illness (*see page 137*) is an ancient form of healing for humans too. However small your garden, you can plant some of the most useful hardy herbs, such as rosemary, thyme, nettles, lemon balm, and one of the many sorts of mint (with its roots confined in a pot or small bed, so they don't spread too far).

Alternatives to a garden If you don't have a garden, take advantage of all of the other ways of being close to nature.

FOR EXAMPLE:

◆ Visit your nearest park or nature reserve.
◆ Spend time in a friend's garden.
◆ Grow plants in containers on a balcony or patio, or in a window box.
◆ Nurture indoor plants.
◆ Walk along the streets so that you can enjoy other people's gardens.

Herbs grow well in a window box or even in individual pots on a sunny windowsill.

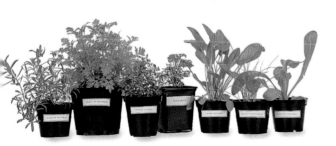

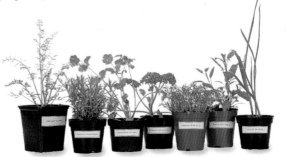

PERIODS AND OVULATION

Just as many young girls whose periods have just begun don't produce eggs each month until a year or two have passed, having periods without ovulating is increasingly likely to happen again once a woman approaches her 40s. Ovaries contain only a finite number of eggs (*see page 74*). This number gradually dwindles throughout your reproductive life. This is mainly because many eggs ripen each

YOUR OVARIES AND WHAT AFFECTS THEM

Ovulation and periods can be affected by many things other than the number of remaining eggs in your ovaries.

One of these is being very underweight. This affects the hypothalamus and can reduce the production of pituitary hormones so that they no

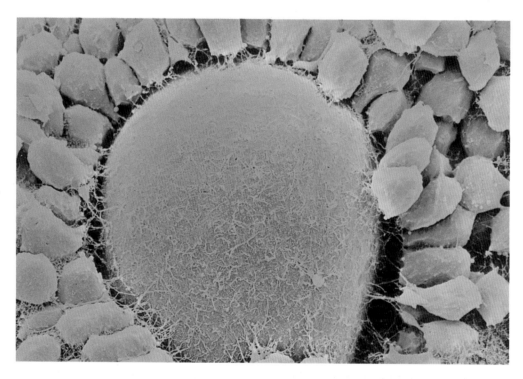

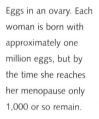

Eggs in an ovary. Each woman is born with approximately one million eggs, but by the time she reaches her menopause only 1,000 or so remain.

month, and while one ripens fully, the rest are wasted. The smaller your remaining store of eggs, the more likely it is that you won't ovulate reliably. You'll go on having periods until the number of eggs reaches a certain critical level (*see page 104*). But your periods may become less regular than they were when you always ovulated in the middle of each cycle. And a period following an anovular cycle (one without ovulation) may be lighter than one during a cycle in which one of your ovaries did release an egg.

Some women think that when their periods start becoming irregular and scantier, their menopause must be imminent. But this usually isn't so. It's simply a natural part of this time of life, and may well continue for five or ten years.

longer stimulate the ovaries well enough. As a result, there may be neither ovulation nor periods.

Being overweight because of regular binge-eating and eating a poor diet can cause other hormone changes which lead to multiple cysts developing on the ovaries (polycystic ovary syndrome, *see page 193*).

Stress can interfere with ovulation by playing havoc with both hormone levels and ovaries. Feeling stressed can also encourage heavy periods by, for example, preventing ovulation, or altering the balance of the prostaglandins that help control bleeding.

Too much exercise can make periods scantier by preventing ovulation, and can sometimes even stop them completely.

Smoking encourages regular monthly ovulation to stop earlier than it otherwise would. The chemicals in cigarette smoke age blood vessels prematurely. This probably interferes with ovulation by preventing enough of the blood that is needed from reaching the ovaries.

Hormonal methods of contraception – including the Pill, the progestogen-releasing coil, and a progestogen injections or implants – may act partly by preventing ovulation. This is why so many women find that their periods become lighter when using them.

Lastly, any surgery to your ovaries or fallopian tubes, or even just in their vicinity, may so damage the ovaries' tiny blood vessels that ovulation ceases. This is a particular risk during a sterilization or a hysterectomy.

THE LIKELIHOOD OF PREGNANCY

The average woman's chances of getting pregnant start plummeting in her late 30s. However, when you do produce an egg, conception is perfectly possible.

CONTRACEPTION

Now is a good time to reassess contraception. If you've had all the children you want, you may want to opt for a type of contraception that prevents pregnancy more effectively or, perhaps, completely (*see page 109*).

◆ The health risks from the combined Pill (one containing estrogen and progestogen) rise as you get older, especially if you're a smoker. And taking it in your 40s means you won't know when you reach your menopause until you swap it for a non-hormonal method. There are three reasons for this. First, the Pill makes you bleed each month, even after the menopause. Second, its estrogen prevents menopausal flashes and sweats. And third, you can't have FSH (follicle-stimulating hormone) and estrogen tests to see if they've reached menopausal levels until two weeks after you've stopped the Pill. (Around the menopause FSH tends to rise dramatically, and estrogen falls.) However, you may be happy to continue on the Pill until you're 53 or 54, because by then you'll probably be past the menopause anyway.

◆ The progestogen-only Pill provides slightly less protection against pregnancy and can disrupt periods. But it doesn't prevent flashes and sweats, or interfere with FSH and estradiol tests.

◆ Your doctor can discuss your personal pros and cons of continuing with the Pill. But once you're 50 you may want to use another form of contraception anyway, because there are no safety data for the Pill beyond this age.

◆ A progestogen-releasing coil, or a progestogen implant or injection, is another possibility.

◆ You could use a diaphragm and spermicidal jelly. However, some women dislike having to remember to insert and remove the device afterward, and some men say the rim bothers them.

◆ Your partner could use a condom plus a spermicide. However, if he doesn't get an

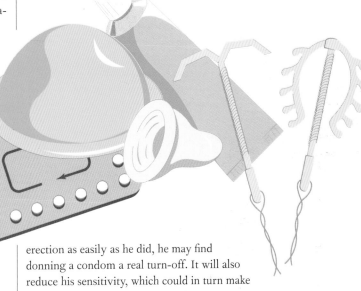

If you've decided when your family is complete – or if you are undecided about whether to have any more children – you may need to reassess the contraception you are using.

erection as easily as he did, he may find donning a condom a real turn-off. It will also reduce his sensitivity, which could in turn make him less able to maintain an erection.

◆ Neither a diaphragm nor condoms are as reliable as the Pill, but you may be happy to take the risk as you become older and less fertile.

◆ Natural family planning (*see page 43*) becomes less reliable as you get older because you no longer ovulate or have periods regularly. This makes it more difficult to identify "fertile" mucus, or to predict ovulation by estimating hormone levels (using urine dipsticks and an electronic monitor).

◆ Having a copper coil won't prevent you from knowing when you're menopausal. Leave it in until a year after your last period.

◆ Sterilization removes any anxiety over unwanted or unplanned pregnancy. However, it tends to advance the menopause by around two years, probably because the operation so frequently interferes with the delicate blood supply to the ovaries.

99

CARING FOR YOUR SKIN

When considering what's worth buying, remember the three skin-care rules:

◆ Boost its natural cleansing ability.
◆ Keep it adequately moisturized.
◆ Protect it from excess ultraviolet (UV) light.

CLEANING

Soap and water may be perfectly fine, but if they make your face tight for more than a few hours, it means your skin isn't replacing its natural oils and lipids fast enough. So instead use either some sweet almond oil (patted off with kleenexes), or a soapless cleansing bar, or a cleanser. This is also wise if your water is hard. Experiment until you find a cleanser that removes make-up and dirt effectively and rinses off easily with water. You don't need to bother with a toner.

MOISTURIZING

Your skin's sebum is a good moisturizer. This contains oils, lipids, hyaluronic acid, urea, amino acids, and lactose (a sugar). So avoid any soap or cleanser that removes so much of your natural secretions that your skin feels taut ten minutes later.

Sweet almond oil makes a gentler alternative to soap and water.

Some women benefit from this inbuilt moisturizer by wiping a fingertip along the creases beside the nose and above the chin, and transferring what they pick up to dry areas on their face.

However, most mature women benefit from extra moisturizer. Commercial ones contain a number of ingredients.

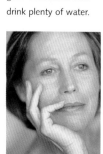

Mature skin tends to be drier, so invest in a good moisturizer and drink plenty of water.

MOISTURIZER INGREDIENTS INCLUDE:

◆ Essential fatty acids (linoleic and alpha linolenic acids, sometimes, confusingly, called vitamin F) – these nourish cells and help prevent inflammation.
◆ Oils – these waterproof the skin.
◆ Silicone – this mimics oil by waterproofing, but doesn't clog pores.
◆ Glycerine – this attracts water.
◆ Collagen – this attracts water.
◆ Hyaluronic acid – this is a more expensive water attractant.

◆ Vitamin C (ascorbic acid) – helps prevent photo-aging (damage from free radicals – unstable particles of oxygen generated by UV light).
◆ Vitamin E – acts like vitamin C.
◆ Retinoids (vitamin A derivatives such as retinol) – help smooth wrinkling caused by UV damage. Tretinoin, found in products such as Retin-A, Renova, and Retinova, is a prescription-only ingredient but is not as effective as first thought.
◆ Alpha-hydroxy acids (fruit acids) – smooth, moisturize, and firm the skin by helping it to shed any dead cells, retain water, and make collagen.

SUN PROTECTION

Protect your skin from UV-damage by avoiding too much sun, applying a sunscreen in the sun, and using a daytime moisturizer containing sunscreens and antioxidants. Photo-protective ingredients in moisturizers include antioxidant beta carotene and vitamins A, C, and E; physical UV blocking agents such as micronized zinc oxide and titanium dioxide; and certain UV-absorbing chemicals.

Look for a product with both UVB and UVA protection. UVB protection alone doesn't protect your skin from the aging effects of UVA rays. And by allowing you to stay in the sun longer, it actually encourages UVA damage.

Remember that a product's SPF (sun protection factor) is only an indicator. If, for example, being in the sun for ten minutes normally makes you burn, using a product with an SPF of 15 means you can stay out for 15 x 10 minutes – 150 minutes.

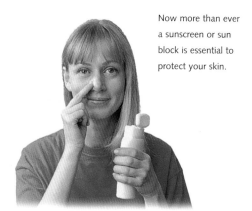

Now more than ever a sunscreen or sun block is essential to protect your skin.

NATURAL ALTERNATIVES TO PLASTIC SURGERY

Some women at this time of life decide they want to do something about their eye-bags, drooping lids, tiny vertical lines above their upper lips, frown lines on their foreheads, or the general sagging of their faces. Others feel unhappy about wrinkles and age spots on their faces in particular. The idea of having plastic surgery, to remove eyebags or tighten the skin of the face, for example, can be tempting, and may indeed have wonderful results. However, such operations are pricey, make you bruised and uncomfortable for some weeks, can have side effects, and often need redoing at least once in the years to come.

It is often far more preferable for a woman to enhance the quality of her skin and the tone of the muscles that flesh out the contours of her face. And these natural alternatives to plastic surgery are often very successful:

Adjusting your diet and avoiding swings of body weight Eat a healthy diet with plenty of skin-friendly nutrients (*see page 24*); drink lots of fluids; and take a daily half-hour of exercise to help keep your weight stable and to avoid the folds of skin that often follow repeated crash dieting.

Exercise, massage, and circulation boosting These all help disperse tissue fluid, and facial exercise keeps muscles fit and helps prevent sagging. Smile more all day to lift your cheek muscles and help prevent drooping around the sides of your mouth. Open your eyes wide while you count to ten, then relax and repeat four times twice a day to help you look and feel more wide-eyed all day. And gently tap your face with the pad of your middle finger along your cheekbones, from the corners of your mouth up the sides of your nose, and along your jaw to bring a glow to your skin.

Creams, cosmetics, and clothing Choose a moisturizer containing humectants (substances that attract water), antioxidants, such as vitamins A, C, and E, and retinoids. Ask a beauty expert to help you choose and use cosmetics to brighten your face, draw attention to your good features, and hide your less attractive ones. And take some useful tips from image consultants by choosing clothes in colors that will flatter, brighten, and enliven your skin.

Increasing your self-esteem and adjusting your attitude Altering your customary facial expressions can make your face brighter and less likely to droop. One key is to avoid the facial tension that accompanies stress. You may not be able to eliminate the stresses in your life, but you can focus on discovering and using more effective stress-management strategies (*see page 34*). The other key is simply to keep reminding yourself to look happier, just as you might have to keep remembering to stand up straighter when aiming to improve your posture.

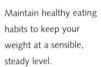

Maintain healthy eating habits to keep your weight at a sensible, steady level.

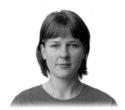

Open your eyes wide. Count to ten.

Relax your eyes, then repeat four times. Do this twice a day.

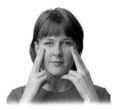

Gently tap your face with the pads of your middle fingers along your cheek bones, and upward from the corners of your mouth.

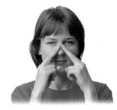

Continue tapping up the side of your nose and along your jaw.

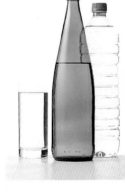

Drink plenty of fluids to keep your skin well hydrated. Bottled or filtered water is best.

EMOTIONAL WELLBEING

Rarely do health experts talk about the effects of people's relationships on their health. Yet we all know that the state of our closest relationships has a huge influence on how well we feel. Sometimes you may find that a relationship problem affects your physical health, making you more likely to come down with a cold, headache, or upset stomach.

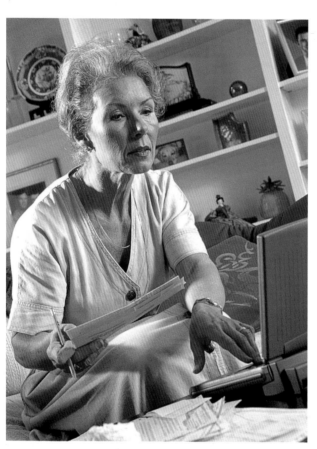

With the advent of e-mail, keeping in touch has never been easier. Rekindle old friendships and widen your horizons by starting new ones.

FRIENDS

Good and lasting friendships are precious, so what are the best ways of safeguarding them?

The starting point is simply to stay in touch. But it's surprising how challenging this can be as you near mid-life. You may, for example, be employed full-time and have little spare time. You may be busy with children or grandchildren. You may have moved away from your friends. You may find you are growing apart from the friends you do have around you. Or you may increasingly prefer a quiet life. But maintaining friendships doesn't have to take much time. You can keep a friendship polished, even if you don't see each other very often, simply by taking the occasional ten minutes to phone, write a card or letter, or send an e-mail. One of the benefits of being on the Internet is that it's so easy to send a message to a friend, even if she's on the other side of the world.

Empathic listening, encouragement, and conflict resolution

Relationships with friends benefit from empathic listening skills and encouragement and perhaps, sometimes, from conflict resolution skills too (*see page 41*). The same goes for your relationships with your partner, children, relatives, colleagues, neighbors, and most other people. Sometimes, when there has been a conflict, it's difficult to pick up the strands of a friendship again. But working through a conflict can eventually strengthen the bonds of friendship, so it's well worth doing.

Getting the balance right

Sometimes it's wise to monitor relationships, especially if they aren't as rewarding as they used to be. If, for example, you tend to feel upset after seeing a particular person, it may be that your dealings with each other have become based on "crossed transactions". This term comes from transactional analysis, a type of psychotherapy based on analyzing whether each person is dealing with the other in their "parent," "adult," or "child" mode at any one time. (Each of us can function with any of these hats on. Normally, though, a mature, emotionally balanced adult functions in "adult" mode most of the time.)

A crossed transaction with someone means you're at cross-purposes because, for example, one of you is expecting your "transaction" (interaction or communication) to be on an adult-to-adult basis, while the other is reacting to you as if they were a child. Sometimes simply stepping aside from a pattern of crossed transactions can turn a difficult relationship around.

FULFILLING YOUR POTENTIAL

Creativity A woman whose children are becoming more independent may feel she now has time for new outlets for her creativity. You might, for example, sign up for a class (or teach one yourself), redesign part of your home, give your image a makeover, or enter into local politics.

Work A mature woman often makes an excellent employee in that she's likely to be reliable, experienced, and responsible. Yet you may have come to a time in life when you want to spread your wings and start your own business or, perhaps, break out and practice professionally on your own. You might like to talk to a career guidance consultant, or have a detailed psychometric test, to see how your personality and abilities could be best used.

Intuition Many women become more in touch with their intuition – their sixth sense – in their 30s and 40s. This can be a powerful tool. And by using and trusting it, intuition becomes even more valuable.

and 40s become increasingly concerned about other people's morals and motivations too.

The media contributes to the ongoing moral debate. The dilemmas that are posed by TV soap storylines, for example, spark many animated discussions. News reports of war, murder, rape, mugging, burglary, and other conflicts and misdeeds trigger more worrying concerns. They may make you yearn for other people to behave better. For some individuals seem to be bound only by their own limited personal morality and, may not even be inhibited by the laws of the land. These people lack the inspiration they need if they are to act for everyone's benefit, let alone for their own.

What we all need if we are to live together in harmony is a deepening of our spiritual dimension. We need hope, wisdom, and the belief that there is more to life than just the meeting of our own needs. Religious teachings can be very helpful.

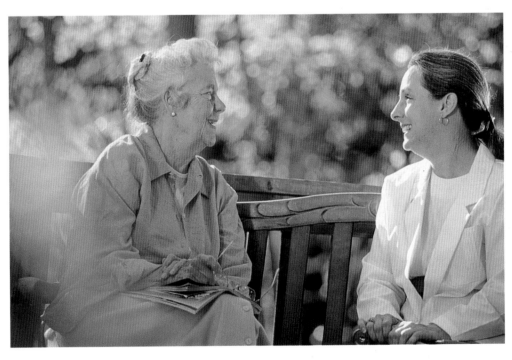

Being an active member of the community can give more meaning to your daily life. Rediscover your creativity and make the best possible use of your talents.

SOUL AND SPIRIT

The Swiss psychologist Carl Gustav Jung observed that many people take more interest in the emotional and spiritual sides of themselves as they grow older. This is because people often realize in mid-life that a vibrant, questing inner life is vitally important to their health, wellbeing, hope for the future, and freedom from anxiety and depression. Besides being interested in their own inner lives, many women in their 30s

They allow the community to be strengthened by the sense and wisdom of a moral code that has been refined over generations, and depicted in user-friendly stories, songs, dramas, and prayers that appeal to children and adults alike.

New-age ideas can be inspirational too. James Lovelock's *Gaia Hypothesis*, for example, reminds us that everyone and everything on the planet is interdependent, and that the connections between us are of vital importance.

THE MENOPAUSE

The menopause is when your periods finally stop, though the changes leading to the end of a woman's natural reproductive ability begin, for the average woman, at around 35. Your periods may come to an abrupt halt. Or they may become lighter, less frequent, and increasingly often completely missed in the two years or so before they finally stop.

A few women have very heavy and, perhaps, frequent, periods for a few years before the menopause. This is usually associated with estrogen becoming too important. This results from a low progesterone level (because there's no corpus luteum, see page 70). Another factor, perhaps, may be a diet lacking in plant hormones, essential fatty acids, and other "hormone-friendly" nutrients.

Changes in hormone levels can cause short-terms signs, such as hot flashes. They can also contribute to long-term problems, such as osteoporosis. But dealing with these using natural methods, plus having the confidence and inner wellbeing that so often accompany this time of life, will help you see your menopause not as a nuisance, or the end of an era, but as the gateway to a whole new time of enrichment and opportunity.

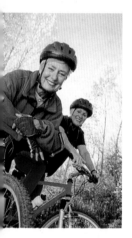

Try to look at the menopause as the start of the next stage of your life, rather than the closing of a chapter.

WHEN WILL IT BE?

If six months have elapsed since your last period, you've probably had your menopause. But you can't be sure for a year.

The average woman has her last period at age 51 (the normal range being 45 to 54). The timing depends mainly on how many eggs remain in her ovaries. By 45, the average woman has so few that her periods become irregular. When only around 1,000 eggs remain, she has her menopause.

One woman in 100 has an early menopause; before she's 40. Triggers for this include: smoking; sterilization; hysterectomy; chemotherapy, radiation therapy, or surgery for ovarian cancer; and removal of the ovaries for some other reason. Women without children tend to have an earlier menopause, as do those who eat poorly.

HOW YOU FEEL ABOUT IT

Some women experience a sense of loss about their inability to have more children – even if they don't want any more. This is also a time of life when you may have other losses, such as children leaving home, parents dying, and a lay-off, early retirement, or other job loss for you or your partner. Not surprisingly, some women become depressed.

However, many more are pleased that they no longer have to be concerned about getting pregnant. Some take early retirement out of choice, so they can have more free time. And most have mixed feelings. Far from moping and going into a decline, a large proportion of mature, post-menopausal women today actively look forward to the years ahead. And this is good, because for many this next life stage will last for a third or even a half of their whole lives.

PHYSICAL SIGNS

Four in five women have hot flashes and night sweats around their menopauses. Most find them little problem and simply, if necessary, find natural ways of dealing with them (*see pages 108–9*). Some, though, seek medical assistance.

Other possible signs include interrupted sleep and mood swings. The skin may become thinner and drier. And some women suffer from headaches, dizziness, or palpitations.

FUTURE HEALTH

The combination of naturally aging cells and lower hormone levels may gradually make your vagina drier. Some women also suffer from oversensitivity of the bladder, and irritation of the opening of the urethra (the passage from the bladder). Your risk of osteoporosis (fragile bones, *see page 179*) rises, as does the likelihood of heart disease (*see page 177*), arthritis (*see page 178*), and cancer (*see page 208*).

However, the good news is that simple lifestyle measures such as a healthy diet that's rich in plant hormones, sufficient exposure to natural unfiltered daylight, daily exercise, good relationships, plenty of pleasure, and adequate stress management, minimize these risks. And you can use a wealth of natural remedies and therapies to help yourself overcome any problems.

CONTRACEPTION

Although a woman's fertility falls ever lower as she approaches her menopause, ovulation – and therefore conception – remain possible for many. This is why you need effective contraception unless you don't mind having another child.

Some women who unexpectedly conceive find having and bringing up a child as an older mother a source of fulfillment and joy. Many, though, find it extremely tiring. They may also be frustrated by having to give up freedoms they previously took for granted. The child of an older mother can have many advantages, such as being brought up by a woman with more experience, worldly wisdom, time, and material security. But as that mom gets older she may not be as fatigue-proof or tolerant as a younger woman; the father is likely to be of much the same age; and the lifespan of each parent is likely to be relatively limited.

But obviously you don't want to go on using contraception longer than necessary, so when is it safe to stop?

It's wise to continue until:

◆ Two years after your last period, if this was before 50 (because sometimes then the ovaries stop ovulating completely for a year, only to start up again).

◆ One year after your last period, if this happened after you reached 50.

It's easy to know when to stop if you don't use hormonal contraception and therefore have normal periods. But if you're on the Pill you'll bleed regularly whether or not you've had your menopause. So every year or so it's sensible to stop for several months (and use condoms or a diaphragm for contraception instead) so you can either wait to see whether your periods return, or have a hormone test. This could be a blood test for FSH (follicle-stimulating hormone, a pituitary gonadotrophin) and estrogen, organized by your doctor, or a mail-order saliva test for estrogen and progesterone levels. Alternatively, you could stay on the Pill until you're 54, when you're highly likely to have had your menopause, though you'll need to use condoms or a diaphragm until you're sure. It's worth noting that the health risks from staying on the Pill after 50 aren't yet known.

An alternative to regular breaks from the Pill is to switch to a hormone-releasing coil. If you're bothered by unacceptable menopausal symptoms, you can take estrogen in tablets, patches or gel. And when you're 53 to 54, you can have the coil removed knowing that you're highly likely to be far enough past your menopause to be infertile. You can stop the estrogen too, unless you want to take hormone replacement therapy (*see page 106*).

YOU AND YOUR PARTNER

Even the best relationships are sometimes challenged by various life events that so often coincide with the years immediately before and after the menopause. However, the actual cessation of periods means relatively little to those who've spent most of their lives together using contraception. Indeed, the freedom from having to bother with contraception can be a big bonus.

The menopause certainly doesn't signal the end of the physical relationship you have enjoyed with your partner. Indeed, freedom from contraception can bring a whole new lease of life.

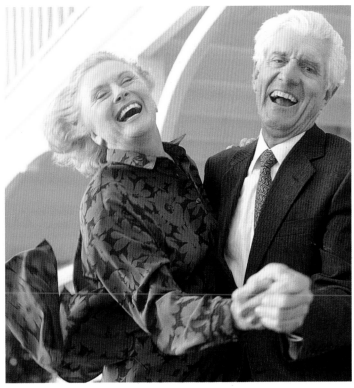

THE HRT DEBATE

More and more women are turning to hormone replacement therapy (HRT), but can this really help keep us in shape, well, and "young" after the menopause … or are we chasing a dream?

The already reduced levels of estrogen and progesterone fall faster after the menopause. The aim of HRT is to raise the levels of estrogen and, perhaps, also to mimic a woman's natural progesterone with man-made substances called progestogens. Estrogen on its own encourages womb cancer, so is recommended only for women who have had a hysterectomy.

Some of the pros and cons of HRT are clear. Others will become more so in 2008, when the National Institutes of Health study of 25,000 US women and the WISDOM study of 34,000 UK women begin yielding results. Until then, you just have to make the best decision you can.

IS HRT FOR YOU?

There is no easy answer. You need to weigh up the pros and cons and consider your health, past medical history, feelings about medication, and any risk factors for osteoporosis (*see page 179*), heart disease (*see page 177*), and breast cancer (*see page 208*). Your doctor will help you.

The answer may be "Yes" to HRT if you have:

◆ Flashes and sweats that are unacceptably disturbing.

◆ A high risk of osteoporosis. Risk factors may be in the past or present (*see page 179*). If your risk is high, your doctor will probably check on the current state of your bones with a special urine test or an X-ray called a bone-scan.

◆ A high risk of heart disease or strokes. Risk factors include a poor diet, high blood pressure, smoking, being overweight, and not exercising

---

THE PROS AND CONS OF HRT

PROS

◆ Prevents flashes and sweats in nine women out of ten.

◆ Thickens skin and boosts production of the skin's natural oils.

◆ Helps keep the vagina and urinary passage healthy.

◆ Halves the risk of osteoporosis by delaying mineral loss from bone.

◆ Some studies suggest it may protect women with a raised risk of heart disease and strokes; one suggests it adds three years to the lifespan of some of these women. Further research will prove whether it really is protective, or whether the women studied were less likely to develop arterial disease simply because they had relatively healthy lifestyles (women who choose to take HRT tend to eat healthier diets, exercise more, and have more health checks than the average woman).

◆ May delay the onset of Alzheimer's disease, though this, too, is unproven.

◆ May make cataracts less likely.

CONS

◆ Most types of HRT cause period-like bleeding, though there is a "bleed-free" type.

◆ More than five years of HRT very slightly raises the risk of breast cancer. More than ten years markedly increases this risk, though some – but not all – research suggests women on HRT who find they have breast cancer are less likely to die from it (possibly because they are encouraged to have regular mammograms, and because the type of cancer tends to be less aggressive).

◆ Makes blood clots in veins three times more likely, especially in the first year. At worst such clots are fatal.

◆ Can cause tender breasts (which usually settle in a few months), headaches, nausea, fluid retention, skin irritation (from patches), and a vaginal discharge (if on estrogen alone).

◆ May increase the risk of ovarian, liver, and skin cancers.

◆ May suppress immunity.

◆ May encourage depression.

◆ May trigger asthma.

enough, drinking too much alcohol, and a family history of such diseases. However, HRT is not yet licensed to prevent heart disease, strokes, or other arterial diseases.

◆ Alzheimer's disease in your close family. However, HRT is not proven to prevent Alzheimer's.

The answer may be "No" if:
◆ Your mother or sister has had premenopausal breast cancer.

WHAT TYPE OF HRT?

Estrogen can come as tablets, skin gel, skin patches (these are changed every three to seven days, depending on the brand), and implants. Progestogens come as tablets and patches.

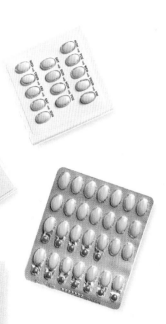

There are many forms of HRT available. Discuss the options with your doctor, and don't agree to anything you are not completely happy with. HRT is not suitable for everyone.

Most doctors prescribe progestogens instead of progesterone. This is because progesterone isn't well absorbed from tablets, and it isn't yet clear whether it's reliably absorbed from cream. (Also, to be realistic, manufacturers can patent progestogens, because they are purely synthetic substances, but they can't patent the synthetic progesterone they would use because this is nature-identical.)

If you start HRT while still having natural periods, as some women do, it's best to start with sequential combined HRT. This provides daily estrogen, and added progestogen for 10–13 days – either each month or once every three months. You'll probably bleed toward the end of the progestogen tablets, or soon after.

If you've been free from natural periods for a year, if your periods stopped before you went on sequential combined HRT, if you've taken sequential combined HRT for one or two years, or if you're over 54, your doctor may suggest continuous combined – or "bleed-free" – HRT. This provides estrogen and progestogen every day. Any initial bleeding usually stops after about six months.

How long to take it If you decide on HRT to prevent flashes, sweats, or other menopausal problems, you'll probably need to take it for one or two years, then stop gradually. If you take it to reduce your risk of osteoporosis, you'll need to continue for at least seven years for it to have any useful protective effect. However, as bone loss accelerates when HRT is stopped, some women stay on it for the rest of their lives.

MAMMOGRAMS

Whether or not you take HRT, you should have a regular mammogram (breast X-ray) every three years at least from the age of 50.

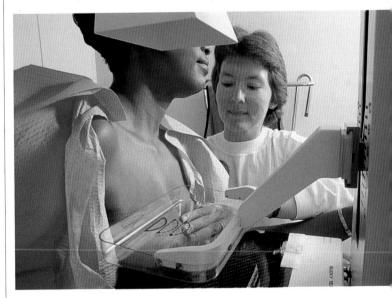

A mammogram is an X-ray of the breasts which can detect early cancer.

NATURAL ALTERNATIVES TO HRT

Natural alternatives to HRT include various remedies and lifestyle measures (which are also important for women who do take HRT). A healthy diet, adequate relaxation, exercise, effective stress management, and not smoking, for example, increase the body's production of estrogen.

A HEALTHY DIET

The estrogen-like effects of plant hormones (*see page 25*) can reduce flashes and sweats and may also lower the risk of breast cancer. Beans are a particularly rich source of the ones that are most active in the human body.

flashes. A good supply of vitamin E can reduce flashes and ease vaginal dryness, especially if your diet also contains plenty of vitamins B and C, flavonoids, and selenium. Vitamin A-rich foods help prevent dryness of the eyes, mouth, and vagina. Thiamine (vitamin B1) and niacin (vitamin B3) help prevent headaches; riboflavin (vitamin B2) reduces vaginal itching; and vitamin B6 can counteract cramp. And your body needs folic acid – another B vitamin – to produce estrogen.

Foods rich in calcium and magnesium, and food sources rich in the amino acid tryptophan help prevent depression (*see page 202*).

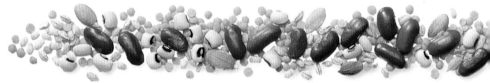

After the menopause, the levels of certain blood fats called low-density lipoproteins (LDLs) tend to rise. The continuing presence of free radicals (unstable oxygen particles) can change LDLs to the oxidized-LDLs that encourage arterial disease. Lower your LDL level by avoiding too much of any food containing saturated and trans fats. Help prevent oxidation of LDLs by eating foods rich in vitamins C and E and flavonoids (*see page 25*), and managing stress well.

A good supply of foods rich in essential fatty acids, vitamins C and E, and flavonoids helps keep the vagina moist (*see page 182*).

Foods containing minerals such as calcium, magnesium, and boron help prevent osteoporosis. Foods rich in calcium can also reduce hot

Tannins in tea reduce mineral absorption from the gut. Caffeine in coffee, tea, cola, or other caffeine-containing drinks, promotes calcium loss in the urine. Too much animal protein does the same, which is why meat-eaters get osteoporosis more often than do vegetarians.

Too much fat and added sugar can reduce stomach-acid production, but you need sufficient acid to absorb calcium. You'll also need zinc-rich foods to produce stomach acid.

Having one unit of alcohol each day will boost estrogen production; this helps prevent osteoporosis without affecting your risk of breast cancer.

Food supplements It may be worth taking a multimineral and vitamin supplement especially formulated for this time of life.

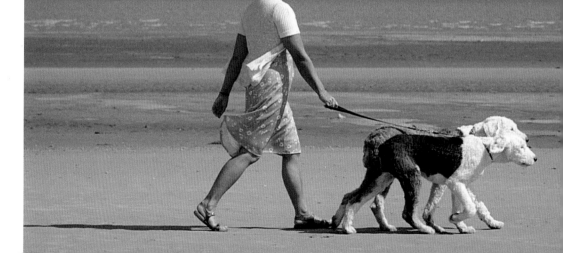

Other food supplements to consider are borage (starflower), blackcurrant or evening primrose oil, and fish oil. These contain certain polyunsaturated fatty acids (PUFAs) that are helpful if your body no longer successfully converts essential fatty acids to other PUFAs needed for hormone production. This can happen with aging, or physical or mental stress.

If you don't like beans, or soybean products such as tofu or soy milk, you could get additional plant hormones called isoflavones from a supplement containing soy or red clover extract.

These help because when there's a shortage of your own estrogen, plant hormones can latch on to your cells' estrogen receptors and act as weak estrogens in their place.

helps you produce vitamin D, estrogen, and "feel-good" hormones called endorphins.

Being a non-smoker Smoking reduces estrogen production and encourages flashes, sweats, a low libido, osteoporosis, and heart disease.

HERBAL REMEDIES

Herbs that encourage hormone balance and lessen flashes, sweats, and other menopausal problems often work best in combination. Herbalists prefer to prescribe them on an individual basis, often choosing from chasteberry, black cohosh, false unicorn root, yarrow, ginseng, motherwort, sage, wild yam, and dong quai (Chinese angelica). To treat hot flashes yourself, take half a teaspoon of chasteberry tincture and half a teaspoon of motherwort.

Consider drinking one unit of alcohol a day to protect your estrogen levels.

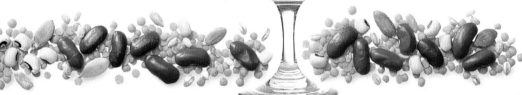

EXERCISE AND OTHER ACTIVITIES

All exercise is good, but daily aerobic exercise is particularly beneficial. This encourages the adrenal glands to manufacture an estrogen called estrone from a hormone called androstenedione. Exercise also raises your stress threshold; boosts your energy; and makes flashes, sweats, cramps, and depression less likely. It aids digestion, sleep and weight control, and may make you feel sexier.

Sexual activity Sexual arousal encourages vaginal secretions and helps prevent the vaginal dryness that troubles some postmenopausal women.

Daylight exposure Enough exposure to bright light helps prevent winter depression (SAD, *see page 202*), while light on your skin and in your eyes

Take this combination twice a day. Alternatively, take a teaspoon of black cohosh twice a day. For vaginal dryness, *see page 182*.

Warning: Don't use hormone-balancing herbs if you're on HRT or the Pill.

THERAPIES

Aromatherapy Several essential oils can help alleviate flashes and other menopausal signs. They include geranium, clary sage, jasmine, neroli, chamomile, rose, ylang ylang, sandalwood, and bergamot. *See page 133* for information about how to use these oils.

Hydrotherapy Reduce the frequency and the intensity of hot flashes with a daily cold sitz bath (*see page 130*).

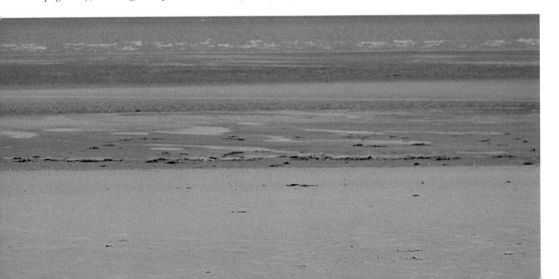

109

BEING A SENIOR

Most women experience a gradual, seamless transition between maturity and "old age." But as you pass through your 60s and 70s you may indeed feel you are entering a different dimension. You are coming to the top of the pile and may have one, two, or more generations beneath you. And because you've had much more experience of life than younger people, you have a lot to contribute.

To make a useful contribution, you'll need to optimize your health and fitness so they're less likely to let you down in the years ahead. You'll also need to polish up your communication skills – those of empathic listening, encouragement, and conflict resolution (see page 41). And you need confidence to fulfill your valuable potential.

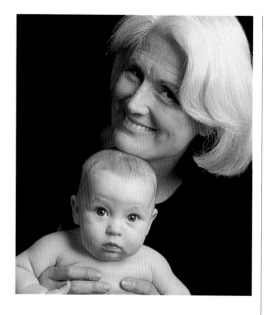

The wisdom you have built up during your life so far can be of great benefit to your children and grandchildren.

RECOGNIZING THE BENEFITS OF EXPERIENCE

It's easy to arrive at this time of life without ever pausing to consider the fruits of your experiences. Yet doing so can boost your confidence and enable you to enjoy your achievements. It can also throw light on what you still want, or need, to do.

A regular assessment of where you are and where you've come from is especially sensible in your 60s, 70s, and beyond, as the average person today can expect to live a good many years as a senior. Focus on what you've learned so far and what you will want to do, including:

◆ Practical skills (driving, cooking, typing, accounting, etc.).

◆ Communication skills.
◆ Professional skills (many elders continue to use such skills).
◆ Spiritual disciplines – such as compassion and service (*see page 49*).
◆ Organizational skills.
◆ Artistic, musical, and other creative skills.

TAKING YOUR PLACE AS AN ELDER

Older people need their needs met just as do those of any other age. Unfortunately, though, this doesn't always happen. But as the generations that were in their teens or 20s in the rock-and-roll decade of the 1950s or the flower-power era of the 1960s join the gray panther brigade, I think they'll insist on the proper provision of leisure, health, residential, and other community facilities for seniors. This is right and proper. For it's only by treating ourselves with the respect we deserve that we can do the same for others.

GRANDCHILDREN

Many grandmothers assist their children by helping to look after grandchildren. This has many benefits. It's a huge asset for their children. Their grandchildren can benefit hugely from getting to know their grandmothers intimately. Undoubtedly you'll have a lot of fun too. And many grandmothers say that their grandchildren help keep them young. This is especially true if they make the effort to keep up with the music, soaps, and trends that interest the younger generations; learn their friends' and teachers' names; and take an interest in what they're doing at school.

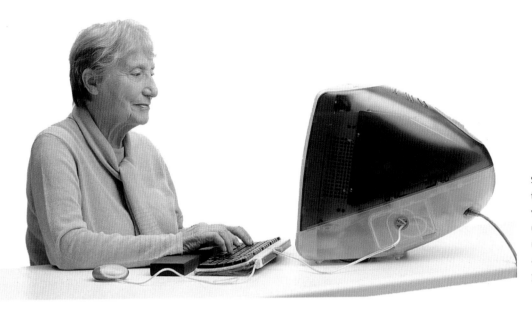

Share your wisdom with the wider community via the Internet. Or use a computer to make recording stories and experiences from your life easier.

You will also be able to pass on some of your experience, wisdom, and sense of humor and help your children to lay the foundations of a moral code that will stand your grandchildren in good stead for life.

BUILDING ON THE PAST

The inventions of the wheel and printing press changed the face of history. The advent of modern telecommunications, including the Internet, is another such quantum leap, as now we needn't rely on personal contact, or the written word, to pass on knowledge. Instead, everyone with a telephone can share in centuries of accumulated wisdom, not to mention an ongoing international debate about current events.

But the existence of enormous, accessible, worldwide databases doesn't detract from the importance of what each individual can offer. Even today, neither children nor adults learn most of what they need to know from electronic sources, let alone strangers. In practice, we learn life's essentials from our family, friends, teachers, colleagues, and neighbors. It is this one-to-one contact that has the biggest impact on who we are and what we do.

So whether as a mother, grandmother, sister, friend, daughter, neighbor or colleague, you can contribute more to your loved ones and, perhaps, others who come into contact with you, than can any computer or book.

You can provide personal opinions, views, and anecdotes that will enrich those around you and give them a vital sense of continuity and belonging. Knowledge, pure and simple, isn't nearly as valuable to an individual as are the insights and wisdom from someone they love, admire, or respect. And your presence, comments, listening ear, interest, and humor are worth more than any computer as you and your family work out how best to cope with today's challenges by building on the wisdom of the past.

Valuing your memories Your memories are a precious store from which to bring past experiences and emotions back to light. They can help you and those around you to learn from and build on the past. And they can also entertain and teach.

However, you may increasingly find that recent events are harder to recall than those that took place years ago. If so, try this tip. Look back at the end of each day at anything that's important to you, and go through it again in your mind's eye to help imprint it in the circuitry of your brain. You could also keep a journal and a regularly updated photo album. And you might like to do the same at the end of each month and year.

Looking at photographs helps keep your life history alive and vivid in your mind.

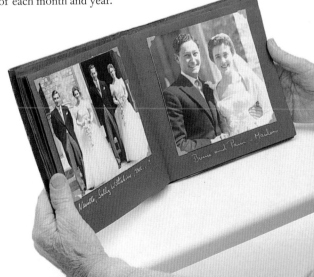

AGING WELL

Choose fresh, whole foods rather than processed ones to maximize your nutrient intake.

Much of aging is genetically predetermined but research over the last decade has cast considerable light on how we can maximize our lifespans. Most of the findings spotlight the value of simple lifestyle measures. And they indicate that the three most important factors involved in feeling young and delaying premature aging are physical exercise, mental exercise, and sex with someone you love (*see page 115*).

PHYSICAL AND MENTAL EXERCISE

Doing daily muscle-strengthening and stretching exercises, along with a daily half an hour of aerobic exercise, will help you feel well. This also has many other benefits (*see page 28*), including lowering the risk of osteoporosis and arterial disease. And researchers say it may even increase the number of brain cells.

Keeping mentally alert is very important too. Examples of how to do this include having stimulating conversations, keeping up with current events, reading, doing crossword puzzles and memory games, and using memory-enhancing tips such as memorizing a name by associating its syllables with related images.

FOOD AND DRINK

As we grow older, we tend not to absorb nutrients so well. This means it's especially important to choose "nutrient-dense" wholefoods rather than to fill up on highly refined "junk" foods. Studies show that many older people could benefit from eating more vegetables and fruit. Some exist on a very poor quality diet, one that saps their energy and wellbeing and raises the risk of infection, cancer, heart disease, and many other disorders.

Choose brightly colored fruits and vegetables – these contain flavonoids and carotenes.

Researchers report that the nutrients most likely to be in short supply at this time of life include calcium, zinc, iron, magnesium, vitamins C, B6, B12, D, and E, and folic acid, so check that you are eating enough of these (*see page 25*):

FOODS YOU SHOULD EAT:

◆ Green, red, orange, yellow, blue, and purple vegetables and fruits. These contain flavonoids and carotenes – brightly colored plant pigments. Our bodies make beta carotene into vitamin A, which among other things is good for the eyes. All the flavonoids are potent antioxidants and work hand in hand with vitamin C to strengthen connective tissue and blood vessels. For example, the anthocyanidins and proanthocyanidins in blue-black fruits (such as blueberries, elderberries, cranberries, black cherries, and black grapes) encourage good night vision, strengthen small blood vessels (so improving poor circulation and reducing bruising), help prevent urine infection by stopping *E. coli* bacteria from sticking to the bladder wall, and help prevent infection, arthritis, and night blindness. Black grape seeds, strawberries, and cherries contain flavonoids called polyphenols (which may fight cancer), and black grape skins also contain an antioxidant called resveratrol, which researchers believe may help prevent cancer and lower a raised cholesterol level. And tomatoes, red bell peppers, and red grapefruit contain a carotenoid called lycopene that can fight cancer. Cooked tomatoes may be more effective than raw ones in this respect.
◆ Onions and garlic (for their sulfur compounds).
◆ Yogurt (for its lactobacilli which help promote a healthy balance of microorganisms in the gut).
◆ Cabbage-family vegetables such as broccoli, brussels sprouts, and cauliflower (for their glucosinolates, which have cancer-fighting properties).

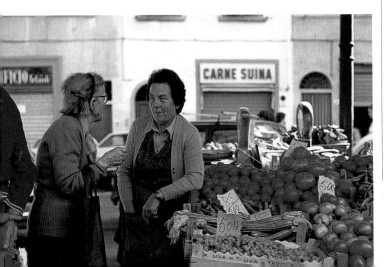

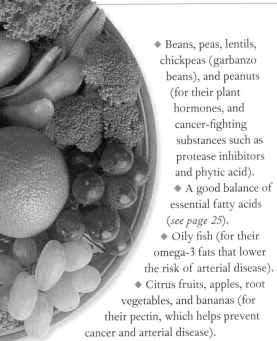

◆ Beans, peas, lentils, chickpeas (garbanzo beans), and peanuts (for their plant hormones, and cancer-fighting substances such as protease inhibitors and phytic acid).

◆ A good balance of essential fatty acids (*see page 25*).

◆ Oily fish (for their omega-3 fats that lower the risk of arterial disease).

◆ Citrus fruits, apples, root vegetables, and bananas (for their pectin, which helps prevent cancer and arterial disease).

◆ Celery, parsnips, and carrots – umbelliferous vegetables (for their excellent mixture of substances that fight cancer and heart disease, including flavonoids, carotenes, coumarins, and phenolic acids).

Food supplements If you are concerned about your food intake and want to take supplements, choose a good quality multimineral and vitamin preparation. It may also be wise to take a daily dose of vitamin E; some evidence suggests that this vitamin helps stave off heart disease, cancer, and osteoarthritis, though this is unproven. (*Warning:* Avoid vitamin E if you take aspirin or other blood-thinners.)

Body weight There's good evidence that avoiding being overweight may help prolong life.

HERBAL AND OTHER ANTI-AGING REMEDIES

Several remedies may promote healthy aging (not proven as such but they will do you no harm):

◆ Aspirin – discuss with your doctor whether it's wise for you to take a daily half-tablet of aspirin to reduce your risk of arterial disease and cancer.

◆ Potent antioxidants – such as coenzyme Q-10, and quercetin – may reduce your risk of arterial disease and cancer.

◆ Ginkgo – may improve a poor memory and boost the circulation.

◆ Ginseng – may improve your wellbeing and fight cancer.

◆ Melatonin – may improve sleep; preliminary studies suggest it may also fight cancer and promote longevity.

Fresh air and smoking Breathing fresh, clean air helps prevent respiratory illnesses. Smoking remains bad for your health and that of those with whom you live. But, even now, if you stop smoking (or cut down) you'll reduce your risk of getting cancer of the lung and certain other organs.

Daylight Exposure to daylight helps counteract the continuing mineral loss that began in your 30s and accelerated after the menopause. So each day get some unfiltered daylight on your skin (taking care not to burn). Light on your face alone is enough. Exposure to bright daylight also helps prevent depression and sleep problems. However, as with most things in life, balance is everything. Getting too much of the sun's ultraviolet light on your skin encourages the formation of skin cancer and age spots (*see page 152*).

HEALTH SCREENING

Recommended screening tests at this stage include:

◆ A mammogram every two to three years in the USA and every three years in the UK, and a Pap (cervical) smear annually in the USA and every three to five years in the UK. Continue with these until you're 64.

◆ A urine test every five years, to assess the risk of osteoporosis (*see page 179*). If this suggests your risk is raised, and if you already have a healthy lifestyle, consider HRT or related drug therapy.

◆ A blood test (for sugar) every two years or so, for unrecognized diabetes.

◆ An eyesight test (for glaucoma, high pressure in the eye; and damage from unrecognized diabetes) every two years, or every year if you are over the age of 75.

◆ A fecal-blood test (for colon cancer) every year if you have a family history of this cancer; or any time if you have a lasting change in your bowel habit. You can buy test kits from the drugstore.

◆ A blood pressure check (and, perhaps, a blood-cholesterol test) every two years or so.

Take plenty of walks in the fresh air and heighten your sunshine exposure, particularly if you are feeling down or are having trouble sleeping.

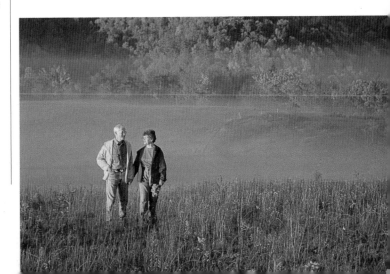

YOUR HOME ENVIRONMENT

Although some people continue to live in the same place at this time of life, a good many move to somewhere smaller, easier to care for, cheaper to run, or nearer family, friends, stores, or other community facilities. But whether you stay put or move on, you'll want your home to fulfill a number of important needs. Not only should it be comfortable, secure, and free from avoidable hazards, but it should also reflect your personality and interests and provide a welcoming background for entertaining friends and family.

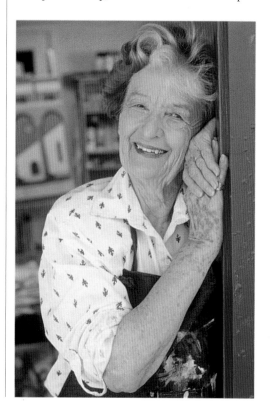

Old age doesn't mean you can't enjoy a good social life.

COMFORT AND SAFETY

Everyone, of every age, wants their home to be comfortable and safe. Here are a few of the considerations that are particularly important now:

◆ The first is your bed or, more specifically, your mattress. Many people keep their mattresses for far too long, then wonder why they don't sleep well. A mattress will last longer if you get help to turn it upside down every year. Every six months, turn it head to tail. As soon as it becomes lumpy or fails to support you properly, discard it.

◆ Pillows, too, have only a limited useful life, so replace them if you think they may be contributing to disturbed or unrefreshing sleep.

◆ Other items of furniture that may need replacing include the easy chair or couch on which you usually sit, and the chair you use for desk reading, writing, or keyboard work. You need the best to reduce the risk of problems in your back, arms, and shoulders as you grow older.

◆ Take time to improve the comfort and safety of the bathroom. Ideas include replacing a hard, slippery floor-covering with carpeting; buying a bathtub with grab-rails on each side to help you

get up easily; and putting non-slip tiles or a rubber mat in the shower.

◆ If you are unsteady on your feet, invest in a cell phone or pager so you can easily alert someone if you have a fall.

Reflecting your personality Ask yourself whether you really like the colors, furnishings, pictures, books, and CDs or tapes in your home. If not, now's a good time to start making changes, especially if, at this time of your life, money has ceased to be a problem. There's no reason why things that gave you pleasure years ago should necessarily continue to do so. Many people find that change is energizing, enjoyable, and keeps them young.

Hospitality Some older people increasingly shut themselves away and rely on ever-shrinking circles of friends for their social lives. Others continue to make new acquaintances and friends of all ages throughout their lives. Age is no barrier to a good social life – all you need is the health, the will, and the confidence to make it happen. You may also need practical help, such as elevators. for example.

At this stage in your life you may have to find a home more suitable for your needs, but you can have fun redecorating.

Having a partner who is also a friend helps many women feel young. But what about sex? It's amusing that when we're adolescent, we're shocked to think that our parents – who at the time are probably in their late 30s – may still be having sex. We realize our foolishness only when we become parents ourselves. There's also often a reluctance in young and middle-aged people to believe that those in their 60s, 70s, and beyond are still interested in sex. But one study found that four in five married women and one in two unmarried women aged 70–79 were still sexually active. So, clearly, sex continues to fascinate, even if its practical expression may change. You and your partner may, for example, take longer to become aroused, though patience, good humor, and inventiveness will probably conquer any problem.

One study suggests that the pleasure of having sex with someone you love is a major factor in keeping people looking and feeling young.

LIVING WITH SOMEONE OR ON YOUR OWN

Women's lives differ enormously according to whether they live with their partners, families, or friends, in rest homes, or alone. Sometimes what happens is out of our control – for example, if a partner dies, or we become ill and need hospital or residential care. Whatever happens, it's never too late to make the most of the relationships we have. Relationships can change and grow in surprising ways, and this is all the more likely if we polish our communication skills (*see page 41*). This is true even for relationships that are set in their ways. Although it's sometimes more of a challenge to change patterns that have evolved over several decades, the results can be particularly rewarding.

Living on your own – perhaps for the first time – can be a shock, especially after a bereavement or divorce. Once you feel able, try listing the positive aspects. Things to consider include being able to get up and go to bed when you like, having more time to yourself, having less to do domestically, and not having to think of someone else all the time. Of course it's possible to view each of these in a negative way, but learning to change your attitude and think positively may be very beneficial.

If your visitors, excursions, phone calls, and letters don't make up for the lack of company, consider connecting to the Internet and joining a chat group. This can be a great source of entertainment and may even produce lasting friendships.

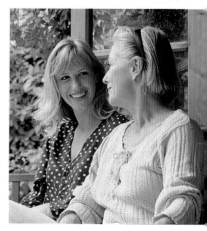

A friendship with a younger woman can be very rewarding for both of you.

YOUR IMPORTANCE TO OTHER WOMEN

As an older woman, what you say and do can be very significant to the younger women you meet. You are further forward than they are on the physical journey through life, and it's quite possible that you'll have gathered many useful insights and creative methods for managing life events on your way. You can share the stories of what's happened in your life, what's going on now, and how you deal with challenges rooted both in the past and in the present. And, in turn, you may find yourself enriched by suggestions and ideas from your younger friends.

You can also have a significant input into the lives of your peers and those older than you by sharing your wisdom and humor in this way.

Romance and sex certainly don't have to stop once you get older, you can continue to enjoy them at any age.

115

Although the bloom of youth, the reproductive fruitfulness of maturity, and the years of paid employment may have passed, there are many ways in which to fulfill your potential and stay young at heart. Indeed, researchers say that enthusiasm, optimism, creativity, and curiosity about new ideas are among the traits that make some older people appear younger than they are.

FULFILLING YOUR POTENTIAL

Work Increasing numbers of people work past retirement age simply because they don't want to stop. Others find their skills and abilities are needed by friends, family, or others. Some older women enjoy helping, advising, teaching, consulting, or encouraging younger people working in their skill areas. Whether on a formal or a casual basis, this can be hugely rewarding to both parties. And you may find that brushing up on new findings and seeing things from the point of view of a younger generation gives you a sense of excitement that may have eluded you for some time.

Education How about branching out and learning new subjects, taking up new hobbies, or brushing up on ones you always enjoyed but never had time for when you were younger? With modern educational facilities – including community colleges, distance-learning packages, and facilities for buying books from Internet bookstores – and with enthusiasm for your chosen subject to motivate you, you could end up learning more during this part of your life than you ever did before. And you might even enjoy it more too.

Creativity The sky's the limit when it comes to practicing new techniques, polishing up others, and learning about your art, whatever form it may take, on your own or in a like-minded group. When it comes to artistic expression, your experience and knowledge of life can be enriched only by the willingness to be fully in touch with your feelings and let them color what you create.

PERSONALITY

It can happen that people become "more like themselves" as they grow older. Their personalities seem to crystallize, showing more clearly who they are. This is partly because we tend, consciously or unconsciously, to lose our inhibitions as the years pass. This enables us to be more truly ourselves rather than always wanting to please others. This is fine as long as it's mutually constructive. If, however, you notice that the newly released

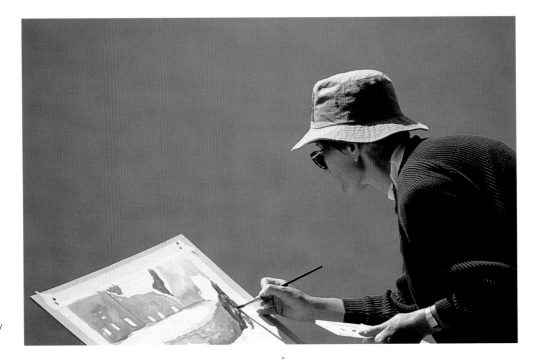

Many an older person has discovered the enormous pleasure to be had in taking up a new activity, especially an artistic one.

expression of certain aspects of your personality belittles or hurts others in any way, it's best to put them firmly back where they came from! There are no medals for wounding people.

MAXIMIZING YOUR ENERGY

Looking after your health (*see pages 112–13*) and fulfilling your potential (*see above*) should be energizing. If you need an extra boost, try having a break from your usual life by going on vacation. Being away from your everyday environment can put life into perspective and give you helpful new insights into how to view things and how to choose what to do next.

SOUL AND SPIRIT

Anyone who has ever come to know a large number of elderly people, either through living or working with them, will have realized that old people remain very different from each other not only in their looks, behavior, personalities, and the ways they view life, but also in something much less tangible – their souls and spirits. Those who retain a sense of hope and purpose stand out like beacons. They have a deep faith that makes them sure there is vastly more to life than our minds and bodies and the obvious material world around us. Like millions of others worldwide, they take comfort from the belief that each of us has an extra dimension – a soul and spirit.

If you've never developed your spiritual life, it's not too late to start. And if you once had an active spiritual life, but have let it slip, it's never too late to return.

You can start by investigating some of the spiritual practices on *page 49*. For example, you might try meditating (*see page 142*), or develop your gift for teaching, or compassion. Simply giving yourself the opportunity to be still and, perhaps, contemplate the beauty around you – in nature, art, or music, or the incomparable miracle of new life, for example – could give your soul and spirit wings. And you could enhance your spiritual awareness by reading about religious and new-age ideas, or exploring them in other ways.

You may be unfamiliar with new-age beliefs. The surge of interest in the subject over the last few decades is partly because so many people yearn to develop their spiritual dimension. Many were brought up without a formal spiritual education, so have no experience of how to access the spiritual riches of the religious practices and teachings once universal in most communities. However, information about new-age ideas and healing methods is often readily accessible, for example, in workshops and magazines.

A lot of people look forward to a time when new-age ideas will more often be used to enrich religious ones, and vice versa. The powerfully mystic and user-friendly nature of certain new-age concepts could enliven religious practice and teaching, and make their insights into dealing with the challenges of life and death much easier for people to access. At the same time, the experience, wisdom, and beauty of religious practice and teaching could add breadth and depth to many relatively unformed new-age ideas.

Whatever you choose to help you on your way, don't delay. You can start an important and lifelong journey along your spiritual path today.

It's never too late to develop your spiritual life. Meditation helps you to connect with your spiritual self, and is excellent for your mental and physical health also.

117

TOWARD THE END

From the moment we're conceived we're all inexorably moving toward the end of our lives. Indeed, death is the only thing of which we can be certain. Yet none of us knows exactly when life will end. Some have a pretty good idea – perhaps because they are extremely old, or are suffering from a terminal illness – but death can take us by surprise at any age or stage of life. The old adage goes, "Today is the first day of the rest of your life". But today may also be the last. Hence the sense of the hymn that urges us to live each day as if it were our last.

BREAKING OUT

Have you ever wondered what you would do today if you knew it were to be your last? Why not have a go now? First, make a list of your ideas and study it. Now divide them into those you could do anyway (such as telling someone you love them), and those you'd contemplate only on your actual last day because they're potentially risky to you or others (such as resigning from your job). The point is to see whether there's anything you could do to enrich your life – or that of those around you – *now*, rather than waiting until you know you're about to die.

Perhaps you'll realize there are things you've always wanted to do, ways of being that you've always wanted to be, and things to say that you've always wanted to say. *And, most important, that you needn't put them off any longer.* Even things that might at first sight appear potentially destructive could carry the grain of something

important inside them for now. Suppose, for example, you'd spend the morning admiring the garden or going out birdwatching if it really were your last day, yet you feel other more mundane things need your attention on an everyday basis. Then how about using this realization as a catalyst for taking more time today to stop and stare, and to enjoy the beauty of the natural world around you?

THE WAY YOU ARE

People's behavior and emotions as they approach their death often tend to reflect their behavior and emotions at other challenging times. We are, in a sense, "living our dying" all life long. It may sound strange, but even now, you can take steps to change your attitude and your approach to others, perhaps through focusing on your communication skills (*see page 41*).

Life is a journey, and it can sometimes seem like an uphill struggle. Take good care of yourself along the way, physically, mentally, and spiritually and you will enjoy both the traveling and the arriving.

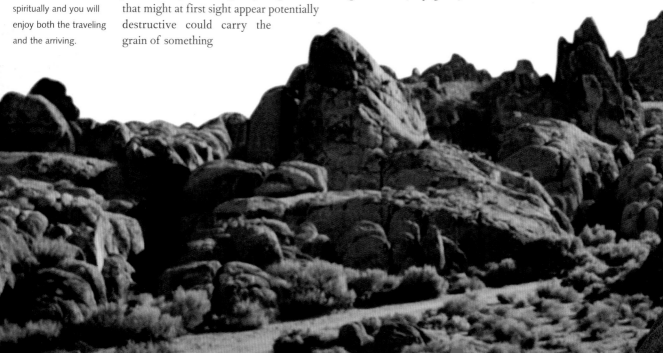

ATTITUDES TO DYING

Many things color people's thoughts, behaviors, and feelings about their lives coming to an end. Depending on what these are, an individual may or may not feel ready to face her death. Yet feeling prepared practically, emotionally, intellectually, and spiritually can so enhance the last years, months, days, or even hours that they can become a time of opportunity and blessing. The good news is that we can all learn to see this time of life in a different way.

Feeling very emotional Many people experience some combination of sadness, fear, anger, and despair about dying. And some also experience a positive, hopeful state of mind. They feel content that the time is right and that things are working out as they should. Whatever the emotions, they are usually best shared. Sharing makes uncomfortable and challenging emotions easier to live with; encourages hope; enables those around to offer support in a more focused way; and is sometimes even inspirational to others.

A few people decide to direct strong emotion about their situations outwardly to fuel change. They may, for example, take steps to improve local or national health-care facilities for others who will one day be in their situation.

Thoughts of suicide are generally triggered by despair. The pain or numbness can make it seem as if there's no other way out, *yet there is always — for everyone, no matter how dreadful they feel — an alternative*. If you feel suicidal and can't see any alternative, get skilled help at once. You need someone else to carry you, metaphorically, through the worst part of this wilderness experience. When you are able, you can then walk with them by your side and together find the path ahead.

Depression Someone who feels depressed (*see also page 202*) may have a welter of unrecognized emotions disturbing her unconscious mind, or may, for example, be responding to the effects of drugs or physical incapacity. There are three ways of dealing with this.

THESE ARE:

◆ Find someone who'll listen empathically, such as a good friend, close relative, nurse, counselor, or minister. Once recognized, painful feelings can be dealt with constructively. This relieves the depression and opens the door to making the most of remaining opportunities.

◆ Take antidepressant drugs or remedies. These take some weeks to work but can be very helpful.

◆ Improve your diet, take exercise, get out in bright sunlight, arrange to do things you enjoy, and find something to laugh about (*see page 200*).

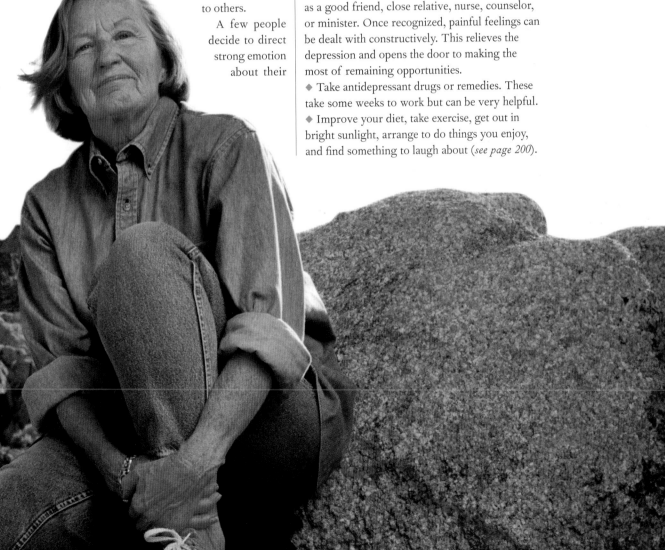

BEING READY

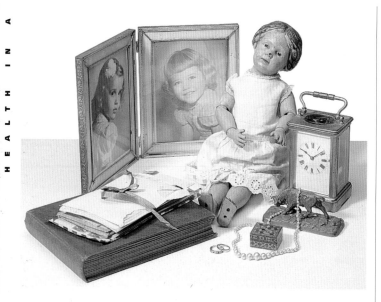

left unmade, all clutter life and impair your ability to concentrate on other things. Clearing clutter could enable you to use the last part of your life in the ways you really want.

Sometimes, too, affairs that are in disarray are a sign of being overburdened and over-busy. At any stage of life this can be uncomfortable and make a person feel worse. Being too busy can be a defense against uncomfortable emotions such as fear or anger, in which case it's well worth addressing these feelings directly (*see page 119*).

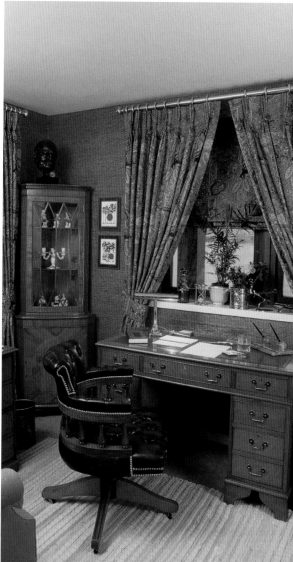

Leaving a relative or loved one one of your most precious mementoes, along with a warm, personal letter, is a positive experience for both you and the person receiving the gift.

Some people, realizing death is imminent, decide to leave letters and mementoes for their loved ones. Such a letter could be a personal message that conveys your deepest feelings about the person and your wishes for the future. A letter from a parent to a child, for example, might outline what you, as a parent, have most enjoyed about him or her, and about your life in general, as well as any special encouraging thoughts just for your child to warm him or her in the future. The positive thinking involved in choosing what to put in such a letter could give you great pleasure and help ease any stress you're going through. And the same goes for choosing what to bequeath to whom in your will.

TYING UP LOOSE ENDS

It's a great help to those we leave behind if we sort out the legal and practical aspects of our lives before we die. Obviously this isn't always possible. You may ask what this has to do with health. The answer is that people who allow their affairs to remain in disorder throughout their lives may, at some level, feel weighed down or burdened by them. Clutter in any sphere of life – whether it's piles of newspapers waiting to be read, closets full of clothes that don't fit, or an address book full of people you no longer see – can drain your energy. And accounts not done or filed, investment notes, property deeds and loan details lost, or your will

Sorting out your life before it ends can make it much easier for others to sort out the practicalities of what you leave behind.

It makes sense to set yourself a target for clearing up your affairs, perhaps one file a week, and getting whatever professional help you need. Then take the time to write a simple note outlining where important documents such as your will are to be found, along with the names and numbers of your accountant, lawyer, bank manager, and any others you think would be useful for your executors.

WHAT HAPPENS NEXT?

A person's belief about what happens once her physical body dies inevitably shapes her feelings, experience, and even her behavior throughout the time leading up to her death. There are basically three possibilities. These are:

◆ Either nothing happens – the individual's mind, spirit, and soul die along with the body, and only the memory of her lingers on.

◆ Or there is reincarnation, with a person bringing to each new life her *karma* – a word used by Buddhists and Hindus to indicate the effect of their deeds in past lives on their present lives.

◆ Or there's some other sort of life with or without God.

The experience of dying sometimes crystallizes an individual's belief or hope about what comes next. Alternatively, it can make one reexamine doubts and, perhaps, open the door to the possibility of enlightenment. Or it may simply enable her to give someone else permission to hope and pray, on her behalf, that her soul will continue to exist and that she will meet her maker.

SEEKING ENCOURAGEMENT

Whatever their beliefs, many dying people feel comforted by the involvement of a minister of religion, or someone who will act as a spiritual counselor. Such a person may speak about issues that others around them dare not or cannot. This sometimes allows the dying person to voice questions or ideas she's never been able to ask or discuss before, or to enter into the sort of dialogue she may never have thought possible. If talking is impossible, simply having such a person there can be comforting and help ease the passage from this life; talking isn't necessary to experience a real connection with someone special.

FAREWELLS

Saying goodbye, like saying hello, is very important. This is why it can be so devastating when someone we love dies suddenly, without us there. But it must also be very sad for the person who realizes she is going to die suddenly without the chance to say goodbye, or without feeling that she has put as much into her relationships with others as she might have wished.

Thankfully, many of us have at least some warning. This gives us the chance to enrich our departure by taking our leave of each person that is dear to us, and to say to them, before we go, "God be with you" (goodbye), and "Fare well".

As our lives end we all have different beliefs, hopes, and expectations as to what, if anything, lies ahead.

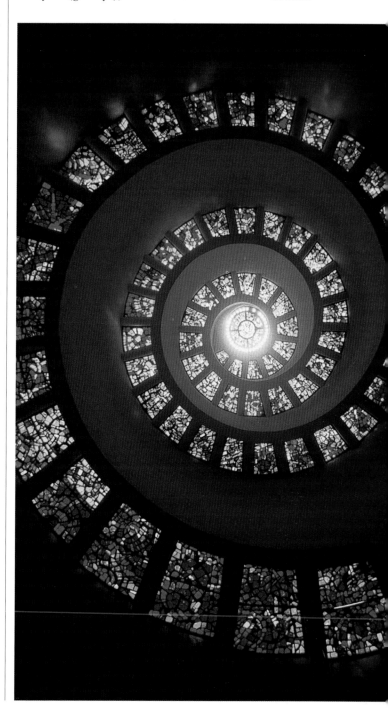

121

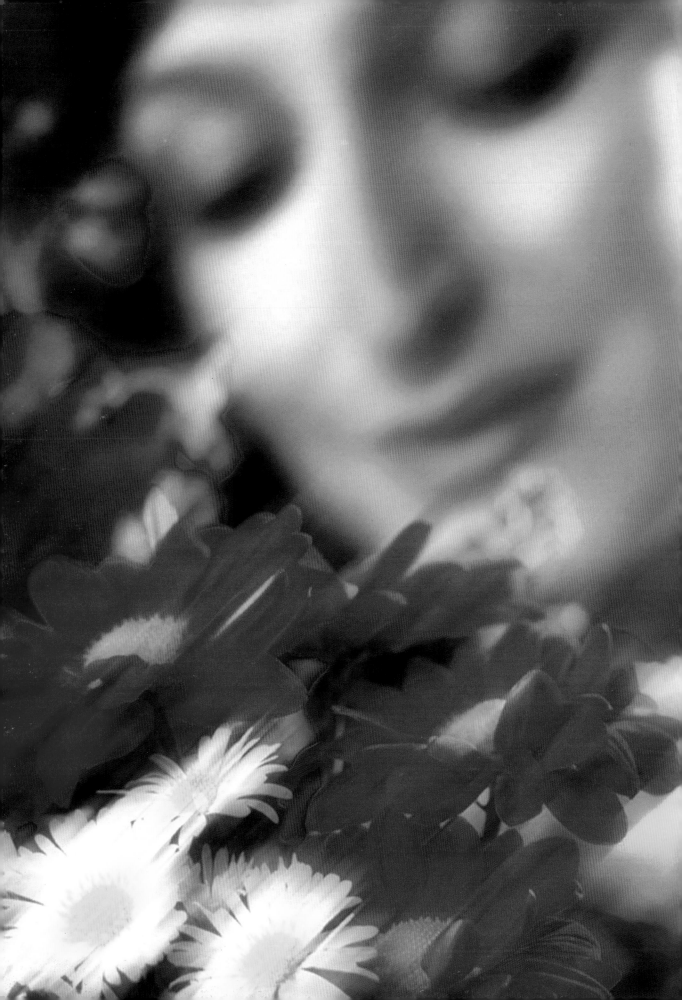

PART 3

Complementary Therapies and Remedies

INTEGRATED MEDICINE

The new hope for health care is that more and more people will benefit not only from the best of tried-and-tested modern medicine, but also from those traditional remedies and therapies, and new healing approaches, that can be used either in combination with modern medicine, or alone. This marriage of orthodox and complementary medicine is called integrated medicine. And it's already extremely popular in much of Europe and, increasingly, in the USA and other countries too.

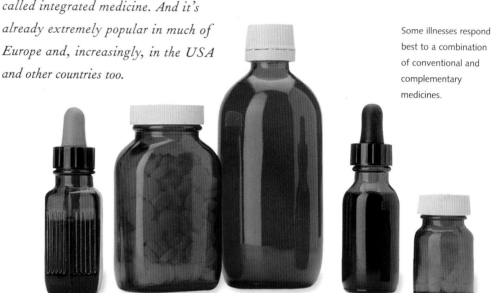

Some illnesses respond best to a combination of conventional and complementary medicines.

ORTHODOX AND COMPLEMENTARY MEDICINE

The sort of medical help and health care known as "orthodox medicine" has become ever more oriented toward pharmaceutical drugs and surgery. However, this approach has major drawbacks. It often doesn't work, it's usually expensive, and certain treatments have considerable side effects. In addition, many medical studies reveal that a meaningful proportion of all healing results simply from a person's belief that she is going to get well, and from trusting the professional who provides her health care.

Few complementary methods have undergone rigorous research to see whether they work. However, they are cheaper than orthodox medicine. They tend to be much less invasive. They are often much more pleasant to use. And most have far fewer, if any, side effects. All this is important, because the majority of common ailments are self-limiting: you will find that they eventually get better on their own.

MAKING THEM WORK TOGETHER

Clearly the ideal is to use the best of both systems, when necessary but this requires communication and cooperation between all concerned.

◆ *From your point of view* – you need to know when to get orthodox medical help. You also need to tell both your doctor and any other therapist about any drugs or remedies you are taking, and any treatment you are having.

◆ *From the doctor's point of view* – a doctor has a duty to care for her patients and she wants you to have the best possible help. She needs to know what other health-care methods you are using in case any might conflict with her treatment. If necessary, and if she is familiar with a particular complementary remedy or therapy, she can advise you about its suitability.

◆ *From the other practitioner's point of view* – some therapists, for example, medical herbalists and homeopaths, prefer to know about a person's drug treatment, if any, before prescribing their own remedies.

WHERE ALTERNATIVE MEDICINE FITS IN

Several types of alternative medicine, including ayurveda (traditional Indian medicine), homeopathy, herbal medicine, and acupuncture, are sometimes used as systems of healing that are complete in themselves. However, most practitioners and patients are happy to add or substitute orthodox medical diagnosis and treatment if extra help becomes desirable.

WHEN TO SELF-TREAT

It's human nature to find ways of looking after your own health and that of your family. Most of the time we instinctively know when it's wise and safe to treat a problem ourselves – which for most of us is the vast majority of the time.

One advantage of treating yourself is that you can easily do it as soon as you notice anything wrong. Our state of health and wellbeing varies from hour to hour, let alone from day to day, week to week, or month to month. If we are alert to our bodies and our feelings, we can start using simple lifestyle measures and home therapies or remedies as soon as anything goes wrong. This way we can often provide help before things get worse, or we may be able to lessen the severity or the duration of many of our common illnesses.

This way of looking after ourselves on a daily basis and in a sensitive and subtle way is very different from the "don't do anything until it's really bad, then hit it with a sledgehammer" approach to health care.

Self-help is more about staying well than treating illness. Some alternative health practitioners (such as homeopaths, and traditional Chinese medicine and ayurveda practitioners) welcome the opportunity to help people stay well rather than to treat them only when they are ill. Of course, treating yourself at home whenever possible is easier and cheaper than visiting a practitioner although it may take a little more thought and planning.

CHOOSING THERAPIES AND REMEDIES FOR HOME USE

A huge variety of remedies and other treatments is suitable for home use. Newly independent young people tend to go for approaches that are familiar because they were used as they grew up at home. But whatever your age and stage in life it's good to experiment so as to discover ways of looking after yourself in health and illness that suit you best.

The methods you choose will probably vary as time goes by, and as your needs and preferences change. Some, for example, sitz baths (*see page 130*), require more time than others, which might not suit someone going through a particularly busy patch. Others, such as a back massage (*see page 132*), require someone else to become involved, which could be a problem if you live on your own.

When using orthodox, complementary, and alternative therapies and remedies to help you stay well or to treat yourself, the choice lies between using one, or some combination of them all. Several elements of treatment, such as the healing power of good food, exercise, and relaxation, are common to all three.

Left: Therapies will only be effective if you combine them with a healthy diet.

Massage in its various forms is a complementary remedy that has never gone out of favor in recent years for treating stress and physical ailments.

WHEN TO SEE A HEALTH PRACTITIONER

Sometimes it's obvious when you need to see a doctor or other health practitioner. But if things aren't clear-cut and you're finding it difficult to decide, it's better not to take risks. Discuss the problem with your doctor on the phone, if possible, to see if you need to make an appointment (or even, in an emergency, to have a home visit, call an ambulance, or go straight to hospital). Alternatively, simply arrange for an appointment to get some advice.

There are certain times when it's always worth seeking help from your doctor.

WARNING SIGNS AND SYMPTOMS

Certain problems are best seen by a doctor even though you may subsequently use home treatment in conjunction with the recommended medical therapy, or, perhaps, visit a complementary or alternative health practitioner.

Don't hesitate to ask for advice if you are worried about a health problem.

SEE YOUR DOCTOR WHEN YOU HAVE:

◆ A new problem that doesn't respond to home treatment within two weeks or so.

◆ A new problem that's worrying because it's unfamiliar.

◆ A serious or worsening problem.

◆ An unexpected adverse reaction to treatment.

Other reasons for visiting your doctor include having screening procedures or routine health checks, such as vaccination, Pap (cervical) smears (*see page 72*), and regular antenatal check-ups (*see page 74*).

PHYSICAL WARNING SIGNS AND SYMPTOMS:

SKIN CHANGES
◆ Unexplained rash.
◆ Any rash in pregnancy.
◆ Yellowing of eyes or skin.
◆ Bluish fingertips or lips even when you aren't cold.
◆ Unusual and persistent reddening of the face.
◆ Ulcer or other sore on skin, in mouth, or on vulva for more than three weeks.
◆ Mole or freckle that grows, ulcerates, itches, develops irregular border, bleeds, or changes color.

GYNECOLOGICAL CHANGES
◆ Unusual lump in the breast.
◆ Bloodstained or other discharge from the breast.
◆ Unexplained vaginal bleeding between periods.
◆ Increased vaginal discharge.
◆ Unfamiliar pain during intercourse.

DIGESTIVE CHANGES
◆ Unexplained difficulty in swallowing.
◆ Unexplained indigestion continuing for more than two weeks or for the first time after 50.
◆ Persistent vomiting; seek help if a baby vomits for more than a few hours; older child for more than half a day; or adult for more than a day.
◆ Severe, unexplained, or continuous abdominal pain.
◆ Unusual diarrhea or constipation over two weeks.
◆ Red or black blood in the feces.

EYESIGHT CHANGES
◆ Halo around lights at night.
◆ Seeing double.
◆ Unexpectedly blurred vision.
◆ Pain in the eye.
◆ Red eye.

OTHER CHANGES
◆ Unexplained weight loss.
◆ Unexplained hoarseness for more than two weeks.
◆ Continuing cough.
◆ Unexpected shortness of breath.
◆ Chest pain or pain down the left arm.
◆ Persistent or repeated headaches, or worsening severe headache other than a usual migraine.
◆ Persistent, high, or unexplained fever.
◆ Unusual thirst in spite of drinking normally.
◆ Passing urine too frequently; and painful urination.
◆ Repeated fainting or dizziness.
◆ Unusual tiredness or weakness for over a week.

WHEN TO SEE
ANOTHER PRACTITIONER

People choose to visit health practitioners other than doctors for many reasons. One is that they want to try therapies that aren't based on drugs, surgery, or other invasive treatment (*see page 124*). Another is that they want a more holistic approach in which they are each seen as a whole person with a lifestyle that may need adjusting to aid healing, not just as someone with an illness which needs treating independently.

However, you don't have to opt for either medical treatment or something else. Increasing numbers of us now choose a combination of professional practitioners to look after our health. There's an interesting and growing tendency for people who are unwell to visit their doctors for medical diagnosis so they know what they're dealing with, and for suggestions about treatment, then to seek opinions about treatment from complementary health practitioners as well. Complementary treatments often work well alongside medical ones, though it's worth being sure that both practitioners know if drugs, food supplements, or herbal or homeopathic remedies are involved.

ASSESSING DOCTORS
AND OTHER PRACTITIONERS

It's essential to have confidence and trust in your doctor or alternative health-care practitioner. But another growing trend is the desire to see one whom you like, feel you can discuss your health with in a relaxed way, and can deal with as one human being to another on an equal footing.

It's important to see someone who's prepared to work with you, rather than simply tell you what to do (unless you prefer the authoritarian approach, which some of us do). So ask around about what sort of a person the practitioner is. Clearly it's also vital that he or she is well trained.

All doctors have a high level of training; some have postgraduate or specialist training too; and continued in-service training and updates are usual. Complementary and alternative practitioners are a different matter. Some are highly trained, perhaps even with a background in medicine as well as their complementary or alternative area. But because anyone can set up as any sort of complementary practitioner without training, you need to check, because there are some frauds around. Don't be embarrassed to ask the receptionist or practice manager – or, if necessary, the practitioner directly – about qualifications, length of training, and accreditation with a professional body. Your health deserves no less.

WHICH THERAPY TO CHOOSE

Familiarize yourself with a choice of therapies and remedies to use at home so you can use one that's appropriate for your symptoms and circumstances. One way of making your choice is to read the outlines of the 16 types of therapy on *pages 128–143* and see what appeals. As you use them, you'll soon learn what you like and what you don't – as well as what's likely to work for you.

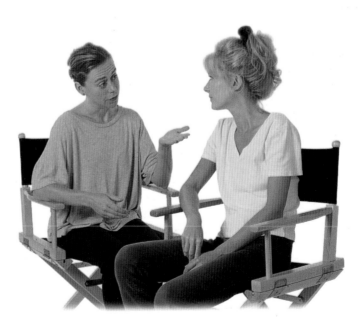

Have a full consultation with a doctor or complementary therapist before beginning any course of treatment. Mention any concerns you have and reassure yourself that your symptoms are being fully and properly interpreted.

NUTRITIONAL THERAPY

Enhancing your health, resistance to disease, and speed of recovery by altering what, when, and how you eat is an ancient therapy. Animals do it instinctively and to some extent humans do too. The most important part is adjusting the balance of the nutrients in your diet. This means eating more of certain foods, less of others, and, perhaps, adding new ones and totally avoiding others. The size of a meal is important, as is how quickly you eat, how well you chew, and the level of your stress while you are eating. The type, volume, and timing of drinks can also play an important part.

A secondary part of nutritional therapy involves taking food supplements, or aids to digestion such as digestive enzymes or acid. While food normally provides all the nutrients a person who is healthy needs, there may be situations – such as during illness or stress, or if you're a smoker, drink a lot of alcohol, or are elderly – when nutrients aren't properly absorbed or used. And at certain times, such as during pregnancy, or if you exercise a lot, you may have a raised requirement that is difficult to meet from your diet. Also, some foods aren't as nutritious nowadays; modern farming methods, for example, mean that wheat now contains much less selenium. So a good quality supplement is sometimes advisable even if you are eating well.

Stir-frying cooks food quickly, with the minimum loss of flavor and nutrients.

IDEAS TO TRY

Get the most nutrients from your food by:
◆ Choosing the freshest of the vegetables and fruits available. Shop in places with a rapid turnover; where possible go for seasonal produce; and be warned that supermarkets may store items such as apples for many months.
◆ Storing food carefully at home and aiming for a rapid turnover. Lettuce, for example, can lose a quarter of its beta carotene and vitamin C during several days in the refrigerator. And spinach kept at room temperature loses half of its vitamin C in three days.
◆ Choosing fresh vegetables and fruits when possible, rather than preserved (canned, dried, bottled, or frozen) ones. Although careful preserving retains high proportions of most nutrients, fruits and vegetables are more nutritious when fresh. They are often best if grown organically, without artificial pesticides.
◆ Cooking for only as long as necessary. Boiling vegetables, for example, reduces their content of the water-soluble vitamins B and C; and frying at high temperatures lowers the amount of essential fatty acids in foods of animal and vegetable origin.
◆ Chewing well, taking time over meals and minimizing stress at mealtimes.

When choosing a food supplement remember:
◆ A multivitamin and mineral product is often best because many nutrients work better in combination. An alternative is a multivitamin and mineral product formulated for a particular condition or stage of life. Sometimes it's wise to supplement individual nutrients too – *see Part 4.*
◆ Always take any supplement according to the packet instructions. Store in a dark, cool place, and use within its sell-by date.

Take a food supplement if you have good reason to believe a particular nutrient is missing from your diet.

LIGHT, COLOR, AND OTHER ELECTROMAGNETIC THERAPY

The following refers to the middle part of the electromagnetic (em) spectrum that includes visible light, ultraviolet, and infrared wavelengths.

One way of thinking about electromagnetic therapy is to envisage the various wavelengths of the em spectrum as being akin to the nutrients in food. Just as we need a particular amount of each nutrient to keep us healthy, so too do we need a particular amount of each em wavelength. And just as we may need more (or less) of certain nutrients when ill, so too may we need more (or less) of certain wavelengths. Another similarity is that just as we may sometimes need more food in general, so too may we sometimes need more exposure to radiation from the whole spectrum.

Another aspect of em therapy is the use – or avoidance – of em fields (emfs). The earth has an emf, but there are also those from simple magnets, as well as from power lines, transmitters, and domestic and other electrical appliances.

◆ Put a colored gel (acetate sheet) safely in front of a light source in order to provide a wash of colored light.
◆ Install a brighter bulb or tube to receive more intense light.
◆ Buy one of the "light boxes" – units containing several fluorescent tubes – specially made for treating SAD (*see page 202*).

Other color in your environment
◆ Choose colors of wallpaint, soft furnishings, and clothing to meet your requirements.
◆ Consider drinking water that you've put in a colored glass container and left in the sun. Some alternative practitioners believe that the water is somehow altered by exposure to particular wavelengths; they describe it as being "solarized," and suggest that there are certain health benefits to be gained from this.

Effective light therapy using warm, red light.

IDEAS TO TRY (*See also page 18*)
Daylight
◆ By going outside each day you expose your eyes and skin to the sun's colored rays, as well as its infrared and ultraviolet (UV) ones. You also benefit from the intensity of the light passing into your eyes and stimulating your hypothalamus and pineal gland. Ordinary window glass does not filter our much UV radiation. Many of us spend a lot of time indoors and may not get enough bright light, or light of certain wavelengths, even if we have big windows and good electric lighting. Some plants thrive only in a greenhouse made of "horticultural glass" – glass that allows a better balance of light through. Humans too need a good light balance, so time spent outdoors is really important (as long as you don't burn).

Electric light
◆ Buy a "daylight" or "full spectrum" bulb or tube for a good color balance.
◆ Buy a "warm" (relatively red) or "cool" (relatively blue) bulb or tube if you need more radiation from one or the other end of the visible part of the em spectrum.

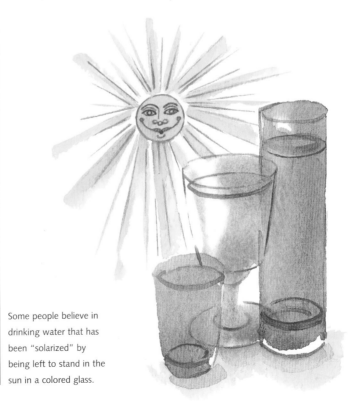

Some people believe in drinking water that has been "solarized" by being left to stand in the sun in a colored glass.

129

HYDROTHERAPY

The use of water to cure ailments or boost recovery is a very ancient therapy. Given that 80% of the body is water, we need to drink enough to keep well hydrated. The amount we need depends on our size, health, and activity level, as well as the ambient temperature and flow of air. Sometimes water makes us feel good simply because it looks lovely. The power of the sea, for example, or the beauty of a stream, waterfall, or rainbow – even dewdrops on a sparkling spider's web – can fill us with awe.

We can also benefit from being cooled or warmed by baths, showers, swims, jacuzzis, foot baths, sitz baths (*see left*), or compresses. Our bodies can be stimulated by jets, sprays, or waves. We can inhale hot steam from bowls, in steam rooms or saunas, or when in hot baths. And we can enjoy the feeling of water on our skin when bathing, showering, or swimming.

Water can hold substances that heal the skin, such as mineral salts, oatmeal, essential oils, and herbal extracts. It can carry nutrients such as spring water minerals, or added nutrients. And it's even possible that its healing potential may be enhanced by certain wavelengths of light (*see page 129*).

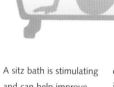

A sitz bath is stimulating and can help improve circulation.

IDEAS TO TRY

◆ Make a compress by folding a piece of cotton material (such as a tea towel), immersing it in hot or cold water, and squeezing out the excess. Lay it on the body part to be treated, cover with a towel to keep the heat in, and secure with a bandage.

◆ Have a steam inhalation or a steam face-sauna: fill a pint bowl three-quarters full with boiling water; add herbal extracts or essential oils if desired; lean over the bowl with a towel over your head and the bowl, and let the steam do its good work for ten minutes.

◆ Take a sitz bath. Put a container such as a baby bath, or any plastic basin or storage box that is large enough to sit in, at one end of the bathtub, and then fill with water. Fill the bathtub with water, leaving plenty of space below the container's brim. Sit in the bathtub with your feet in the container. For a *hot sitz bath*, use comfortably hot bathwater and cold container-water; continue for two minutes the first time, and up to ten minutes as you become used to it. For a *tepid sitz bath*, use tepid bathwater and cold container-water; continue for ten minutes. For a *cold sitz bath*, use cold bathwater and tepid-to-hot container-water. Continue for five minutes or as long as comfortable. For a *contrast sitz bath*, have a hot sitz bath for two minutes, then turn around so you sit in the basin with your feet in the bath for two minutes. Repeat twice.

Warnings: Take care not to slip. Avoid hot baths, and hot sitz baths, if you are suffering from high blood pressure or if you are pregnant.

A steam inhalation will help relieve congestion. You can also add essential oils or herb extracts to the water.

HEAT AND COLD THERAPY

We often instinctively use heat or cold to make ourselves feel better or to comfort pain. We benefit from warming ourselves if we feel too cold, or cooling ourselves if we feel too hot. And we enjoy the simple delight of basking in the warmth of a sunny day, or breathing the cold crisp air of a winter's day.

In general, heat tends to be relaxing, and cold stimulating. We can take advantage of these properties in many ways. For example, every day we use heat and cold by having hot or cold food and drinks. Another use is hydrotherapy – the various forms of hot, tepid, or cold water treatment (*see page 130*). We can warm our bodies by taking exercise; exposing ourselves to direct heat from the sun or heaters; breathing warmed air and wrapping up well with clothing and other covers. And we can cool down by keeping relatively inactive; exposing ourselves to cooler, breezy, or otherwise moving air; using fans or air conditioning; or taking off some layers of clothing.

Certain items of clothing are particularly valuable, yet they are often forgotten, if you need to keep warm. One is a hat – because a relatively large proportion of body heat can escape from, for example, a bare head in cold weather, or in a cold room when in bed at night. Others are scarves and wrist warmers. Warmth trapped within a scarf around the mouth and nose will warm cold inhaled air, and reduce the risk of cold-sensitive asthma.

Additional forms of heat include infrared radiation from a lamp. This is said to be particularly penetrating and good for many muscle problems. We can also benefit from specially shaped electric heating pads, electric blankets, hot-water bottles and microwaveable hot packs or glove warmers. Another type of glove warmer or hot pack is a small plastic container of liquid which crystallizes when pressed, and which releases heat that remains for some time. Breathing warm air can be beneficial for certain respiratory disorders, but the benefits vary according to whether the air is moist or dry.

The use of a homemade or commercially produced ice pack is an additional form of cold therapy.

IDEAS TO TRY

Be ready to treat ailments, or to help yourself relax or wake up, by having the following ready:

◆ Ice cubes. Make an ice pack by putting some cubes into a plastic bag, well tied so it can't leak, and wrapping it in a towel so it can't burn the skin. Alternatively, always keep a spare packet of peas in the freezer ready for use as a cold pack.

◆ A hot-water bottle – or microwaveable equivalent.

◆ Cold weather clothes, including hats, scarves, gloves, and boots.

◆ Extra blankets or other covers.

◆ Alternative heaters in case of power cuts.

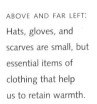

ABOVE AND FAR LEFT: Hats, gloves, and scarves are small, but essential items of clothing that help us to retain warmth.

ABOVE CENTER: Keep the freezer stocked with plenty of ice cubes so you can make a cold pack when required.

LEFT: As well as keeping you warm, a hot-water bottle can help relieve period pain.

A large scarf wrapped around mouth and nose will warm any bitterly cold air before you inhale it.

131

MASSAGE

Massage is the art of stroking, rubbing, kneading, or touching the body in other repeated ways with the hands. It encourages relaxation, stimulates the circulation of blood and lymph, and makes muscles more supple. Massage is an age-old art, and something we do instinctively – perhaps when we want to ease someone's pain, comfort someone in distress, or show affection. The touching involved isn't just a way of releasing physical aches and pains; it is also a way of showing concern, love, and support which can be far more effective than words.

Experiment with different massage oils to discover which you find most beneficial.

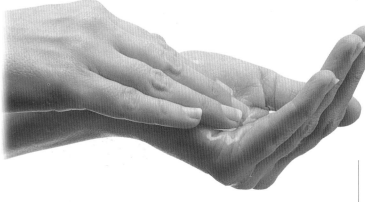

When a muscle feels tense, its fibers are in spasm and can't relax. This leads to an accumulation of waste substances which makes the muscle hurt. Massage encourages the contracted fibers to relax by lengthening them, increasing their blood supply (which helps remove the accumulated substances), and heating them up, both by increasing their circulation and simply by the physical friction of the hands as they move on the skin.

BELOW: Touching shows love and support, and massage soothes tension and relieves pain.

If an area is painful, two possible causes may respond to massage. These are muscle tension (*see above*) and injury. Gentle massage (not on broken skin) can reduce pain by sending touch signals to the spinal cord; these prevent pain messages from getting through. This technique can also ease labor pains (*see page 84*).

If tissue fluid accumulates in an area and causes swelling, a combination of exercise, elevation of the part, and massage can often help disperse it.

You can easily massage many parts of yourself, but for difficult-to-reach areas, or to promote relaxation, ask someone else to do it for you.

IDEAS TO TRY

◆ It's possible to learn special massage techniques from a teacher, a video, or a book, but it's often best to do what comes naturally, and if you're massaging someone else, to remain alert to the reaction of the person you're massaging.

◆ Before you start, check that the room and your hands are warm. Have a large towel available to cover any exposed skin.

◆ Lubricate your palms with oil. You can use any oil, such as baby oil, but diluted essential oils are best. Certain oils smell better than others; they may also have special properties (such as encouraging relaxation), or be more effective lubricants (*see page 133*).

◆ Get comfortable and relax as much as possible. Some people like music.

◆ When massaging someone, always keep one hand on him or her, even when adjusting the towel or getting more oil. This makes the person feel safe and cared for.

◆ Start by smoothing the area gently, with long strokes, one hand at a time, or one hand after the other. Then gradually work up to more vigorous movements, such as deeper stroking, kneading, and even patting. Finish with long, gentle, slow strokes again. Afterward the person you've massaged may want to sleep, or just be quiet.

AROMATHERAPY

Aromatherapy uses oils extracted from plants — their "essential oils" – to lift the spirits, promote relaxation or stimulation, or heal illness. The combination of naturally occurring chemicals in each essential oil accounts for its particular smell and effects on the mind and body.

We can access an oil's healing qualities in several ways. One is by inhaling its aroma. Aromatic molecules waft into the nose and stimulate tiny nerve endings that feed messages to the brain. This encourages relaxation or stimulation. Some molecules also pass through the lining of the nose and other breathing passages into the bloodstream, to exert healing effects around the body.

Molecules from an oil can also enter the body through the skin, for example, during a massage; however, the effects of inhalation are more pronounced than those of passage through the skin.

IDEAS TO TRY

◆ Choose a few oils for home use. Some good ones to start with are lavender, ylang ylang, geranium, neroli, cypress, rosemary, and tea tree. Other useful ones include bergamot, clary sage, cardamom, frankincense, juniper berry, petitgrain, rose, grapefruit, bay, and eucalyptus.
◆ Buy a "base" oil with which to dilute your essential oils. Sweet almond oil smells pleasant and lubricates well during massage; alternatives include apricot-kernel, grapeseed, jojoba, macadamia nut, peach-kernel, and wheatgerm oils.

◆ For massage: add 3–5 drops of your chosen essential oil to two teaspoons of base oil.
◆ For the bath: run the water, then add up to 15 drops of the essential oil, or one teaspoon of blended massage oil (*see above*). If you mix this oil with a teaspoon of moisturizing cream, it'll disperse well in the water.
◆ For a compress (*see also page 130*): shake 1–2 drops of the chosen essential oil into the water; agitate gently; lay the cloth flat on the water to absorb the oil film; let excess water drip away; then place the compress, oily side down, on the area to be treated.
◆ For an oil burner: add up to 5 drops of your chosen essential oil to the water in the container, and light the night-light.
◆ For perfume: use some massage blend (*see above*) on the pulse points of your wrists, temples, and throat.
◆ For a steam inhalation (*see also page 130*): add 3–5 drops of the essential oil to the water in the bowl.
◆ For easier night breathing (*see page 168*): put 2 drops of the essential oil on a tissue and tuck this by your pillow.

Warnings: In pregnancy, choose only from lavender, citrus (neroli, bergamot, grapefruit, petitgrain, orange, lime), frankincense, and ylang ylang oils. Dilute all oils except tea tree and lavender.

Lavender is renowned for its relaxing aroma that comes either from its dried flower heads or from the oils extracted from them.

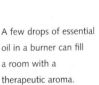

A few drops of essential oil in a burner can fill a room with a therapeutic aroma.

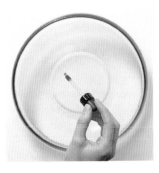

To make a healing compress add a few drops of your chosen oil to a bowl of warm water.

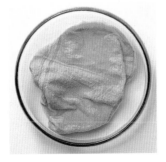

Place a washcloth on the water so it absorbs the film of oil on the surface.

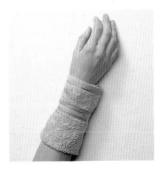

Let the excess water drip away then place the oily side of the compress on the area to be treated.

ACUPRESSURE

This therapy has a long history of use in traditional Chinese medicine and, while closely allied to acupuncture, involves using thumb or fingertip pressure instead of needles. The theory is based on the ancient proposition that energy (chi – pronounced "chee") flows up and down the body along channels called meridians. There are said to be 12 major meridians, each named after a particular organ, plus two others.

The flow of energy is sometimes blocked, overactive, or weak. However, stimulation of various points on the skin overlying the meridians is believed to encourage its normal circulation. These points are called acupuncture points – or acupoints.

Acupoints are thought to be "gateways" for influencing the level of energy in the meridians. Stimulation of acupoints

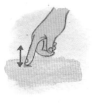

If the energy flow is blocked, use an up-and-down pumping motion on the acupoint.

Another technique for removing an energy blockage involves making continuous circular movements on the acupoint, without losing contact with the skin.

If the energy flow is weak, apply stationary pressure to "tonify" the energy.

CENTER, ABOVE AND BELOW: According to traditional Chinese medicine, the body contains meridians, or channels through which energy flows. When these energy channels become

can be done with long fine needles that pierce the skin (acupuncture); an electric current ("electro-acupuncture"); a laser beam or magnet; a heat source (such as burning herbs – a method known as moxibustion); or – as with acupressure – fingertips. Scientific research has found that acupoints have a lower electrical resistance than surrounding skin, which suggests that acupoint stimulation for health problems may have a sound scientific basis.

It's interesting that many acupoints correspond with what doctors now call myofascial trigger points (and used to call fibrositic nodules) – tender places in muscles, fascia or tendons which sometimes feel like tight bands or knots. Stimulating these trigger points by massaging, heating, chilling, stretching, using a counter-irritant

(such as a liniment), stimulating electrically, or inserting a needle can sometimes relieve both local tenderness and radiating pain.

You can do acupressure on yourself, or have someone else do it on you. Experts say the latter is more effective. Most important is to let yourself relax when you have acupressure. It doesn't matter whether it's done on bare skin or through a layer of light clothing.

Acupressure is easy and safe; only occasionally is the treatment of a certain point best avoided; when necessary this is discussed under individual entries in Part 4. For acupressure to treat pregnancy sickness, *see page 80.*

IDEAS TO TRY

Learn the three basic ways of doing acupressure, so you can work on the acupoints recommended in Part 4.

blocked or the flow is weak, it affects our health and wellbeing. Acupressure uses ancient techniques to help remove blockages and promote good energy flow throughout the body.

◆ If the energy flow may be weak, stationary pressure is believed to increase it. This is called "tonifying" the energy. Do this by pressing vertically down with the tip of your thumb or finger for two minutes, and imagining the acupoint as a funnel that is filling up with energy.

◆ If the energy flow may be blocked, release it with one of two types of finger pressure for two minutes. The first is an up-and-down pumping pressure with thumb or fingertip on the point, never losing contact. The other consists of continuous little circular movements, again made without losing contact.

◆ If the energy flow may be overactive, calm it by gently stroking over the point with your palm.

THE ALEXANDER TECHNIQUE

Australian actor Frederick Matthias Alexander became interested in the phenomenon of muscle tension after losing his voice on stage. He discovered that certain movements and postures lead to unnecessary muscle tension, and that this tension can play havoc with our health. Using his insights and the skills he learned for himself, Alexander went on to teach others how to relax and eliminate their excess tension. His useful methods, known as the Alexander technique, are now taught and practiced around the world.

Of course, our muscles normally tighten and relax as we go about our daily lives, but if our posture and coordination are poor, the muscles tighten more than necessary. This state of affairs – from habits such as slumping when sitting, walking with a bent back and throwing our legs out sideways when running – can begin all too easily, without us realizing what is going on. These habits feel natural because we're used to them, but the associated muscle tension saps energy and vitality, tends to make breathing shallow, and can even alter the voice. As the years pass, overworked muscles stiffen and ache and it becomes more difficult to relax. And continued tension can gradually throw certain joints out of alignment. Not surprisingly, all this sometimes leads to depression, anxiety, and bad temper, as well as to accidents and illness. Headaches, backache, stress, and exhaustion are common problems that are often caused by muscle tension. And taut, tense, tight muscles can also

contribute to high blood pressure, indigestion, and many other common illnesses too.

The Alexander technique re-educates the body with a variety of exercises, maneuvers, and tips. Many people, for example, benefit from learning to walk the Alexander way, concentrating on lengthening their spines by moving, forward and upward from a point on the top of the head, and not rolling their shoulders or tilting the pelvis. These small changes can make walking so smooth that you almost feel you're floating.

Various Alexander tips can help streamline everyday movements like getting in and out of a car, using a vacuum cleaner, and bending over a wash basin. Even something as seemingly simple as sitting on and rising from a chair becomes more graceful when done the Alexander way.

IDEAS TO TRY

For maximum benefit, incorporate the Alexander technique into the way you habitually move your body. Alternatively, if you are less than well, you may find some of the tips mentioned under certain entries in Part 4 particularly useful.

◆ Buy a book on the Alexander technique and practice its tips for streamlining common movements every day; alternatively, have lessons from an Alexander teacher.

Learning to walk the Alexander way involves moving forward and upward, keeping the spine lengthened without shoulders rolling forward.

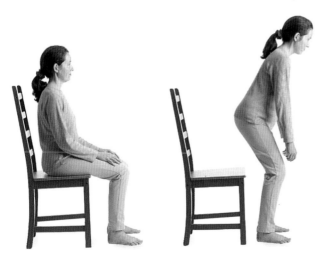

The Alexander technique teaches us to put less strain on our bodies while performing simple maneuvers such as getting up from a chair. Here, the pupil is encouraged to bend her knees and lengthen her back as she gets up.

135

EXERCISE THERAPY

Exercise therapy comes in many forms. The most familiar is the basic program of aerobic, strengthening, and stretching exercises (*see pages 28–31*). This is something every healthy person, able-bodied or disabled, should do on at least five days of the week. If you haven't been doing this, you may find it helps to ease any one of many of the common ailments outlined in Part 4. Always remember when starting an exercise program to exercise within your capabilities and to take all the safety precautions (*see pages 30–31*). Certain types of exercise are especially useful for particular conditions, some of which are dealt with in Part 4.

But apart from this basic exercise program, several others can be very useful. One of these is pelvic floor exercises. These strengthen the pelvic floor – the hammock of muscles which supports the womb, bladder, and urine passage. Having a strong pelvic floor helps prevent or treat problems such as incontinence or a prolapsed womb. It can also enhance a couple's enjoyment of sex. Another is a group of exercises for the eyes called Bates eye exercises; these can help prevent or treat short sight and other common eyesight disorders (*see below*). You can easily do pelvic floor and Bates exercises at home.

TO STRENGTHEN YOUR PELVIC MUSCLES:

◆ Check first that you can recognize them by squeezing to stop the flow of urine; do this for a few seconds until you've registered what it feels like, then let the urine go again.

◆ At least five times a day, sit or lie with your knees slightly apart, and tighten these muscles for two seconds, working up to ten seconds when they are fitter. Relax for the same time, then repeat the cycle up to ten times.

◆ Remember that you can do these exercises at almost any time without anyone knowing.

SOME BASIC BATES EYE EXERCISES:

◆ Screw your eyes up tightly several times a day and make sure you blink frequently.

◆ Splash or bathe your eyes twice a day with alternately warm, then cold, water.

◆ Rest your eyes by "palming" them every half-hour when you've been doing a lot of close work. Slightly cup your hands. Place your cupped palms over your closed eyes without touching them, and with your fingers lying on your forehead, tightly together so as to exclude the light. Check that your elbows are supported and you are relaxed. Continue for two minutes.

◆ For information about more advanced eye exercises, read a book or consult a Bates teacher.

1. Blink your eyes frequently to wash them and to prevent dryness.

2. Bathe your eyes in warm, then cold, water twice a day.

3. Refresh tired eyes when doing close work by palming them every 30 minutes.

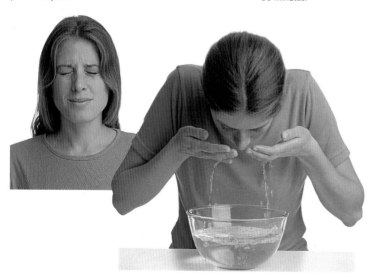

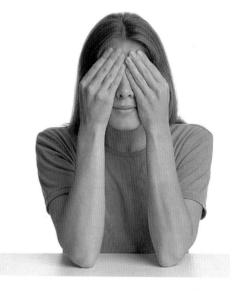

HERBAL REMEDIES

Herbal remedies contain extracts of healing substances. These are extracted either from whole plants, or from roots, stems, leaves, flowers, seeds, or bark.

To make a herb tincture (concentrated herb extract), ground up plant matter is steeped in a solvent of alcohol and water (or glycerine) for around two weeks. Then the alcohol, laden with the plant extract, is filtered off. One teaspoon of herb tincture has roughly the same strength as one strong cup of herbal tea.

Herbal teas are simpler to prepare (*see below*); a decoction is simply herbal tea made from hard roots or woody parts. Healing substances can be extracted from herbs by steeping plant matter in oil heated to 212°F (100°C) for up to three days (turning the heat off at night). Fresh or dried herbs can be used in poultices, eaten, or added to bath water.

When treating an illness, continue a herbal remedy until the symptoms go, or for two weeks, unless directed otherwise.

IDEAS TO TRY

◆ Grow medicinal herbs – such as feverfew, comfrey, stinging nettles, lemon balm, mint, and aloe vera – in the garden, in pots on a terrace or balcony, in a window box, or grow them indoors on the windowsill.

◆ Buy ready-made tinctures from a drugstore or health store. If you'd like to make your own, learn from a book on herbal medicine. If you need to use several herbs, you can mix tinctures together. The usual dose is a teaspoon of tincture in a little water two or three times a day, with or after meals for chronic conditions, or every two hours for an acute illness.

◆ Make tea from plants you have grown, or from store-bought herbal teabags. Put 2oz (60g) of fresh, or 1oz (30g) of dried, plant parts in a cup, fill with boiling water, cover, steep for ten minutes, then strain and drink the tea, sweetened with a little honey or brown sugar if you like. To make tea from hard roots (including carrots), bark, or seeds (a decoction), chop or crush the material; put the above amount in a pan, add two cups of water, simmer for 15 minutes, strain, and sweeten if desired.

◆ Make a poultice: finely chop half a handful of dried herbs, or crush a handful of fresh ones, then moisten with a little warm water. Lay out a strip of cotton gauze (enough to cover the area to be treated). Smooth the herbs over an area in the middle of the gauze, then lay an equal-sized piece of gauze on top. Lay the herb sandwich on the part, keep in place with a crêpe bandage secured with a safety pin, and place a hot-water bottle on top. Leave in place for several hours and repeat twice a day.

◆ Make a herbal oil: put a handful of the herb in a screw-top jar, cover with sweet almond oil, then screw on the lid. Leave the jar on a sunny windowsill and shake every day for two weeks. Strain the oil into a bowl through a muslin cloth and squeeze out the rest from the herbs in the cloth. Put the herbal oil into a dark bottle and keep it in the dark.

Peppermint leaves made into a tea aid digestion.

Feverfew tea can help relieve migraine.

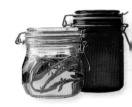

Herbal oils are useful for making compresses and for massage.

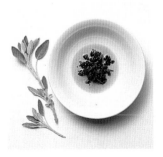

To make a poultice, moisten a small handful of chopped dried herbs or a handful of crushed fresh ones.

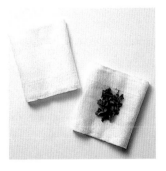

Make a herb "sandwich" with herbs between two strips of gauze.

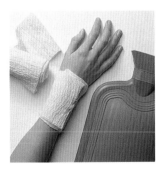

Hold the "sandwich" in place with a crêpe bandage, and place a hot-water bottle on top for several hours.

137

FLOWER ESSENCES

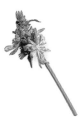

ABOVE: Chicory flower essence can help encourage independence.

RIGHT: Wild rose flower essence can be taken to treat depression.

Just seeing and smelling a beautiful flower can be a therapy in itself.

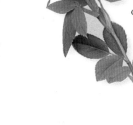

Flowers are among nature's most precious gifts and can be used as healing remedies in many ways. Flowers can be beautiful, startling, or even funny. Their scent usually allures, sometimes repels. Their colors span the rainbow. And not for nothing is Paradise depicted as a garden: flowers can be balm for the soul, healing for the heart and mind, and soothing or stimulating for many ailments.

Simply seeing, feeling, or smelling flowers can be enchanting. This, in time, relaxes you, allowing muscle tension to ease away. Since tension and anxiety underlie many mental and physical disorders, including high blood pressure, depression, heart disease, and cancer, it is easy to see the real benefits of flowers for healing.

The healing power of flowers can also be harnessed via their essential oils (*see Aromatherapy, page 133*) and via specially prepared tinctures (alcoholic extracts) called essences.

Flower essences are said to embody the healing power of blossoms. They include the well-loved Bach (pronounced "Batch") remedies. Edward Bach was a prominent doctor and homeopath. He lived in the UK in the 1930s and was particularly interested in people's moods and feelings. Using his powers of intuition and observation, he developed 38 floral extracts that he called flower remedies. These are made by two methods.

In the first, the blossoms are gathered at their peak, put in a glass bowl of spring water in the sun, left for three or four hours, then removed. The resulting liquid is preserved with 40% alcohol. This is called a mother tincture, and is diluted with water before use. In the second method, used for spring-flowering plants – mostly trees – the blossoms are simmered in water for 30 minutes, then removed and the liquid preserved as above.

Essences made from indigenous flowers are also available in the USA, Australia, and some other countries. These essences are available in health food stores and by mail order; some drugstores stock them too.

Because Bach devised a system of seven emotional groups split into 38 negative states of mind under which people could be classified before finding the right flower remedy, it is possible that one important way in which flower essences work is simply by providing us with the opportunity to recognize, name, and accept our emotions as we choose which essences to take.

IDEAS TO TRY

Benefit from flower essences by:
◆ Choosing one or more flower essences according to your predominant emotions or state of mind. For example, Aspen for fear; Holly for jealousy or anger; Larch for a lack of confidence; Honeysuckle and Star of Bethlehem for depression caused by sad or negative thoughts; Mustard and Wild Rose for depression for no obvious reason; and Olive for tiredness or stress.
◆ Putting two drops of your chosen essence in a glass of water and sipping throughout the day. Alternatively, put two drops each of up to seven essences in a 1fl oz (30ml) dropper bottle. Add one teaspoon of brandy or glycerine, and top up with spring water. The dose to take is four drops, four times a day.
◆ Buying combined flower essences formulated for particular conditions, rather than choosing individual essences according to your emotions.
◆ Stocking your first aid box with Rescue Remedy, a mixture of flower essences chosen to help with emotional upheaval.
◆ Finding out more from a book (*see page 218*).

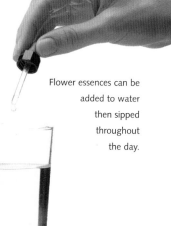

Flower essences can be added to water then sipped throughout the day.

HOMEOPATHY

This is a gentle system of medicine that aims to boost the body's natural healing power. The word comes from the Greek *homos* (same) and *pathos* (suffering). Homeopathy uses traces of substances known to cause particular symptoms in a healthy person to heal similar symptoms in an ill one. The principle is that "like cures like," and history helps us understand it a little more.

Homeopathy was used in ancient Greece, and the philosophy of healing with the afflicting agent is mentioned in the ancient Jewish bible. Various physicians referred to curing with "similars" over the centuries, but most doctors continued to practice allopathic medicine (*allos*, other; *pathos*, suffering). This suppresses symptoms by fighting them with medicines once known as "contraries." It wasn't until the 18th century that homeopathy became more popular.

German doctor Samuel Christian Hahnemann gave up his practice because he didn't want to "incur the risk of doing injury." While translating a book on drugs, he felt unhappy with its explanation of the action of Peruvian bark, a source of quinine (a treatment for malaria). He decided to see what Peruvian bark would do to him. The results were astonishing. It caused the very symptoms it cured in malaria. He then recorded the symptoms caused by large numbers of substances in healthy people. Next, he used each as a remedy for people with symptoms identical to those the substance caused in a healthy person.

He soon realized that the more dilute a remedy, the greater its strength. The most potent contain no molecules of the original substance. Their efficacy is put down to being shaken ("succussed") each time they are diluted. It has been suggested that a remedy enables healing by increasing a person's electromagnetic field at the frequency needed (like a tuning fork makes another of identical frequency vibrate, creating resonance). Some physicists suggest that molecules in the liquid in which the substance is shaken may become electrochemically charged by this shaking, thus "remembering" the vibratory properties of the original substance.

Homeopathic remedies come as tiny round lactose (milk sugar) pills (pillules), granules, solutions, creams, and ointments. A "constitutional" remedy is chosen for an individual and stays the same for life. Other remedies are best chosen according to the precise nature and combination of a person's symptoms, which means there may be a choice of many possible ones for each common ailment. This said, using a remedy marketed as suitable for one particular ailment sometimes helps.

NOTES FOR USING HOMEOPATHIC REMEDIES

◆ Discover your constitutional remedy by reading a book on the subject (*see page 218*) or consulting a homeopath when you are well.

◆ Seek professional help for skin problems.

◆ Keep remedies away from light, heat, and smells, and try not to touch them.

◆ Remember that symptoms may worsen soon after taking a remedy. This may be a "healing crisis" that shows it's working. However, stop the remedy until the crisis subsides.

◆ If you'd like to use homeopathy, find out about treating common ailments from a book or a homeopath.

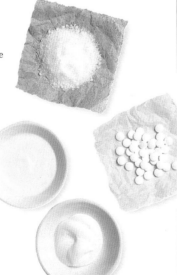

Homeopathic remedies are available as lactose pills, granules, solutions, creams, and ointments.

Try not to touch homeopathic pills before you take them. Dispense them into the lid of the bottle.

139

YOGA

BELOW: Relax in the corpse pose, focus on your breathing and picture energy flowing into your body.

RIGHT: The child pose is useful for resting between postures, when back muscles are tense.

RIGHT: Keep your hips on the floor when doing the cobra pose to relieve tension in a tight back.

FAR RIGHT: Tilt your pelvis before you arch your back in the cat pose.

Yoga began in the Orient more than 5,000 years ago and has gradually become popular in many other regions. Many people don't realize that yoga developed not just as a form of exercise and relaxation, but also as a way of recognizing and developing the spiritual part of a person's being. There are many types of yoga, but hatha yoga is the best known in the West. This consists of five ways of encouraging health and wellbeing: a series of postures (*asanas*), breathing exercises (*pranayama*), hand positions (*mudras*), locked muscle poses (*bandhas*) said to control the flow of energy, and meditational practices (*kriyas*) that promote relaxation and are said to encourage harmony of body, mind, and spirit. Indeed the word "yoga" is Sanskrit for union.

Yoga can benefit anyone, from the complete beginner to a yogi – someone who has spent years becoming adept at its disciplines. Practicing yoga helps many people relax and deal with stress more effectively. The exercises counteract muscle tension and are said to promote the free flow of energy – "*prana*" – roughly equivalent to *chi* (*see page 134*) in the body. Certain postures increase the blood flow to particular abdominal organs, such as the pancreas.

Regular yoga can ease a variety of health problems, including some cases of high blood pressure, sleep problems, depression, migraine, and back trouble. It can also encourage those types of brainwaves (theta waves) associated with creativity.

Because of its Hindu origins, some people of other religions avoid yoga (or at least some of the philosophical explanations offered by some teachers), while others adapt these to their own faith.

Many non-yoga exercise teachers include in their classes postures similar to if not identical with certain yoga postures. And it's perfectly possible to incorporate yoga postures into your daily exercise routine and to add the breathing exercises and meditation only if you wish.

Many postures have interesting names, for example, the:
◆ Corpse pose.
◆ Child pose (good for resting between postures and stretching back muscles).
◆ Cobra pose (useful for a stiff back and for period problems).
◆ Cat pose (useful to keep the back flexible and for stress relief).
◆ Salutation to the sun, a series of 12 postures that stretch and invigorate the whole body.

IDEAS TO TRY

(For breathing exercises, *see page 141*; for meditation, *page 142*.) You can incorporate yoga exercises into your daily life by:
◆ Learning an exercise routine from classes, or a book (*see page 218*).
◆ Using the corpse pose to help you relax when stressed. Lie on an exercise mat for five minutes. Rest your hands, palms up, by your sides, feet slightly apart, and close your eyes. Relax, imagining your smooth, rhythmical breaths bringing energy. Get up slowly.

RELAXATION EXERCISES

Promoting relaxation with breathing and muscle relaxation exercises encourages good health. These exercises are grouped together because a poor breathing technique (rapid, shallow breathing) often goes hand in hand with muscle tension.

Stress makes muscles tense. Besides encouraging rapid, shallow, irregular breathing, this is tiring and leads to aching from the accumulation in muscles of lactic acid and other waste substances. Tense muscles restrict the blood flow in neighboring arteries and veins, which can cause distant health problems by reducing the circulation in the organs and tissues supplied by these blood vessels.

People who breathe unnecessarily rapidly (hyperventilate) puff out so much carbon dioxide that their blood becomes too alkaline to release oxygen efficiently. Besides triggering muscle tension, this lack of oxygen in the tissues causes many other symptoms (*see page 13*). A Russian scientist, Professor Konstantin Buteyko, believes hyperventilating while resting encourages asthma by making airways oversensitive. A small Australian trial suggests that breathing in a slower, more controlled way can lead to some people with asthma being less dependent on their medication. (*Warning:* Don't reduce asthma medication without first discussing this with your doctor.)

IDEAS TO TRY

Benefit from breathing and relaxation exercises by:

◆ Learning to recognize your breathing style (*see page 12*).

◆ Practicing deep breathing when under pressure. Do this standing, sitting, or lying down. Put your hand on your stomach and take a slow, deep breath, making your hand rise a little. Exhale slowly, letting your hand subside. Take around six of these deep breaths, then breathe normally for a minute to reduce the chance of becoming dizzy. Repeat the cycle if necessary.

◆ Setting time aside each day to practice progressive muscular relaxation (*see page 33*).

◆ Doing a stress-relieving yoga exercise called alternate nostril breathing. It's interesting that at any one time we usually breathe through only one nostril anyway, and we unconsciously alternate the side we use. This exercise has five steps: 1) Sit comfortably and put your right index and middle fingers between your eyebrows; gently press your thumb on the right nostril (in yoga, the "dynamic" side); and lightly rest the tips of your ring and little fingers on the left one (the "passive" side). 2) Take a slow, deep breath through your left nostril and notice how this feels in your nose and head. 3) Now block your left nostril instead and breathe out slowly and completely through the right nostril, noticing how this feels. 4) Next, breathe in through your right nostril and repeat the cycle. 5) Repeat the cycle five times, always ending by breathing normally for at least a minute.

◆ Consider seeing a Buteyko teacher for guidelines on breathing if you think habitual hyperventilation may be contributing to your attacks of asthma.

Learn to recognize when your breathing is shallow. Practice deep breathing to calm yourself in stressful situations.

1. Breathe in slowly and deeply through your left nostril.

2. Breathe out through your right nostril. Repeat the cycle the other way.

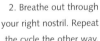

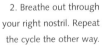

MEDITATION AND VISUALIZATION

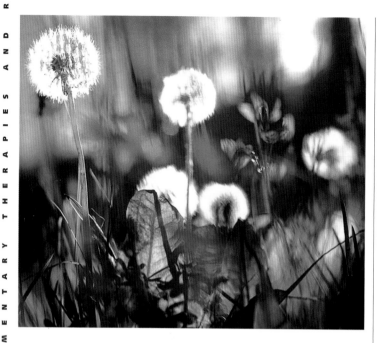

When meditating, try to picture a comfortable place, perhaps somewhere you have been happy, or a neutral site such as a peaceful summer meadow.

Meditation is a practice that encourages relaxation and refreshment of body, mind, and spirit. Regular meditation lowers blood pressure, enhances the circulation and immunity, relieves pain, and alleviates stress-related disorders (including headaches, sleep problems, asthma, and addiction). It reduces the heart and metabolic rates, and increases creativity by altering the brainwave pattern. Learning to be still also helps us to remember we needn't rush headlong into actions.

Various religions encourage meditation as an aid to spiritual development. Meditation plays a part in Christianity, Judaism, and Islam (*see page 48*), as well as yoga (*see page 140*), and Zen Buddhism. The origins of transcendental meditation (TM) are Buddhist, though simple TM can be done without reference to Buddhist philosophy (just as simple yoga exercises need have nothing to do with Hindu beliefs).

Visualization is a mental exercise in which a person imagines one of the following, for example:
◆ Being in a relaxing environment.
◆ Overcoming a challenge.
◆ Dealing with a difficult situation in a new and helpful way.
◆ Willing an increased flow of healing antibodies to a diseased body part.

IDEAS TO TRY

Consider:
◆ Meditating somewhere quiet, sitting with feet flat on the ground, closing your eyes, relaxing, and allowing your mind to clear. Some people focus on something beautiful, such as a flower, picture, view, swimming fish, candle flame, scent, sound, or story. Ignore worrying thoughts and focus on your breathing. Aim to meditate for 10–20 minutes once or twice a day.
◆ Visualizing by lying comfortably in a quiet place, relaxing, and imagining, for example, a barefoot walk through a peaceful garden at dawn, with dew on the grass, the birds singing, the warmth of the sun on your back, and the scent of the flowers.
◆ Consulting a stress counselor about visualization, a minister, or meditation teacher about meditation (some meditation courses have a religious content; if this is unacceptable, go elsewhere).

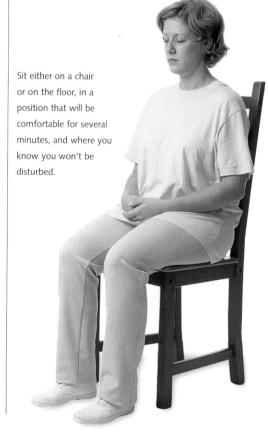

Sit either on a chair or on the floor, in a position that will be comfortable for several minutes, and where you know you won't be disturbed.

HEALING

Healing in its general sense helps a person become well in body, mind, and/or spirit. Doctors, nurses, ministers, counselors, and complementary therapists are professional healers, but parents, friends, lovers, and many others frequently offer healing with a variety of treatments, including medicines, massage, and good food, as well as with a listening ear and tender loving care. However, there is also a particular form of healing in which certain people – sometimes known as spiritual healers – encourage health and wellbeing by willing a so-called "healing power" to affect the person in question. Some healers do this by mental concentration, others by laying hands on the individual or placing their hands very close to them.

Healers are something of a mixed bunch. Some claim God's healing power works through them. Others believe they use an unidentified source of energy from a higher power, or believe in the healing potential of their own "mind energy". A few assert they are channels for healing power from the spirits of those who have died and "passed over to the other side". But whatever the supposed source of their power, does any of their so-called healing actually work?

A multitude of anecdotes suggests it may. Perhaps more important, nearly half of the many carefully controlled scientific studies of healing agree. And healing seems especially useful for long-term complaints for which orthodox medical therapy has few solutions.

Most people who receive healing are positive about its benefits; some describe experiencing a feeling of heat from the healer's hands and others a sensation of coldness or tingling. Many people being healed become deeply relaxed; this state may in itself alter their levels of stress hormones and immune factors enough to promote wellbeing. Mind over matter, perhaps, but no less valid for that. Many healers also report a sensation of heat in their hands. Their intense concentration often slows their brainwave patterns to that seen during meditation and contemplative prayer. And they may feel tired afterward and need to replenish their energy.

IDEAS TO TRY

You can ask for healing from another person, or try healing yourself. Suggestions include:

◆ Cupping your face or holding the sides of your head gently in your hands, then asking God – or a beneficent healing power, depending on your belief – to make you well. Alternatively, place your hand over the area requiring help. Relax, and be confident that healing will happen if the time is right and it is meant to be. Be aware that any healing you receive may not be in the form you expect. Some people, for example, find the healing they experience is a positive acceptance of the problems caused by their illnesses (rather than a negative and passive sense of resignation), together with feelings of contentment and peace.

Healing through touch is popular, but some healers just put their hands very close.

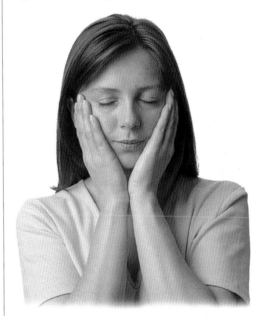

By focusing your mind on the healing you need, you may be able to alleviate your own symptoms.

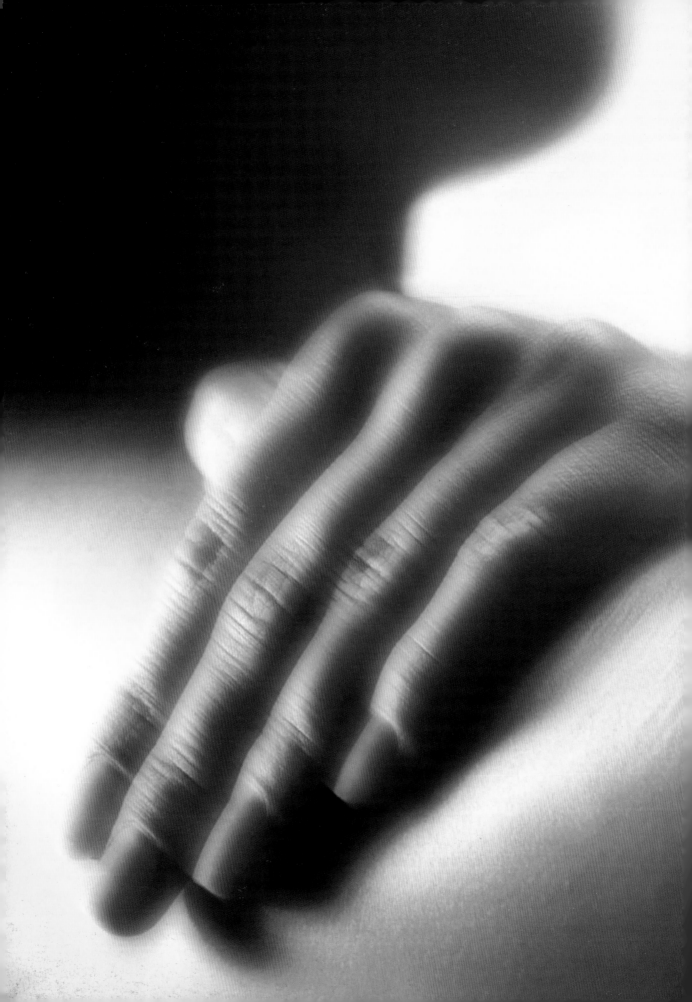

PART **4**

Common Ailments

BODY SYSTEMS AND CONNECTIONS

Good health depends not only on a well-functioning body, but also on the state of our mind and spirit. Staying well often means favoring the best possible health behaviors. We can readily treat most common ailments at home. By understanding how our body systems function we can see how they are interconnected and how they can be treated.

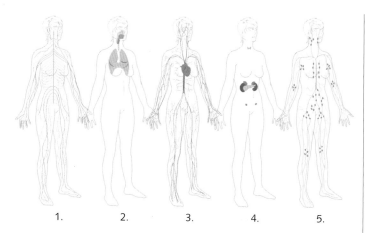

1.   2.   3.   4.   5.

The human body is a complex network of interdependent systems. When you have a problem with one it is likely to have a subsequent effect elsewhere. Similarly an ailment caused by, for instance, too much stress is likely to affect respiration, the immune system, the nervous system, and the endocrine system.

1. THE NERVOUS SYSTEM

Message transmission along nerves depends partly on the levels of neurotransmitters. These are substances such as adrenaline (from the adrenal glands); noradrenaline (from the adrenals and certain nerve endings); endorphins, enkephalins, and GABA – gamma-aminobutyric acid (from certain nerve endings); and serotonin (present in many tissues, including blood platelets, digestive lining, and the brain). Some neurotransmitters act locally to where they are produced, but others behave as hormones and travel to distant parts of the body.

Our lifestyle can have important effects on neurotransmitter levels. A healthy diet, for example, encourages normal levels of serotonin. Another is stress: effective stress management has a major influence on many neurotransmitters.

2. THE RESPIRATORY SYSTEM

Our breathing rates and styles (*see pages 12–13*) are influenced by the needs of our cells, together with the levels of neurotransmitters, hormones, and other important substances. And while most of the time we breathe automatically, we can also control our breathing styles consciously. The resulting levels of blood and tissue gases can affect our health.

3. THE CIRCULATORY SYSTEM

On its way around the body, the blood collects nutrients from the digestive system; oxygen from the lungs; immune cells and antibodies from the lymph nodes, spleen, and thymus; and neurotransmitters, hormones, and hormone-like substances (such as endorphins and prostaglandins) from the endocrine organs, brain, and other tissues. It then distributes these substances to all the body's cells. Most important, it also collects waste products and delivers them to the right place for disposal.

The heart and blood vessels respond to the levels of nutrients, gases, hormones, and neurotransmitters by increasing or decreasing the blood flow. These responses are often readily reversible. But sometimes – as with the build-up of fatty deposits on the insides of the artery walls – they are long-lasting or, unless circumstances change, permanent.

4. THE ENDOCRINE SYSTEM

Hormones produced by endocrine glands (pituitary, pineal, thyroid, parathyroids, pancreas, adrenals, ovaries and testes) travel in the blood to exert their effects throughout the body. They are affected by a variety of lifestyle factors, including diet, exercise, light-exposure, mood, and sleep.

5. THE IMMUNE SYSTEM

The healthy working of antibodies and immune cells, and the protective nature of the skin and mucous membranes lining the body's openings, are influenced by many ordinary lifestyle factors. These include your diet, stress, sleep, light exposure, exercise, and both the nature of the air you breathe and the way you breathe.

Too much stress – be it physical, mental, or spiritual – occasionally even makes the immune system turn on an individual's own body cells. This causes one of a variety of illnesses known as autoimmune diseases.

HOW TO USE THE COMMON AILMENTS SECTION

Using self-knowledge and self-help is not to deny the sometimes enormous and, at times, lifesaving value of medical diagnosis and care, but to acknowledge that we can readily treat most common ailments ourselves at home. Most poor health consists of simple "diseases" that respond to straightforward, cheap, pleasant-to-use treatments that are free from harmful side effects. The ailments in this section are divided into groups that reflect the various parts and systems of the body. Each entry has three sections: "What it is and what causes it," "Treatments," and "What else doctors may suggest".

The causes outlined in "*What it is and what causes it*" include certain things you may be able to prevent.

Before reaching for the medicine chest, it might be possible to alleviate the symptoms by modifying your lifestyle in some way.

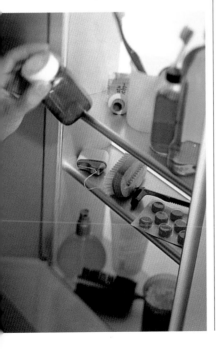

"*Treatment*" includes lifestyle changes, therapies, and remedies for use at home. These may be based on the complementary or alternative methods outlined in Part 3 (*see pages 128–143*), or on well-known home treatments, including some that your doctor may suggest. When necessary there is guidance on how long to use home treatment. Otherwise simply continue the treatment for as long as is needed to relieve your symptoms.

However, we are all individuals, and our ailments respond in an individual way. This means that treatments that work for one sufferer might not be effective for another. This is why it's often worth experimenting to see which remedies and therapies suit you and your ailment best. If you decide to use any homeopathic remedies, choose them from a recommended homeopathy book that outlines the best remedy for the precise nature and combination of your symptoms.

You'll find a list of the nutrient content of foods on *page 25*.

"*What else doctors may suggest*" includes advice on when to see the doctor only when relatively minor symptoms and signs could be hiding a more serious problem that might merit medical diagnosis and treatment. Otherwise the decision over when to seek medical advice is up to you. It will depend on the severity of the ailment, your ability to tolerate it, and whether it responds to home treatment.

To use the medical suggestions you must discuss your problem with a doctor. This allows the doctor to diagnose what is wrong, using any tests or investigations needed; to recommend treatment; and to supervise treatment for you if necessary. Many doctors are warm toward complementary therapies.

The possible side effects or dangers of home treatments are noted under "*Warnings.*" There may also be some warnings in Part 3 under each individual therapy, so it's worth checking there before using any therapy or remedy with which you are unfamiliar.

ACNE

❓ WHAT IT IS AND WHAT CAUSES IT

Acne can include blackheads, whiteheads, pimples, pustules, and, at worst, cysts. Seven out of ten teenagers who suffer from acne grow out of it in four or five years, but it can persist, or reappear, for example, around the menopause. One cause is an increased production of sebum (an oily fluid) due to oversensitivity of the sebaceous glands to normal levels of testosterone. Another is the stickiness of hair-follicle cells that then block follicles when dead. Changes in the composition of sebum may also be important. Sebum and cells block and widen pores, allowing skin bacteria to produce infection. Oxidation by the air then darkens oils in sebum, causing blackheads.

Acne triggers include: a falling estrogen level before periods (which encourages the influence of testosterone); the progestogen-only Pill; polycystic ovary syndrome (*see page 193*); hot, humid conditions; stress; certain drugs (especially steroids and phenytoin); and a nutritionally poor diet. A few people are sensitive to certain foods. If you usually crave chocolate before a period, this may be because both your acne and your food craving result from your changing hormone levels.

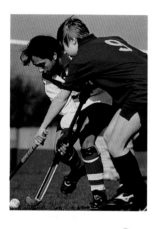

Acne can make a youngster's life miserable, but a combination of home care and medical treatment should do the trick.

✳ TREATMENT

Be sure to take regular exercise, and to expose your skin to unfiltered daylight outside for at least 15 minutes each day (*see Part 1*).

Skin care Wash with a pH-balanced soapless cleansing bar, or facial-wash lotion or gel. Choose oil-free, "non-comedogenic" moisturizer, foundation, and make-up remover gel or lotion. Use astringent for oily skin.

◆ For blackheads, use salicylic acid cream, gel, or wash (to dissolve dead cells), a blackhead extractor, or adhesive blackhead strips.

◆ For mild acne, use benzoyl peroxide cream or gel (to kill bacteria).

◆ Picking or squeezing pimples can encourage infection and scarring; if you must interfere, wait until a pimple comes to a head, wash your hands, pass a needle through a flame, puncture the spot, squeeze gently, and dab with tea tree oil.

Food supplements to try A multivitamin and mineral supplement.

Aromatherapy Use this face-splash after washing: add to a pint of water a tablespoon of vinegar and two drops each of petitgrain, juniper-berry and geranium oils. Vinegar boosts skin acidity, petitgrain reduces inflammation, juniper-berry, may regulate sebum, and geranium is antiseptic.

Apply neat tea tree oil to infected pimples twice daily as a non-drying alternative to benzoyl peroxide (*see below*).

Herbal remedies Sarsaparilla (wild licorice root, *Smilax*) contains substances that seem to block the effects of male hormones by preventing them from locking on to receptor sites on cells, so may be well worth trying. Take a teaspoon of tincture twice a day for one month.

✚ WHAT ELSE DOCTORS MAY SUGGEST

Effective medicinal treatment can make pimples 50 percent better within two months.

MOSTLY BLACKHEADS

Use a retinoid (a vitamin A derivative such as tretinoin, isotretinoin or adapalene) gel or lotion for greasy skin, or cream for dry or sensitive skin. (*Warning*: Unsuitable if you are, or might become, pregnant.) If too drying, try azelaic acid cream.

MILD ACNE

Apply an antibiotic solution, lotion, or gel (twice daily; perhaps alternated with a retinoid). Sometimes vitamin B3 cream is useful.

MODERATE ACNE

Use oral antibiotics. (*Warning*: If on the Pill, use an additional contraceptive method for the first month.) Alternatively, take a Pill (Dianette) containing cyproterone acetate to counteract the effects of testosterone.

SEVERE ACNE

If two courses of antibiotics are unsuccessful, consider oral isotretinoin. *Warning*: Not suitable if you are, or might become, pregnant.

A new treatment being researched is exposure for 15 minutes daily to blue and red light-rays to kill bacteria.

DERMATITIS

❓ WHAT IT IS AND WHAT CAUSES IT

There are several types of the skin inflammation known as dermatitis.

ATOPIC ECZEMA

Affects one in eight babies, often eases in childhood, and occurs on the face, neck, insides of the elbows, behind knees, or the whole body. There is often a family history of eczema, asthma, or hay fever. Triggers include dust mites, dried saliva on a pet's coat, heat, certain foods (rare in adults), infection, molds, smoke, hard water, and stress.

IRRITANT CONTACT DERMATITIS

Causes tiny blisters, often on the palms and between the fingers; irritants include certain detergents, disinfectants, acids, and cement.

ALLERGIC CONTACT DERMATITIS

The triggers for this include nickel (in bra hooks, jewelry, stainless-steel cutlery); glue; rubber; detergents; skin-care products; perfumes; certain foods, plants, and drugs; and chemicals used in the garden, on pets, or at work.

SEBORRHEIC DERMATITIS

See page 153.

❇ TREATMENT

Skin care Moisturize affected skin with unperfumed cream; this minimizes contact with irritants and allergens. Cover weeping or cracked skin to encourage moist healing conditions.

Food Certain nutrients help allergies subside. These include inflammation-soothers (a balanced supply of essential fatty acids – with only three times as many omega-3s as omega-6s (*see page 25*); vitamins A and B; and zinc) and antioxidants (beta carotene, vitamins C and E, flavonoids, and selenium). Spice your food with turmeric, a very potent antioxidant. Psoralens in celery, citrus fruit, figs, parsley, parsnips, and watercress increase the healing effect of sunlight (*see below*).

Light exposure Sunlight benefits some eczema. *Warning*: Avoid overheating, and irritation by sand, chlorinated or sea water, or certain sunscreening products (choose one with titanium dioxide or zinc oxide instead).

Herbal remedies Two or three times each day, apply some cream containing extracts of: *Viola tricolor* (wild pansy), borage (starflower), *Mahonia aquifolium*, marigold, chamomile, St. John's wort (hypericum), arnica, witch-hazel, sage, paracress (*Spilanthes oleracea*) and sanicle (*Sanicula europaea*) seed. This "Seven Herb Cream" is available from Bioforce UK (*see Useful Addresses on page 219*) and yes, it does contain more than seven herbs.

Alternatively, apply a cold compress (*see page 130*) soaked in borage, chickweed, chamomile, marigold, or carrot tea (*see page 137*).

Warning: Many Chinese herbal preparations for eczema contain added steroids.

Aromatherapy Apply a cream containing hemp-seed oil, or use the contents of a hemp-seed oil capsule. This oil helps counter inflammation of the skin because it contains a good balance of omega-3 and omega-6 fatty acids, and a helpful omega-6 fatty acid called gamma-linolenic acid.

Hydrotherapy Either stir two cups of powdered oatmeal into your bath water; or dissolve a handful of salt in a pint of very hot water and add this to a tepid bath; or add a pint of strong chamomile tea (*see page 137*). Soak in the bath for half an hour, dry yourself thoroughly, and then use moisturizing cream afterward.

Warning: Salt water may sting broken skin.

Avoid soap, or use an unperfumed, pH-balanced soapless cleansing bar daily. For bad eczema, wash with emulsifying ointment (from a drugstore).

An ion-exchange water softener removes calcium and magnesium from hard water and makes it lather more easily, so you need less soap.

✚ WHAT ELSE DOCTORS MAY SUGGEST

Mild steroid creams encourage healing. *Warning*: Prolonged use of steroid cream should be avoided; it makes the skin abnormally thin and fragile. Skin-prick tests aid trigger detection. Some eczema responds to UV therapy plus light-sensitizing drugs.

A suspected food sensitivity can be tracked down with a food-elimination and multiple challenge test for food sensitivity (*see page 164*).

Warning: Have professional supervision if altering a child's diet.

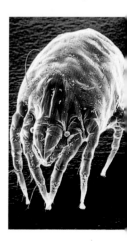

Dust mites are a fact of life and do no harm to the majority of people. However, in some they can trigger severe skin inflammations. Good housekeeping and non-allergenic bedding and furnishings can help.

149

PSORIASIS

❓ WHAT IT IS AND WHAT CAUSES IT

Psoriasis shows on the skin of the knees, elbows, and scalp as itchy, silvery, flaky patches. Scraping flakes away reveals reddened skin. Sometimes the nails are pitted, or the joints are inflamed. Each skin cell lives for only four days instead of the usual 28, and dead cells form flaky patches. Psoriasis often runs in families. The cause of the increased turnover of skin cells isn't usually clear, though stress can be a major trigger. Other triggers include smoking, alcohol, cold weather, sunburn, injury, hormone changes, certain drugs, and sensitivity to gluten. Little spots of psoriasis ("guttate" psoriasis) are usually the result of a respiratory infection.

Turmeric contains skin-friendly antioxidants.

✳ TREATMENT

Relaxation and other stress management
Many therapies and remedies relieve stress. For example, the choosing of flower remedies helps you focus on unrecognized emotions; and massage, yoga exercises, and muscle relaxation can be very soothing.

Herbal remedies Look for creams containing anti-inflammatory herbs such *Mahonia aquifolia* (oregon grape) root, marigold (*Calendula*) flowers, and extracts of oak, or the neem tree (*Melia azadirachta*, from India and Myanmar). Alternatively, use soothing aloe gel, or try a traditional Zulu remedy – bandage a banana skin, moist-side down, to a patch in the morning; remove and replace in the evening.

Light Sunlight eases some cases of psoriasis. (*Warning*: Take care not to burn.) It may be worth experimenting with bathing in electric light filtered through a red gel (a colored transparent acetate sheet) for half an hour a day (*see below*).

Food Eat relatively little meat or dairy foods. Include more green leafy and other vegetables, fruit, nuts, beans, and seeds in your diet, along with other foods containing skin-friendly folic acid, selenium, zinc, and essential fats. Eat oily fish three times a week, and olive and other cold-pressed oils for their anti-inflammatory fatty acids. Spice food with turmeric, a potent antioxidant. Each day eat some foods containing psoralens (celery, liquidized whole citrus fruit, figs, parsley, parsnips, and watercress); these may boost the action of sunlight (*see above*). (*See also page 17.*) Avoid drinking more than a little alcohol. Consider trying a gluten-free diet (no wheat, oats, barley or rye grains, or flour) for four weeks (*see page 25* for alternative sources of nutrients).

Warning: Have professional supervision if altering a child's diet.

Food supplements to try
◆ Folic acid, selenium, and zinc (as individual supplements or in a multivitamin and mineral supplement).
◆ Cod liver oil or fish oil.

✚ WHAT ELSE DOCTORS MAY SUGGEST

Various creams prevent drying: salicylic acid reduces scaling; tar soothes inflammation; and dithranol reduces flaking. Other possibilities include a vitamin D-like drug (calcipotriol) in cream, ointment, or scalp lotion; steroid skin products; a retinoid (vitamin A-like drug) skin product or, for very severe psoriasis, certain oral drugs (*Warning*: Use extra contraception during this therapy, and for two years afterward); and antifungal or cytotoxic (cell-killing) drugs.

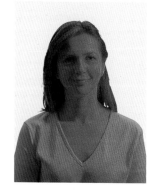

Light therapy involves either exposure to ultraviolet B (UVB) rays; or PUVA – UVA exposure after taking a psoralen drug to make the skin more responsive to light; or exposure to red light two to four hours after painting patches with light-sensitive acid.

Electric light filtered through a red transparent acetate sheet for half an hour a day may help psoriasis.

ROUGH OR DRY SKIN

❓ WHAT IT IS AND WHAT CAUSES IT

Rough skin feels unpleasant and stings when the weather is wet, cold, or windy. Conditions that roughen skin include excessive immersion in water, dermatitis (*see page 149*), psoriasis (*see facing page*), shingles, chickenpox, prickly heat, goose bumps, and flaking sunburn. Another common cause is photo-damage from years of sun exposure. Tiny rough spots (*keratosis pilaris*), resembling goose bumps on face, chest, back, upper arms, and thighs, are worse in winter, and more likely with eczema, and usually go in a person's 20s.

Dry skin is prone to cracks and infection. Deep cracks are very painful, especially on the lips or soles of the feet, which are areas that have a rich nerve supply but no natural oil. Sometimes, too, deep heel cracks can actually bleed.

✻ TREATMENT

Lifestyle More exercise and sleep sometimes improve skin quality and texture. Wear rubber gloves when working with water.

Food and drink

ROUGHNESS

Eat more foods rich in essential fatty acids and beta carotene to smooth skin.

CRACKS

Eat more vitamin B2-rich foods; a deficiency encourages soreness and cracking.

DRY SKIN

Have more water and foods containing the skin-friendly nutrients beta carotene, vitamins C and E, zinc, and essential fatty acids.

Food supplements to try

◆ Borage (starflower) oil and cod liver oil for roughness.
◆ Vitamin B complex for cracks.
◆ A multivitamin and mineral supplement, borage oil, and fish oil for dryness.

Aromatherapy

CRACKED SOLES

Before bedtime, massage with two teaspoons of sweet almond oil containing five drops of frankincense, myrrh, patchouli, or benzoin oil. Slip a polythene bag on your foot, then a sock. The next morning, apply a non-adherent "burns" dressing, bandage, or "heel-crack bandage" to help to keep the moisture in and smooth the skin.

CRACKED LIPS

Mix two drops of rose oil with the contents of two capsules of evening primrose oil, and apply a little of this oil morning and night.

Herbal remedies

CRACKED LIPS

Bathe with carrot tea (*see page 137*); this contains healing vitamins, minerals, and flavonoids.

CRACKED SOLES

Soften callused skin by soaking in strong chamomile tea (*see page 137*) for ten minutes. Alternatively, apply a paste made from six crushed aspirin tablets and half a teaspoon each of water and lemon juice. Encase your foot overnight in a plastic bag, then a sock. The next morning, remove the softened skin with a callus file or pumice stone, and work in some rich cream.

General skin care

DRY SKIN

Wear gloves and barrier cream to protect your hands. Moisturize your skin well, especially after a bath. Use a sunscreening moisturizer or foundation cream by day, and nourish your skin at night with a cream enriched with evening primrose or starflower oil, and vitamins A and E.

CRACKED LIPS

Don't lick sore lips as this encourages even more uncomfortable "lip-licker's dermatitis".

✚ WHAT ELSE DOCTORS MAY SUGGEST

Keratosis pilaris may respond to ten percent urea cream. Rough, photo-aged skin can benefit from a cream containing 0.05 percent tretinoin (a vitamin A derivative). *Warning*: Not if you are, or might become, pregnant.

Carrots and carrot oil are rich in vitamins, minerals, and flavonoids, and can help relieve the symptoms of dry skin, such as cracked lips.

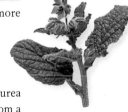

Add borage to your diet if you have dry or rough skin.

AGE SPOTS

❓ WHAT THEY ARE AND WHAT CAUSES THEM

There are three main types of age spots. Flat brown marks called freckles (lentigos) are most likely on hands and face. Red, or skin-colored, lumps called solar keratoses can affect any sun-exposed skin. Rough, yellow, brown, or black, flat marks or warty growths called seborrheic keratoses appear almost stuck on, and favor hands and trunk. Freckles, and solar and some seborrheic keratoses, result mainly from "photo-aging". Skin cells make melanin, which absorbs UV light and counters sunburn and skin cancer. But years of sun exposure exhaust the cells, so melanin no longer produces an even tan but clusters in the areas we call freckles.

✳ TREATMENT

Skin care Shade exposed skin and use a factor 15 sunscreening product. Eat plenty of foods rich in antioxidants (beta carotene, vitamins C and E, selenium, flavonoids) to counter sun damage. Antioxidants in creams and food supplements aren't as effective as those in foods.

Skin creams containing alpha-hydroxy (fruit) acids may help. And you can lighten brown spots with hydroxyquinone cream.

Warning: See a doctor if any spot darkens, grows, itches, or changes in other ways.

Various creams are available to treat age spots but foods rich in antioxidants might be more beneficial.

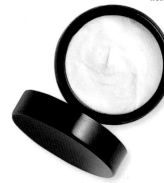

BELOW RIGHT:
Encourage a better blood flow to ridged nails by giving the fingertips a twice-daily, one-minute massage.

✚ WHAT ELSE DOCTORS MAY SUGGEST

Photo-aged skin may benefit from 0.05 percent tretinoin cream. *Warning*: not suitable if you are, or might become, pregnant. Seborrheic keratoses can be treated if necessary. There is a small cancer risk from solar keratoses, so see a dermatologist regularly for observation or treatment with cryotherapy (freezing with liquid nitrogen), laser therapy, scraping, cutting out, cautery (heat), or chemical peeling (with 5-fluouracil).

NAIL SPLITS AND RIDGES

❓ WHAT CAUSES THEM

The commonest reason for nails to flake or split is overexposure to water, which softens a protein in nails called keratin. A knock can separate the layers of nail, leaving a white fleck that eventually flakes off. Detergents encourage splitting, and tight shoes cause horizontal ridges.

A poor diet, or poor nutrient absorption caused by digestive problems, weakens nails. A lack of iron makes them brittle and ridged; too little zinc makes them brittle; and a shortage of essential fatty acids results in splits and flaking. Poor circulation (*see page 174*), and rheumatoid arthritis (*see page 178*), both restrict the nutrient supply and can lead to ridges up and down the length of the nail. Any shock disturbs new cells under the cuticles and creates horizontal ridges. Patchy baldness (*see page 154*) can be associated with rough, ridged, pitted nails; fungal infection (*see opposite page*) causes ridges, pits, and crumbling; and psoriasis (*see page 150*) causes pits, and splits near the cuticles.

✳ TREATMENT

Nail care Keep nails out of water as much as possible and either avoid rubber gloves, or wear cotton-lined ones to absorb sweat.

Smooth in nourishing nail cream each night. And several times a day, with clean hands, wipe your nails along the creases beside your nose and beneath your mouth to benefit from your sebum.
Food Check that you are eating ample protein and eat more foods containing calcium, magnesium, zinc, and essential fatty acids.
Food supplements to try
◆ Calcium, magnesium, and zinc.
◆ Borage (starflower) and fish oils.

Exercise and massage
Twice a day, boost the circulation with a one-minute session of arm swinging, and massage the skin around each nail with small pumping movements of your index finger and thumb.

FUNGAL SKIN AND NAIL INFECTIONS

❓ WHAT THEY ARE AND WHAT CAUSES THEM

These include ringworm (round flaky patches with red rims on the skin); athlete's foot (loose, soggy, or flaky skin on the soles or between the toes); a *Candida* infection of the nipples (see also vaginal *Candida*, *page 192*); thick, crumbly, yellow (or green or black) nails; and patchy baldness (*see page 154*). Dandruff and seborrheic dermatitis (a red, scaly, itchy skin rash) can be associated with a yeast overgrowth. Fungi are spread from infected people, cats, and dogs, and thrive on warmth and moisture.

✻ TREATMENT

All infections Boost immunity with foods rich in beta carotene, vitamins C and E, selenium, zinc, and flavonoids, and raw garlic. Wash bedsheets, towels, and clothes in very hot water, and don't share towels, washcloths, or bath mats. Vacuum well after treating an infected person or animal, as spores can live for years.

Nail infection Keep nails dry. Have a separate file for infected nails, and clean scissors or clippers well. Rub tea tree oil into affected nails for three minutes, three times a day. Alternatively, apply clotrimazole cream two or three times daily.

Ringworm Add eight to ten drops of tea tree oil to bath water, and massage patches twice daily with tea tree, lavender, or myrrh oil, or apply marigold tincture (*see page 137*). As skin heals, use a cream made from five teaspoons of calendula cream and three to four drops each of tea tree, lavender, and myrrh oils.

If this doesn't work, then apply some cream containing miconazole, clotrimazole, or ketoconazole twice a day.

Athlete's foot Have a daily foot-bath in warm water containing five to ten drops of tea tree oil and two teaspoons of vinegar. Use powder for dry skin, and cream or oil for moist or cracked skin. To make powder, mix three tablespoons of cornflour with five to six drops each of tea tree, lemongrass and lavender oils; wait 24 hours before using. Or apply a few drops of tea tree oil twice a day. Alternatively, use powder or cream containing miconazole, tolfanate, or chlorphenesin.

Dandruff and other scalp infections Shampoo frequently with rosemary, horsetail, or nettle shampoo, or tea tree oil shampoo. Add a tablespoon of vinegar to the final rinse, or rinse with half a pint of rosemary or thyme tea (*see page 137*). Massage your head once a week before bed with olive oil, then shampoo in the morning.

You may occasionally need a shampoo containing zinc pyrithione or selenium sulphide, or salicylic acid hair lotion or, for stubborn dandruff, a product containing tar or ketoconazole. Use a ketoconazole-containing product daily for four weeks on seborrheic dermatitis.

✚ WHAT ELSE DOCTORS MAY SUGGEST

Nail infection Nail scrapings reveal the cause of the infection. Applying a lacquer (containing amorolfine or tioconazole), for six months for fingernails, or a year for toenails, can help; if not, use an oral drug (terbenafine) for at least six weeks for fingernails, three for toenails.

Skin infection Cream containing an antifungal agent (such as terbinafine or amorolfine) often works; failing that, oral antifungal drugs.

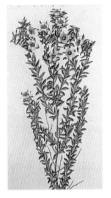

An antifungal oil can be extracted from the tea tree plant.

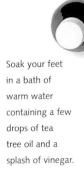

Soak your feet in a bath of warm water containing a few drops of tea tree oil and a splash of vinegar.

153

HAIR LOSS

WHAT IT IS AND WHAT CAUSES IT

Some thinning is a natural part of aging. Other causes include anemia (*see page 172*), thyroid problems (*see page 181*), changing hormone levels after childbirth, a fever, a low-protein diet, and repeated poor quality slimming diets. An unhealthy diet may thin hair by impairing the scalp's circulation. A sensitivity of the hair follicles to normal levels of a hormone called dihydro-testosterone (DHT) affects one in ten women under 40, one in four by 50, and three in five by 70. This is probably inherited, usually occurs on top of the head, and is prevented to some extent by estrogen before the menopause. Stress and shock can stop hairs growing and send them into an early "resting" phase. Then, after three months, many more hairs than usual fall out at the same time. Sometimes only pigmented hairs fall, giving the impression of going white "overnight".

Patchy loss can result from alopecia areata, in which the immune system mistakenly attacks the follicles; hair regrows eventually in three people out of four. Fungal infections (*see page 153*) can be to blame. And some women weaken their hair by pulling it or dragging it into tight bunches.

Molasses and other foods rich in vitamins B and C can form part of the treatment for hair loss.

TREATMENT

Lifestyle Check your stress-management strategies (*see page 34*) and take regular exercise. The process of choosing appropriate flower remedies (*see page 138*) could help difficult feelings surface. Aromatherapy massages (*see page 133*), yoga (*see page 140*), relaxation exercises (*see page 141*), and meditation (*see page 142*) all aid relaxation.

Massage diluted essential oils into your scalp and keep in place with a warm towel to encourage absorption.

Food Eat more foods that are rich in vitamins B and C, PABA (eggs, molasses, wheatgerm, brewer's yeast, wholegrains), inositol (wholegrains, oranges, nuts), iron, and zinc. Eating more foods that are rich in plant hormones might help after a hormonal upset.

Food supplements to try
- Vitamin B complex.
- Vegetable lecithin.
- Isoflavones (plant hormones).

Hair care Use a pH-balanced shampoo; avoid dye, bleach, perms, and blow-drying. Choose a hairstyle that enhances the volume of your hair; use pretty scarves or hats; and perhaps consider a wig or hairpiece.

Aromatherapy, herbal, and other remedies
Gently massage your scalp at bedtime once a week with a warmed mixture of two tablespoons each of wheatgerm and coconut oils, and five drops each of lavender, bay, and rosemary oils. Wear a towelling turban overnight, shampoo your hair the next morning, and then rinse with nettle tea (*see page 137*).

Make a stimulating lotion with one tablespoon of cider vinegar, three drops each of lavender, bay, and rosemary oils, and half a glass of rose or orange-flower water. Shake and massage a little into your scalp each morning. Alternatively, buy a lotion containing silicon (from a drugstore). Licorice may help to prevent male hair loss by preventing the conversion of testosterone to DHT.

WHAT ELSE DOCTORS MAY SUGGEST

Minoxidil lotion stimulates hair growth in one in two people affected by DHT-sensitive hair loss. It takes four months to work, must be used permanently, and can have side effects.

ROSACEA

❓ WHAT IT IS AND WHAT CAUSES IT

One woman in ten aged 30–55 suffers from a facial skin problem called rosacea (pronounced rose-asia). This often begins in the teens, with bouts of intense blushing brought on by one of many triggers – see below. As rosacea progresses, tiny veins enlarge, and the skin swells and becomes permanently red and, perhaps, painful. The next stage is a symmetrical pimply rash. One woman in two with rosacea also has inflammation of the surface of her eyes and eyelids. At worst, the nose thickens and reddens.

The cause isn't clear, though possibilities include irritation by mites in hair follicles, digestive disorders associated with a lack of stomach acid, and oversensitivity of the walls of the small blood vessels. Rosacea can run in families and is commoner in fair-skinned women. Migraine is more likely in women with rosacea. Two common triggers are exposure to sunlight or wind, or to extremes of temperature or weather. Another is certain foods (spicy, fermented, pickled, marinated, and smoked foods; liver; sirloin steak; yogurt; sour cream; cheese (not cottage); chocolate; vanilla; soy sauce; yeast extract; dark vinegar; eggplant; avocados; spinach; citrus fruit; tomatoes; bananas; red plums; raisins; figs) or drinks (alcohol – especially red wine – coffee, cocoa, and tea). Stress is another possibility, with some women finding the reddening so embarrassing that they blush, which makes the problem worse. A few women are so upset by rosacea that they get depressed.

✳ TREATMENT

Keep a careful diary so you can see what makes your rosacea worse. Then avoid these triggers.

Skin care Be gentle with your skin. Avoid products containing fragrances, oils, and alcohols (for example, many toners, hairsprays, hair gels, witch hazel). Use a sunscreen of factor 15, but choose one with reflecting minerals (such as titanium

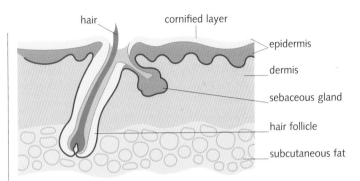

Irritation of the hair follicles by tiny mites is one possible explanation for rosacea.

dioxide or zinc oxide) rather than absorbent chemical filters. Choose a light-textured, green-toned foundation, or a camouflage make-up to help minimize the redness.

Food and drink Eat more foods rich in vitamins B (to nourish the nerves supplying blood vessel walls) and C and flavonoids (to strengthen blood vessel walls). If menopausal hot flashes make your rosacea worse, be sure to eat plenty of foods rich in plant hormones.

Food supplements to try

◆ Vitamin B complex.
◆ Vitamin C with flavonoids.
◆ Betaine hydrochloride (an acid supplement to increase acidity in the stomach).
◆ Isoflavones (plant hormones).

Relaxation and other stress management

Experiment with relaxation exercises, as well as other stress-management strategies (*see page 34*).

Massage Try gently massaging your face with your fingertips, using stroking and tapping movements.

✚ WHAT ELSE DOCTORS MAY SUGGEST

Metronidazole gel applied twice daily to affected areas helps inflamed skin. Long-term oral antibiotics (tetracycline), or a cream that contains isotretinoin (a vitamin A derivative – not suitable if you are, or might become, pregnant) may be advised. Laser treatment is useful for unsightly broken veins and a swollen nose.

Gently massage the skin to release tension that can contribute to a high skin color.

COLD SORES

❓ WHAT THEY ARE AND WHAT CAUSES THEM

Herpes simplex virus infection causes lip sores called cold sores. These viruses can also affect the skin elsewhere, or the vagina, back passage, or (usually only in young babies) eyes and brain. Genital herpes generally results from a different strain of the virus, and is usually caught from sex with a partner who has genital herpes. However, cold sore viruses (*Herpes simplex* type 1) occasionally cause genital infection, and genital viruses (*Herpes simplex* type 2) sometimes cause cold sores.

Most of us have had a herpes infection by the age of 25. You first catch herpes by contact between broken skin and someone else's sore. Blisters erupt within 14 days. They then form ulcers which eventually heal. Some people feel feverish, tired, and headachy, with joint and muscle pain and swollen lymph nodes. The viruses then travel up the nerves and "hibernate" near the spinal cord. Half of all herpes sufferers have recurrent sores, heralded by tingling, itching, or stinging. Triggers that reactivate viruses include stress, periods, infection, skin damage, sun, and fatigue.

✻ TREATMENT

General tips If you have a cold sore, don't kiss anyone (especially if they are very young, unwell or pregnant, or have widespread eczema). And don't perform oral sex on your partner; even using a condom gives scant protection.

Food Eat two raw garlic cloves each day. The balance of two amino acids, arginine and lysine, may affect your susceptibility to this viral infection. So eat more lysine-rich foods (fish, eggs, meat, milk, beans, potatoes). And cut down on arginine (found in meat, nuts, beans, seeds, chocolate, and cereal grains).

Food supplements to try
- Vitamin C with flavonoids.
- Zinc.
- Lysine – an amino acid.

Skin care Avoid touching your sore. If you do touch it, wash your hands well and dry thoroughly on paper towels, or your own towel (laundered at as high a temperature as possible).

FAR RIGHT: Echinacea is widely available in health-food stores. It boosts the immune system and can help treat colds, cold sores, and other infections.

Garlic can help alleviate a cold sore. It is available in capsule form to overcome the odor problem.

A sore usually heals better if kept moist with frequent applications (with a cotton swab) of ointment, cream, or oil, put on when the tingling starts. Other remedies include lavender and tea tree oils, and vitamin A and E oils, obtained by piercing a vitamin A or E capsule. To make a cream, buy 30g of unscented cold cream and add nine drops of lavender oil and six of tea tree oil.

Some people prefer to dry a sore with surgical spirit or witch hazel – or even black coffee. Over-the-counter remedies include ingredients such as iodine, menthol, ammonia, phenol, and alcohol.

Herbal remedies Take a teaspoon of echinacea tincture in a little water twice a day by mouth for two months to boost immunity. Smooth melissa ointment on sores twice a day.

Homeopathic remedies Take your constitutional remedy (*see page 139*), because cold sores often occur when resistance is low.

✚ WHAT ELSE DOCTORS MAY SUGGEST

Cream or tablets containing an antiviral agent such as aciclovir cream can help.

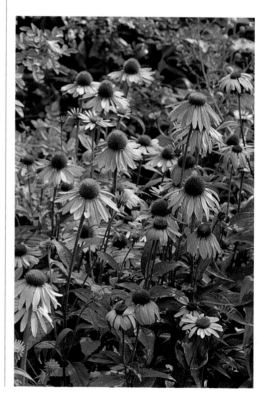

MOUTH ULCERS

❓ WHAT THEY ARE AND WHAT CAUSES THEM

For such small things, mouth ulcers certainly make their presence felt. Even a single one is impossible to ignore. Whenever food, drink, or your tongue touches it, a sharp pain warns, "keep away". Mouth ulcers are shallow, flat-bottomed craters in the mucous membrane of the cheeks, gums, tongue, or roof or floor of the mouth. Often light gray, they have a raised yellow border, sometimes inflamed around the edge.

The commonest, known as aphthous ulcers, remain a mystery and can last for one or two weeks. They tend to come at the very worst times. Any stress, be it tiredness, worry, depression, or repeated infection or other illness, can be a trigger, and these ulcers are often most likely before a period. One person in five with long-term ulcers is sensitive to gluten, a protein in wheat, barley, oats, and rye. Gluten-sensitive ulcers may be more likely before a period, when hormone changes can lower immunity and reduce the protectiveness of mucus.

Accidentally biting the inside of your cheek can pave the way for an ulcer, as can scratching your mouth with a toothbrush or rough piece of toast or other food, having a rough filling, and wearing a badly fitting brace, bridge, or denture.

Other causes include: smoking; food colorings in the E100–155 range (especially when the source is acidic boiled sweets); hay fever and other allergic rhinitis; hand, foot, and mouth disease; anorexia nervosa (*see page 206*), herpes virus (*see facing page*) or *Candida* infection (*see page 192*); anemia (*see page 174*); drug allergy; tuberculosis; leukemia; and mouth cancer. A bacterial infection called Vincent's disease (triggered by poor oral hygiene, smoking, throat infection, and stress) can cause ulcers, bad breath, and a horrible taste.

✳ TREATMENT

Lifestyle Avoid any known triggers, including smoking.

Food and drink Have two raw cloves of garlic each day. Avoid sugary, acidic, and salty foods and drinks such as candy, potato chips, and lemon juice. Experiment with avoiding gluten-containing foods for two weeks.

Mouth care Use an over-the-counter medication such as a painkilling gel or lozenges; a gel containing carbenoxolone (from licorice); or an antiseptic mouthwash.

Herbal remedies Rinse your mouth every two hours with sage tea, or ten drops of myrrh tincture in half a glass of water. Alternatively, chew a piece of licorice root every few hours. (*Warning*: Don't do this if you have high blood pressure.)

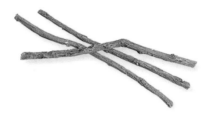

Chewing a piece of licorice root can bring some relief from the pain of mouth ulcers.

Aromatherapy Use a mouthwash every two hours made from two to three drops of lemon, tea tree, chamomile, sage, or fennel oil in half a glass of water.

✚ WHAT ELSE DOCTORS MAY SUGGEST

Hydrocortisone pellets or a mouthwash containing tetracycline may help aphthous ulcers.

Warning: If a mouth ulcer persists for more than three weeks, see a doctor.

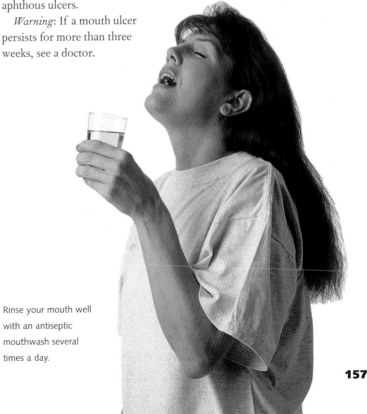

Rinse your mouth well with an antiseptic mouthwash several times a day.

157

TOOTHACHE

❓ WHAT CAUSES IT

Toothache results from exposure of the nerve endings in dentine (the soft part of a tooth beneath the enamel). This happens when a tooth's enamel covering is breached by a crack due to injury, or by dental decay.

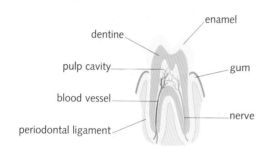

When nerve endings are exposed, toothache results. Soothe the pain by self-help methods, but also see a dentist.

When we eat food containing added sugar, mouth bacteria break down food traces in the sticky material (plaque) in tooth crevices and around teeth. This releases acid within five to ten minutes. A good saliva flow washes this acid away. However, if the flow is reduced because of insufficient chewing, bland foods, aging, or certain illnesses, the high acidity level remains for some time. This then breaks down the enamel's surface by dissolving its minerals. If the high acidity is quickly counteracted (*see below*), minerals reenter the enamel. But if the acid attack is long-lasting, it causes a cavity. With repeated acid attack the cavity wall can break through to the dentine.

Sometimes teeth ache for other reasons. This can happen, for example, when having very hot or cold food or drink (which sometimes suggests an infection in a root canal), or when cleaning teeth (which could indicate gum disease).

❀ TREATMENT

See a dentist, because you need dental treatment (*see below*) to safeguard your tooth. You also need to remove the plaque and strengthen tooth enamel by brushing twice a day with fluoride toothpaste, and by flossing once every day.

Food and drink Eat more foods rich in calcium and other minerals to strengthen your teeth. Naturally occurring sugars in wholefoods such as

fruit are not a problem. Clean your teeth after consuming foods containing added sugar. If this is inconvenient, eat some fibrous food (such as celery) to clean acid-containing plaque away, or have a little cheese or a few nuts to neutralize the acid. Limit sugary foods to mealtimes, because the saliva flow triggered by chewing washes acid away. If you can't clean your teeth or eat cheese or celery, rub your tongue around your teeth and gum margins to dislodge food traces, then swish a mouthful of water around your mouth.

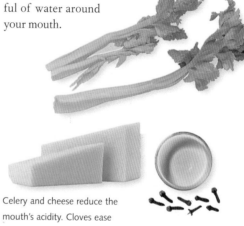

Celery and cheese reduce the mouth's acidity. Cloves ease the pain of a toothache.

Aromatherapy Soak a cotton swab in clove oil and place over the cavity. A substance called eugenol in the oil numbs exposed nerves and kills bacteria.

✚ WHAT ELSE DENTISTS MAY SUGGEST

A dentist can fill a cavity with dental amalgam or other material (such as composite or gold). Amalgam releases very small amounts of mercury into the mouth, and releases more as vapor when fillings are removed. However, dentists insist that amalgam fillings are stronger and longer lasting than are composite fillings, and that fewer healthy teeth are removed for amalgam fillings than for gold inlays. Studies have revealed health problems from amalgam fillings only in those few people who are sensitive to mercury. But for safety's sake it's wise to avoid having an amalgam inserted or removed during pregnancy. If you have an amalgam removed, ask your dentist to use precautions (such as giving you a paper mask, and using a rubber dam) to reduce mercury absorption.

SORE GUMS

❓ WHAT THEY ARE AND WHAT CAUSES THEM

Inflammation (gingivitis) is the commonest cause of tooth decay. Gingivitis makes gums swollen, purple-red and likely to bleed when you brush your teeth or eat hard foods. A film of plaque develops on teeth after eating. This contains food residues and bacteria and accumulates around the gum margins. Undisturbed plaque absorbs salivary minerals and hardens to hard chalky-white calculus (tartar).

Anyone can suffer from gingivitis if they neglect toothbrushing and flossing, or do it roughly. Women are more prone to it during pregnancy, because pregnancy hormones soften gums. Diabetes encourages gum disease. And gum disease is associated with an increased risk of heart attacks, because bacterial toxins absorbed into the bloodstream make the blood more likely to clot.

✳ TREATMENT

Mouth care Ideally, brush teeth (from gum to tooth) after each meal. Alternatively, eat some fibrous food (such as celery), or rinse your mouth well. Floss daily. It's better to use good dental hygiene to prevent calculus accumulating, and to have a regular appointment with a dental hygienist than to try and remove it yourself.

Food and drink Choose foods that need a lot of chewing. Eat more foods rich in vitamin C, flavonoids, and selenium.

Food supplements
◆ Vitamins C and E.
◆ Selenium.
◆ Co-enzyme Q10.

Herbal remedies and massage Rinse your mouth with sage tea, or with ordinary black tea, morning and evening. Massage your gums gently each day with some fresh sage leaves or some aloe vera gel. And take a teaspoon of echinacea tincture twice a day for three months.

✚ WHAT ELSE DENTISTS MAY SUGGEST

Your dentist (or dental hygienist) will remove calculus and do any necessary dental work. A blood-sugar test can reveal hidden diabetes (*see page 180*).

BAD BREATH

❓ WHAT IT IS AND WHAT CAUSES IT

Most people have halitosis occasionally, and for some it's an ongoing problem. It usually results from the same dietary and mouth conditions that underlie tooth decay and gum disease. These encourage certain bacteria to break down food proteins and release sulfurous compounds (such as hydrogen sulfide – the bad eggs smell – and methyl mercaptan, the smell in rotting dung). A dry mouth concentrates bacteria and food residues. And if you kiss someone with bad breath when your mouth is dry, you may catch the bacteria that can induce halitosis!

✳ TREATMENT

Brush and floss regularly, and consider brushing or scraping your tongue. If you can't brush after a meal, swish a mouthful of water around instead. Disinfect your toothbrush once a week in a mild bleach solution and replace it every few months.

Food and drink Eat more raw green leafy vegetables for the breath-purifying action of their chlorophyll. Disguise halitosis after eating garlic, raw onions, meat, tuna, curry, or blue cheese, or drinking alcohol, coffee, or milk, by chewing parsley, caraway seeds, or sugar-free gum, or sucking a mint. Have frequent drinks if your mouth feels dry.

✚ WHAT ELSE DOCTORS OR DENTISTS MAY SUGGEST

See your doctor if you are unwell, as an illness (such as diabetes, cancer, or liver disease) could be responsible. Your dentist can treat dental decay (*see page 158*) and gum disease (*see above*).

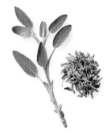

A sage tea rinse helps oral hygiene.

ABOVE LEFT: Chewing crunchy salads helps to remove the slimy layer of plaque.

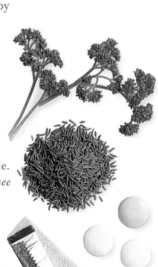

Prevent bad breath by chewing parsley, caraway seeds, sugar-free gum, or sucking mints after meals.

INDIGESTION

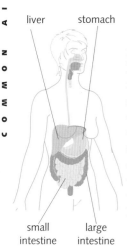

liver   stomach

small   large
intestine intestine

Indigestion has many causes and can result in pain anywhere from the pit of your stomach to your chest.

WHAT IT IS AND WHAT CAUSES IT

Indigestion, with stomachache, gas, nausea, or heartburn (pain beneath the breastbone from acid reflux), may result from an over-filled stomach, gas, or muscle tension or inflammation of the wall of the stomach or intestines. Causes include a poor diet, poor eating habits, stress, infection, food sensitivity, gallstones, and a lack of stomach acid and digestive enzymes (from drinking during mealtimes, aging, stress, illness, food sensitivity, or a vitamin B deficiency). Occasionally other problems are to blame.

TREATMENT

Avoid wearing a tight belt, and don't bend or lie down after meals. Stop smoking, and take regular exercise to reduce weight.

Food and drink Eat more foods rich in vitamins B and C and zinc. This fosters a healthy digestive system and sufficient saliva, mucus, stomach acid, and digestive enzymes. Let your stomach guide you on how often and how much to eat. Boost the flow of digestive juices by savoring the aroma and flavor of meals, having bitter appetizers (such as olives) and aperitifs (such as tonic water – or gin and tonic), flavoring food with rosemary, and eating chicory, watercress, or artichokes. Begin your main meal with a salad as its fiber helps condition the stomach and intestinal lining. And chew food thoroughly. Counteract indigestion with papaya, pineapple, raw cabbage, dill, parsley, or ginger with meals, and afterward sipping chamomile or mint tea or chewing cardamom, fennel, or caraway seeds.

Fatty foods, alcohol, and caffeine encourage heartburn, as do overeating and rushing meals. Avoid foods that upset you (milk, white flour, and added sugar are common culprits), and get expert help with a food-elimination and multiple challenge test (*see page 164*), if you suspect a food sensitivity.

If antacids don't help indigestion after a protein-containing meal, try sipping water containing a teaspoon of cider or balsamic vinegar, or adding such vinegar to meat, fish, eggs, and cheese. This could help if your body is making too little stomach acid.

Include papaya and pineapple in a meal to counteract indigestion.

Food supplements

◆ Digestive acid (betaine hydrochloride) and enzymes (if antacids don't help, and provided you don't have a peptic ulcer).

◆ Vitamin B complex.

Stress management Use more effective stress-management strategies, as stress can make the stomach muscles overactive, and alter acid production. Remember that antacids aren't recommended for long-term use. Relax and enjoy meals as one of life's great pleasures, and avoid using food or drink to smother or drown difficult emotions. Comfort foods and alcohol can't cure what's wrong and may make you tired, unwell, and overweight in addition to worsening your digestion.

WHAT ELSE DOCTORS MAY SUGGEST

If necessary, a doctor can arrange investigations such as a breath test, blood tests, scans, X-rays and endoscopy (a look inside the stomach via a swallowed camera), then use drugs or surgery to treat any problems if necessary.

Warning: Seek help for anything other than occasional mild symptoms, problems beginning after 50, and pain in the neck or arm.

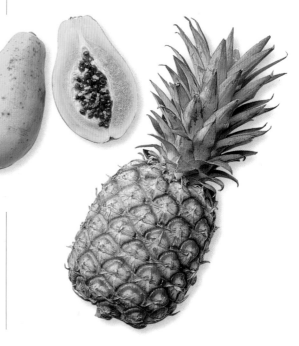

IRRITABLE BOWEL SYNDROME

☯ WHAT IT IS AND WHAT CAUSES IT

One person in three occasionally has an "irritable" bowel. This means that they have some combination of stomachache (usually eased by emptying the bowels or passing gas); constipation, diarrhea (especially in the early morning), or alternating diarrhea and constipation; mucus in the feces; a feeling that the bowels are never empty; and gas and bloating for hours after eating. Diarrhea, constipation, and pain partly result from poor coordination of muscle contractions of the bowel wall which prevents food passing through smoothly; pain also results from an unusual sensitivity of the bowel nerves to stretching.

One in five people with an irritable bowel has frequent attacks and is said to have the irritable bowel syndrome (IBS). Women are twice as likely as men to suffer from IBS. Their bowels react adversely to one or more of certain triggers, such as stress, gastroenteritis, smoking, antibiotics, certain foods, changing hormone levels, excessive exercise, and pelvic surgery.

The three types of IBS have rather unfortunate names. "Spastic colon" causes all the above symptoms. "Functional diarrhea" particularly causes diarrhea with an urgent desire to open the bowels. "Primary foregut motility disorder" (also known as the pain/bloat/gas type of IBS) causes right-sided stomachache, bad bloating, and gas.

People with IBS are more prone to headaches, tiredness, and depression. They may also sometimes have pain in the back or thighs, heavy or painful periods, pain during sex, and a frequent or urgent need to pass water.

✱ TREATMENT

Take regular whole-body exercise to reduce your stress level. Moving your body also encourages good digestion by "massaging" your intestines.

Food and drink Counteract indigestion (*see facing page*) and avoid foods that upset you (such as dairy foods, starches, or alcohol). If you suspect a food sensitivity, go on a food-elimination diet (*see page 164*). Avoid added bran, and cut down on coffee, tea, and cola.

Stress management Choose and practice effective stress-management strategies. Some people find massage with relaxation-inducing essential oils (*see page 133*), meditation (*see page 142*), or yoga exercises useful. Breathing exercises and muscle relaxation (*see page 141*) can help. And incorporating the Alexander technique (*see page 135*) into your movements may ease the nervous tension that often accompanies IBS.

Herbal remedies Help relax your intestines by drinking peppermint, chamomile, or ginger tea (*see page 137*) after eating.

Flower remedies The process of choosing appropriate Bach flower remedies (*see page 138*) helps you identify any difficult feelings and find ways of dealing with them.

Hydrotherapy Take a daily hot sitz bath (*see page 130*) to ease painful spasms.

✚ WHAT ELSE DOCTORS MAY SUGGEST

It's important to exclude other causes of pain (such as lactose intolerance, *see page 164*; pelvic inflammatory disease, *see page 188*; and endometriosis, *see page 189*). Once IBS is confirmed, discuss drugs or other treatments. Some people with IBS benefit from acupuncture.

Warning: See your doctor if your pain is unusual, or you pass blood.

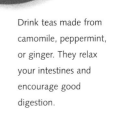

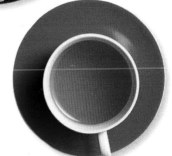

Drink teas made from camomile, peppermint, or ginger. They relax your intestines and encourage good digestion.

CONSTIPATION

❓ WHAT IT IS AND WHAT CAUSES IT

Being constipated means having hard, dryish, difficult-to-pass stools. The Pill and pregnancy (*see page 81*) encourage constipation, as do depression (*see page 202*) and anorexia nervosa (*see page 205*).

❋ TREATMENT

Do daily exercise and pelvic floor exercises (*see page 136*). Use effective stress management. Make a regular time to open your bowels when you won't be rushed. And don't put off going to the lavatory when you first need to go.
Food and drink Drink plenty of water, and see whether eating more high-fiber food helps.

A daily relaxing stomach massage can help alleviate constipation. If symptoms persist, consult your doctor before taking any laxative medicines.

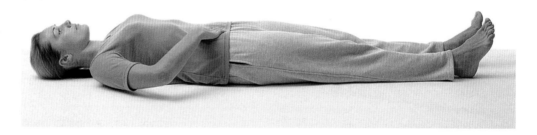

Massage and aromatherapy Give yourself a gentle abdominal massage twice daily. Lie down, relax, and move your hand slowly in large clockwise circles around your abdomen for five minutes. Lubricate your skin with a relaxing essential oil if desired (*see page 133*).
Hydrotherapy and herbal remedies Experiment with a daily sitz bath (*see page 130*) with tepid water containing a pint of chamomile, dandelion, or fennel tea (*see page 137*) in the main bathtub, and cold water in the foot bath.

✚ WHAT ELSE DOCTORS MAY SUGGEST

Your doctor may recommend a simple laxative, such as lactulose, for temporary use, and assess whether other symptoms or a sudden change in the way you open your bowels suggests another problem, such as irritable bowel syndrome (*see page 161*), hemorrhoids, an anal fissure, diverticulitis, endometriosis (*see page 191*), or cancer of the ovary, womb, or bowel (*see pages 208–209*).

GAS

❓ WHAT IT IS AND WHAT CAUSES IT

Burping results from swallowing air while eating quickly, drinking or talking a lot with meals, having carbonated drinks, chewing gum, smoking, or feeling stressed. A rumbling stomach is associated with vigorous intestinal contractions from hunger, anxiety or fear, irritable bowel syndrome (*see page 161*), or certain other illnesses. Abdominal distension (bloating) may be caused by eating a fat rich meal or a lot of high-fiber foods, or by irritable bowel syndrome. We normally pass flatus between 3 and 40 times a day (with an average of 15 times). Flatus arises from the bacterial fermentation of carbohydrate residues in the bowel. It is encouraged by high-fiber foods, cabbage- and onion-family foods, some seeds, and sorbitol (a sweetener in sugar-free chewing gum). It can also result from an intolerance to gluten (a protein in wheat, barley, oats, and rye) and can be a symptom of certain other bowel diseases.

❋ TREATMENT

Stress management Reduce stress-induced belching and stomach rumbling by using more effective stress-management strategies such as breathing exercises (*see page 141*).
Food and drink Relax during mealtimes and avoid eating quickly or talking or drinking too much during a meal. If you are troubled by smelly flatus, try avoiding garlic, onions, spices, fennel, beer, white wine, and fruit juice.

✚ WHAT ELSE DOCTORS MAY SUGGEST

Your doctor can help by assessing whether any underlying problem is likely.

GASTROENTERITIS

❓ WHAT IT IS AND WHAT CAUSES IT

The most likely reason for a surprise attack of gastroenteritis (diarrhea and vomiting due to inflammation of the lining of the stomach and intestines) is irritation from certain microorganisms or their toxins. The usual cause is infected food or drink. Food poisoning resulting from bacterial toxins begins 6–12 hours later; symptoms from infection with Salmonella, typhoid, or dysentery bacteria, or rotaviruses start after 12–48 hours.

Other causes of diarrhea and vomiting include anxiety; antibiotics and some other medications; spicy food; alcohol; sugary drinks; the sweetener sorbitol; and food sensitivity. Repeated attacks of diarrhea may be due to irritable bowel syndrome (*see page 161*), inflammatory bowel disease (ulcerative colitis or Crohn's disease), diverticular disease, an overactive thyroid (*see page 181*), and bowel cancer.

✳ TREATMENT

Rest if you feel weak. Prevent infection spreading by washing your hands well after using the lavatory, keeping towels to yourself, and washing crockery and cutlery in very hot water. Wash sponges and dishtowels well each day in hot water (70°C), or soak in bleach, and dry thoroughly before reusing. Alternatively, microwave on high for 60 seconds or pop them in the dishwasher along with the dishes. Consider using paper towels instead.

Warning: You may need to take extra precautions if you're on the Pill (*see page 71*).

Food and drink Drink water, fruit juice, weak tea, or vegetable broth to replace your fluid losses. If diarrhea lasts for more than one day, have drinks made with oral rehydration salts from a drugstore. These provide energy-giving glucose, replace minerals, and correct your body's acidity balance. Alternatively, make your own rehydrating drink with one level teaspoon of table salt and eight level teaspoons of sugar in one liter (2 pints) of water. Take half a liter every hour. Keep eating, if possible: choose easily digested foods such as stewed apple, a ripe banana, and brown rice, and have some live yogurt each day to help restore a normal balance of your bowel bacteria. Boost your immunity with the vitamin C and flavonoids found in blackcurrants or blueberries.

If necessary, calm your bowel with fennel tea (made from an ounce of crushed seeds, boiled with one pint of water in a covered pan for ten minutes, strained and cooled); or loperamide (Imodium, from a drugstore).

Food supplements

◆ A daily multivitamin and mineral supplement to help replace lost nutrients.

◆ *Lactobacillus acidophilus* – for a daily dose of helpful bowel bacteria, until a healthy population of bowel microorganisms re-establishes itself naturally within a few days or weeks

◆ Grapefruit seed extract – for natural antibiotics to help kill infecting organisms

✚ WHAT ELSE DOCTORS MAY SUGGEST

Contact your doctor if you can't keep fluids down, or if you have severe diarrhea for 48 hours (12 if very young, elderly or weak), or mild diarrhea for 72 hours (24 hours if very young, elderly, or weak); repeated vomiting; or blood in your feces. You may need intravenous fluids, and antibiotics.

When you feel like eating again, try the BRA diet: banana, rice, and apple.

Drink plenty of fluids, especially when you are still experiencing vomiting and diarrhea.

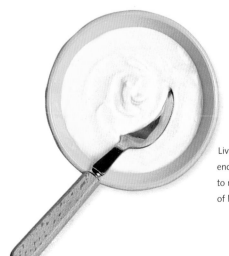

Live yogurt will encourage your bowel to re-establish its levels of helpful bacteria.

163

FOOD SENSITIVITY

❓ WHAT IT IS AND WHAT CAUSES IT

Certain reactions to food are known as food sensitivities. Non-allergic reactions have many triggers. These include the lack of a digestive enzyme; toxins, irritants, additives, or certain other substances; and foods that provoke a slow-onset immune response (thought to result from immunoglobulin G – IgG – antibodies). A slow-onset immune response isn't an allergy, though it's often wrongly referred to as one.

Non-allergic food reactions are common and can cause many symptoms. These include vomiting, diarrhea, stomachache, bloating, gas, joint pain, rashes, headache, fatigue, cough, runny nose, seizures, irregular periods, miscarriage, infertility, depression, nerve disorders, epilepsy, osteoporosis, blisters, mouth ulcers, pitted, discolored tooth enamel, and even cancer.

Lactose intolerance, due to a lack of the enzyme lactase, means that drinking more than a little milk – which contains lactose (milk sugar) – causes nausea, bloating, stomachache and diarrhea.

Slow-onset immune reactions include gluten intolerance, due to a sensitivity to a substance called gliadin in gluten (a protein in wheat, barley, rye, and oats). This means the person produces anti-gliadin antibodies after eating gluten-containing food. These antibodies can damage the bowel, leading to celiac disease (diarrhea, stomachache, gas, and weight loss). They can also enter the blood and be deposited elsewhere in the body, causing irregular periods, miscarriage, infertility, depression, nerve disorders, seizures, osteoporosis, blisters, mouth ulcers, or pitted, discolored teeth. Anti-gliadin antibodies are particularly likely in people with insulin-dependent diabetes, thyroid inflammation, patchy hair loss, lupus (an autoimmune condition leading to arthritis, rashes, and other problems), inflamed kidneys (glomerulonephritis), Sjögren's syndrome (dry mouth, eyes, and vagina) and Down's syndrome.

Foods which commonly cause sensitivity include eggs, wheat, nuts, milk, and strawberries.

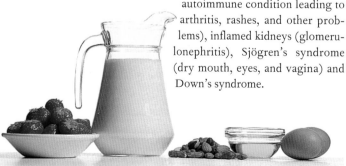

Allergic reactions are caused by a tiny amount of a food that provokes a rapid immune response (by IgE antibodies). The commonest allergens are eggs, fish, shellfish, wheat, milk, nuts and nut oils, seeds, and strawberries. Food allergy can cause urticaria, asthma, hay fever, migraine, vomiting, diarrhea, and, at worst, a potentially fatal reaction.

The following factors encourage immune reactions (both slow-onset and allergic):
◆ A family history of allergy.
◆ Bottle-feeding in the first four to six months.
◆ A damaged ("leaky") gut that allows poorly digested food particles to enter the blood.

❄ TREATMENT

Food and drink Eat more foods rich in immunity-enhancing beta carotene, vitamins C and E, selenium, and zinc, and have a good balance of essential fats (*see page 25*). Eat smaller amounts of the problem food, eat it less frequently, or – for a food allergy – avoid it completely. If you have celiac disease you must always avoid gluten even if symptom-free; otherwise certain cancers become more likely.

Food supplements
◆ A daily multivitamin and mineral supplement.
◆ Vitamin C plus flavonoids.
◆ Acid (betaine hydrochloride) and digestive enzymes with main meals for a three-week trial.
◆ *Lactobacillus acidophilus* – for a three-week trial.
◆ Lactase added to milk to predigest its lactose – if you have lactose intolerance.

✚ WHAT ELSE DOCTORS MAY SUGGEST

A food-elimination and multiple challenge diet will identify most food sensitivities. Avoid suspected foods one by one for up to three weeks each. If the symptoms settle, try the food again. If the symptoms return, stop the food. Repeat this challenge twice, with a week between the end of one and the beginning of another.

If necessary, your doctor will test for lactose or gluten intolerance, or refer you to an allergist for skin-prick or blood tests. Blood tests for non-allergic immune reactions are often not reliable.

Warning: Get urgent medical attention for throat and tongue swelling, wheezing, chest pain, or shock. Carry a shot of adrenaline in the future.

OBESITY

❓ WHAT IT IS AND WHAT CAUSES IT

Being either overweight or obese (*see page 27*) encourages illness. Simply losing weight isn't usually too difficult. The problem is keeping weight off. Many women who do this time and again testify to the discipline and self-denial of each new slimming diet and the disappointment or despair as the pounds pile back on. Ninety-five percent of slimmers regain their lost weight within a year.

Clearly the secret of successful weight management lies in using the following ways of becoming part of the elite five percent who remain slim.

✳ TREATMENT

Exercise Take a daily half-hour of aerobic exercise to feel more in shape and brighter and to burn more calories. Also, move your body more during your daily activities.

Looking after yourself and managing stress Look after yourself so that your body receives a healthy mix of exercise, stress relief, and food. Use a diary to plan physical activity, relaxation and other stress management, and your meals each day. Think of yourself as someone precious who deserves time spent on her care. If comfort eating is a problem, write a list of things you can do instead of reaching for food, and keep this handy at all times. (*See also page 66.*)

Flower essences The process of choosing appropriate flower essences (*see page 138*) may help you to recognize and deal with any underlying emotions that trigger comfort eating.

Food and drink Eat regularly, so you don't get so hungry that you stuff yourself with easy-to-prepare junk food. Permanently change the way you eat, so instead of having to lose a lot of weight every few months or years, you eat healthily all the time. Many people who successfully maintain a healthy weight shed unwanted pounds early, before they mount up and cause a problem that is much harder to shift.

Eat more low-calorie food, especially vegetables and fruit, and less high-calorie food. Choose highly nutritious foods rather than "junk foods" which have a lot of calories, and refined carbohydrates and animal fats, but few other nutrients. Don't eat too little fat, as this could lower your cholesterol level too far and encourage depression and hormone imbalance. As you lose weight, make sure you eat plenty of foods rich in antioxidants to counteract the effects of toxins that are released as stored fat breaks down.

Aim for an average loss of one to two pounds a week. You may lose more in the first week, or after a period starts, because of fluid loss. But if you lose any more on a regular basis, you'll lose nutrients as well as fat.

Make sure you drink enough. Being even slightly dehydrated can reduce your body's metabolic rate and make you burn fewer calories.

Food supplements

◆ A multivitamin and mineral supplement.

Massage and aromatherapy Each day do three minutes of skin brushing over any cellulite (dimpled fat on hips, thighs, and upper arms) to boost the circulation. Alternatively, massage with firm strokes plus light patting, lubricating with sage, rosemary, juniper, grapefruit, celery seed, fennel, geranium, or lime oil. (*Warning*: Don't expose your skin to sunlight after applying any citrus oil.)

Hydrotherapy Work over fatty areas with a loofah or bath-brush in the bathtub as an alternative to dry skin brushing (above). And experiment with the circulation-boosting effects of a daily contrast sitz bath (*see page 130*).

✚ WHAT ELSE DOCTORS MAY SUGGEST

Orlistat is a drug that reduces fat absorption but is suitable only for obese people on a low-fat slimming diet. Side effects include gas and diarrhea.

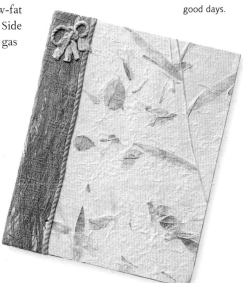

Keep a note of things you can do instead of eating. Record times when you feel particularly tempted, as well as noting down tips from your good days.

HAY FEVER

❓ WHAT IT IS AND WHAT CAUSES IT

Hay fever (seasonal allergic rhinitis) is an allergy to one or more types of pollen. This triggers sneezing, itchy, red, streaming eyes, and swollen eyelids. Tree pollens can be to blame in early spring. Grasses and weeds are the main cause in summer; later the culprits are other plants that continue shedding pollen into the fall. Just a few grains in the eyes or nose trigger the production of pollen antibodies. These, in turn, trigger the release of an irritating substance called histamine.

❄ TREATMENT

Pollen avoidance Keep windows closed, especially at night; close car windows and ventilators too. Damp-dust surfaces and mop floors indoors, and buy an ionizer to clear pollen from the air. Use the pollen count as a guide to planning activities: hot, breezy, sunny mornings and late afternoons are the worst. Stay away from smoky rooms and city centers, as polluted air traps pollen. Don't rub your eyes, and trap pollen with petroleum jelly smeared around your nostrils. Avoid weedy and grassy places and get someone else to cut the lawn. Wear wraparound sunglasses or a cyclist's face mask. When you come indoors, put on clean clothes, splash your face and eyes with cold water, or bathe with salty water. Launder clothing frequently and dry your clothes indoors. Shower and shampoo before bedtime.

Food and drink Eat foods rich in natural antihistamines, anti-inflammatory agents, and immunity-boosting agents, such as beta carotene, vitamins B5, B6, C, and E, selenium, zinc, and flavonoids. Onions and red wine contain a particularly useful flavonoid called quercetin that acts as an antioxidant and a natural antihistamine. Buckwheat contains another strong antioxidant called rutin. Some people benefit from two daily teaspoonfuls of locally produced, non-heat-treated honeycomb (including the wax that caps each cell) for two months before they expect hay fever. This may act as a natural vaccine by encouraging resistance to the local pollens that get trapped from the bees' legs in the sticky honeycomb. The best source is a local beekeeper.

Food supplements
◆ Vitamin B.
◆ Vitamin C.
◆ Quercetin, rutin, or proanthocyanidins.

Acupressure Press lightly with your index finger for one minute on the depression beneath your cheekbone by the side of your nose. Repeat on the other side.

Herbal remedies Drink a cup of nettle, elderflower, or thyme tea two or three times a day, or take regular doses of herbal Pollinosan tablets (*see Bioforce, page 219*).

Homeopathy Experiment to see whether a mixed pollen remedy helps prevent symptoms.

Light therapy Researchers report that bathing the eyes and nostrils with red light reduces symptoms in seven out of ten people. Experiment by placing a red gel sheet safely in front of a light bulb, and sitting with your face one foot away from it for ten minutes twice a day.

✚ WHAT ELSE DOCTORS AND PHARMACISTS MAY SUGGEST

Antihistamine, steroid, or other anti-inflammatory medications can help. Many are available without prescription, and some are best begun before you expect hay fever. Immunotherapy is a newly improved method of desensitizing people by injecting gradually increasing concentrations of pollen beneath the skin. It is safest done in hospital.

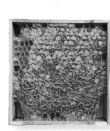

Honeycomb can act as a natural vaccine against an allergic reaction to pollen.

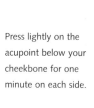

Press lightly on the acupoint below your cheekbone for one minute on each side.

ASTHMA

? WHAT IT IS AND WHAT CAUSES IT

Asthma is an oversensitivity of the lungs' airways that makes them tighten in response to certain triggers. This causes a cough, and also wheezing, which reduces the airflow in and out of the lungs – in some people to a dangerous degree. In childhood, boys are more likely to suffer than girls but the numbers equalize in the teens, and from the ages of 20 to 50 women are more asthma-prone than men, partly because of hormone changes during periods and pregnancy. In pregnancy asthma improves in one woman in three, stays the same in another one, and worsens in the remaining one. Asthma is more likely if a woman is expecting a girl. Asthma may temporarily worsen around the menopause. Only a few women have their first attack in later life.

There are several types of asthma. One, allergic asthma, is most common in people with a family history of eczema, hay fever, or asthma. Common triggers of allergic asthma include dust mite droppings, pollens, pet dander, molds, certain foods, and food mites.

Asthma can also result from: infection; irritation by cigarette smoke, vehicle-exhaust emissions, nitrogen dioxide in burned gas fumes from poorly maintained gas cookers, perfume, chemicals in new clothes, paint, glue, shoe waterproofing or conditioning spray; drugs such as aspirin; stress; cold air; a sudden fall in atmospheric pressure; thunderstorms; and exercise.

❋ TREATMENT

Avoiding triggers Identify and avoid your asthma triggers if possible.

Food and drink Eat more foods rich in essential fats, beta carotene, vitamins B5, B6, C, and E, magnesium, selenium, and zinc. These help guard against allergy and other inflammation. Include plenty of dark red or blue berries and other brightly colored fruits and vegetables (for their antioxidant proanthocyanidins), and onions (which contain quercetin, a natural antihistamine). Remember to have three helpings of oily fish a week.

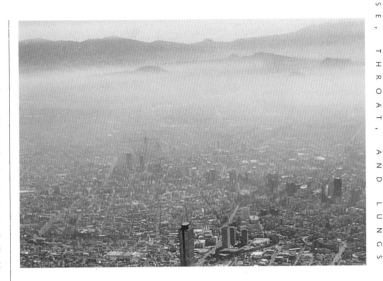

Listen to the pollution forecast and stay in, if you can, on particularly bad days. If you must go out, wear a cycling mask or respirator.

Food supplements
- Magnesium and selenium.
- Vitamin C with flavonoids.
- Vitamin E.
- Quercetin or proanthocyanidins.
- Fish oil.

Breathing exercises Avoiding hyperventilating (*see page 13*) in response to stress. A small Australian study found that three months of controlled Buteyko breathing (*see page 141*) reduced reliever-drug use by 90 percent of trialists and halved the use of "preventer" steroids (*see below*).

✚ WHAT ELSE DOCTORS MAY SUGGEST

A "reliever" inhaler containing a bronchodilator drug (which widens the airways) can be used on an occasional basis for mild symptoms. For more severe asthma a doctor may suggest adding daily treatment with a "preventer" inhaler of steroids or other anti-inflammatory drugs. Such drugs can, however, have side effects; for example, prolonged steroid treatment can lead to osteoporosis (*see page 179*), so it's worth keeping the steroid dose as low as possible, or using alternative drugs if necessary. Skin tests to identify allergy triggers (such as pollen, cat fur, and dust mite droppings) allow you to try to avoid them. Also, if you have severe asthma, you can then discuss whether to have immunotherapy (immunization by injecting gradually increased concentrations of the trigger beneath the skin).

LEFT: Blueberries contain antioxidants called proanthocyanidins which help protect against the allergic reactions associated with asthma.

COLDS AND FLU

❓ WHAT THEY ARE AND WHAT CAUSES THEM

Colds and flu are viral infections caught from the fine spray of saliva that accompanies coughs, sneezes, kisses, laughter, and conversation. You're most likely to be infected if a new viral strain is circulating, if you're very young or old, or if your resistance is poor. There's usually no mistaking a cold for flu. Both can cause similar symptoms but flu is very much more severe and means you have to go to bed. A bad cold can cause an itchy nose, sneezing, and catarrh; a sore throat and cough; aching muscles; and a headache. Flu causes all these, but also causes muscle tenderness, sensitive skin, loss of appetite, painful eyes which hurt to move, irritation by light and noise, slowed reactions, weakness, and exhaustion. Both can last for up to a week. Some people feel weak, tired, and depressed for several weeks after flu.

✳️ TREATMENT

Rest, if necessary. Smear petroleum jelly around your nostrils to prevent soreness.

Food and drink Have more drinks, including homemade lemonade (pour boiling water over a finely sliced lemon and sweeten with honey). Include garlic, leeks, and onions in your diet for their quercetin, which fights infection. Homemade chicken soup is a traditional remedy: boil a chicken for an hour in water containing diced carrots, celery, and onions, and a handful of lentils; remove the chicken, liquidize the soup – and enjoy.

Similarly, homemade soup is an excellent comfort food. Onions and leeks are particularly effective against colds.

Food supplements

◆ Vitamin C (1,000mg two or three times daily) with flavonoids.

◆ Zinc lozenges sucked at the first signs of infection to help prevent the viruses from multiplying.

Hydrotherapy and aromatherapy Have twice-daily steam inhalations (*see page 130*) to loosen your catarrh, reduce congestion, and kill viruses. Add three drops of tea tree oil to the bowl of water to help kill viruses, and two teaspoons of menthol and eucalyptus inhalation mixture to ease breathing. Ease breathing at other times by inhaling the vapor from a few drops of eucalyptus oil on a kleenex.

Herbal remedies Take twice-daily doses of extract of elderberries (from the black elder tree, *Sambucus nigra*), or echinacea (purple coneflower) tincture; flavonoids and other substances in these reduce viral multiplication. Drink a cup of ginger and coriander tea (*see page 137*) twice a day.

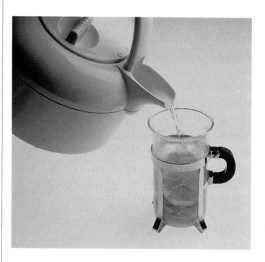

➕ WHAT ELSE DOCTORS MAY SUGGEST

If you are elderly, or have a condition that makes regular immunization advisable (*see below*), see your doctor right away because an antiviral drug, such as amantadine or zanamivir may prevent complications. Otherwise, see the doctor if you are no better after a week or become seriously ill; have chest pain, breathlessness or a stiff neck; or cough up blood or lots of colored phlegm. Antibiotics and other treatments may be necessary.

Regular flu vaccination is recommended for anyone with long-term heart, lung, liver, or kidney disease; diabetes; sickle cell disease; on steroids or immunosuppressant drugs; with no spleen; in a residential care or nursing home; or working in such a home or in a hospital or doctor's office.

EARACHE

❓ WHAT IT IS AND WHAT CAUSES IT

Pain in the ear can stem from the outer ear (the part you can see), the middle ear (the bone-surrounded space that passes sounds as vibrations from the eardrum to the inner ear), or more distant structures such as a tooth, the throat or even the neck muscles. The most usual cause, especially in children, is inflammation of the lining of the eustachian tube and middle ear caused by an allergy or infection. An allergy may be associated with a tendency to have hay fever (*see page 166*) or asthma (*see page 167*). An infection may be part of a cold (*see facing page*) or sore throat (*see below*), or may occur for no apparent reason.

❋ TREATMENT

The treatments below are for an infection.

Pain relief Lie on your side with the bad ear uppermost to encourage drainage of inflammatory fluid down the eustachian tube into the throat. Place a covered hot-water bottle or microwaveable or other hot pack over the ear.

Food and drink Drink plenty of water, and eat foods rich in natural anti-inflammatory agents, including beta carotene, vitamins C and E, flavonoids, selenium, and zinc.

Food supplements

◆ Vitamins B5 and 6, C and E.
◆ Flavonoids.
◆ Selenium.
◆ Zinc.

✚ WHAT ELSE DOCTORS MAY SUGGEST

Your doctor may recommend antibiotics for a middle-ear infection. It's widely considered best to do this only if the symptoms are severe.

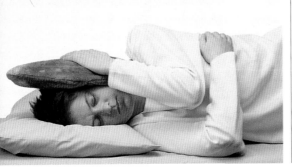

SORE THROAT AND LARYNGITIS

❓ WHAT IT IS AND WHAT CAUSES IT

A sore throat means the throat lining is inflamed; laryngitis means the voice box and vocal cords are inflamed. These conditions usually result from a viral (or, less often, bacterial) infection; allergy; or irritation by inhaled chemicals, hot dry air, or overuse of the voice.

❋ TREATMENT

If you also have a cold, *see facing page*. If you also have hay fever, *see page 166.*

General throat care Buy a new toothbrush, as germs in old bristles sometimes encourage infection. Don't smoke, and avoid breathing smoky air or air polluted by vehicle-exhaust emissions. Keep your throat warm; a red scarf is said to be better than one of another color. If you have laryngitis, rest your voice as much as possible, because speaking – even whispering – vibrates inflamed vocal cords and hinders healing.

Hydrotherapy and herbal remedies Dissolve a teaspoonful of salt in a glass of hot water, cool, then gargle with it twice a day. Wrap a hot sage compress (*see page 130*); around your throat, cover with a thick towel, and relax. Moisten the air you breathe with an electric humidifer, a kettle boiling safely, or bowls of water near radiators. Dry air irritates an inflamed throat or larynx.

✚ WHAT ELSE DOCTORS MAY SUGGEST

Persistent symptoms may benefit from antibiotics or anti-allergy medication. Seek medical help if hoarseness persists for more than two weeks.

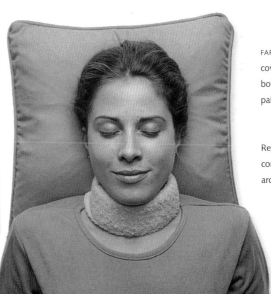

FAR LEFT: Lie with a covered hot-water bottle on the painful ear.

Relax with a sage compress wrapped around your throat.

SORE EYES

⚫ WHAT CAUSES THEM

Sore eyes often result from conjunctivitis – inflammation of the membrane that covers the eyes and lines the lids. Affected eyes look pink, feel gritty, and may itch and have a sticky yellow discharge. Causes include infection and allergy, for example to make-up or pollen (*see page 166*). Tiny airborne particles can irritate eyes and dryness (*see facing page*) sometimes makes them sore.

✽ TREATMENT

Wash your hands after touching infected eyes. Keep washcloths and towels to yourself and launder washcloths, towels, and pillowcases daily at as high a temperature as possible.
Herbal remedies Bathe your eyes with tea made from eyebright (*Euphrasia*), calendula, or chamomile (*see page 137*) twice daily to counteract soreness and infection. Alternatively, ease itching and inflammation with an apple poultice, made by grating a peeled apple, lying down, covering your closed eyes with the apple, and placing a damp cloth on top. Relax for half an hour before removing the poultice.
Food Eat foods rich in beta carotene, vitamins B, C, and E, and zinc to counteract infection and inflammation.

✚ WHAT ELSE DOCTORS MAY SUGGEST

Seek medical help if the soreness lasts for more than two days, if you have a fever or discharge, eye pain or blurred sight, or if you see haloes around things. You may need antibiotics, antiviral therapy, or other treatment.

Relaxing for half an hour with an apple poultice on sore eyes can ease itching and reduce inflammation.

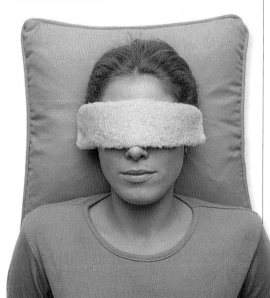

AMD

⚫ WHAT IT IS AND WHAT CAUSES IT

Age-related macular degeneration (AMD) affects the macula of the eye, a small area in the middle of the retina responsible for seeing fine detail in the center of the visual field. It's more frequent in women, and the commonest cause of blindness in developed countries. Studies show it's encouraged by oxidation by free radicals induced, for example, by too much UV exposure, or by smoking. Smoking 20–25 cigarettes a day more than doubles the risk. It takes up to 15 years for a reformed smoker's risk to fall to that of a non-smoker.

✽ TREATMENT

All you can do is prevent further damage. So stop smoking at once (*see page 37*), with help if necessary, and counteract UV rays in bright sunlight by wearing sunglasses.

Protect your eyes by wearing dark sunglasses and boosting your intake of beta carotene.

Food and drink Eat more foods rich in the antioxidants beta carotene, vitamins C and E, and selenium. Include tomatoes in your diet for their antioxidant carotenoid called lycopene; cooking tomatoes in a little fat releases more lycopene. Also eat egg yolks, corn, red grapes, pumpkin, and orange bell peppers (for other important carotenoids called lutein and zeaxanthin).
Food supplements
◆ Beta carotene and vitamins C and E.
◆ Selenium.
◆ Lutein.

✚ WHAT ELSE DOCTORS MAY SUGGEST

Only a very few people can hope for improvement after laser treatment. However, surgeons now report some success with macular translocation, a new operation that doctors think can restore a healthy retina in one affected person in ten.

DRY EYES

❓ WHAT THEY ARE AND WHAT CAUSES THEM

Several things dry up tear fluid. One is not blinking often enough, especially in a hot, dry environment. This can happen while reading, watching TV, or working at a computer. Dry "computer eyes" are encouraged by the screen's electromagnetic field. This creates electrically charged particles (positive ions) that latch on to floating dust which is then attracted to the eyes. Dry eyes can also result from aging, photo-aging, and auto-immune illness (in which immune cells mistakenly attack mucus-producing cells) such as rheumatoid arthritis and Sjögren's syndrome.

✺ TREATMENT

Avoid smoking and breathing smoky air.
Exercises Moisten eyes with daily Bates exercises (*see page 136*): palm for a minute every half-hour, blink frequently, and do ten long blinks each half-hour.
Food and drink Eat more foods rich in essential fats and vitamin A (to protect against free-radical damage and to nourish your eyes).
Hydrotherapy and herbal remedies Twice daily, remove charged dust by splashing your eyes with water or eyebright (*Euphrasia*), or cold chamomile, calendula, or elderflower tea (*see page 137*). Alternatively, soak two cotton pads in this tea, place over closed eyes, and rest for ten minutes to soothe and nourish.

✚ WHAT ELSE DOCTORS MAY SUGGEST

Eye-drops can help if necessary.

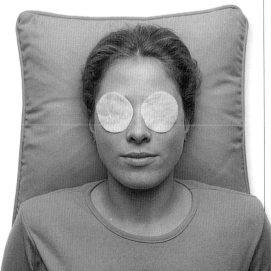

CATARACTS

❓ WHAT THEY ARE AND WHAT CAUSES THEM

A cataract is a clouding of the eye's lens – the flattened sphere behind the iris that helps focus light. This makes things look fuzzy, like looking through a waterfall. To an observer a severe cataract looks like a whitish tinge in the eye's dark center. One in every two of the world's 40 million blind people has cataracts (most of those in developing countries because of infection, see below), and many over-65s have them to some degree. Triggers include a high sugar level from poorly controlled diabetes (*see page 180*), high blood pressure (*see page 176*), free-radical damage from smoking (and, perhaps, UV light), injury, infection, and certain drugs (such as inhaled steroids).

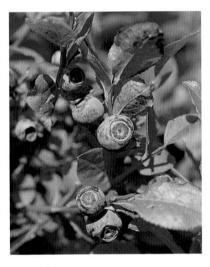

✺ TREATMENT

Avoid smoking and smoky or vehicle-exhaust polluted environments.
Food and drink Nourish eyes and counteract free-radical damage with foods rich in vitamins B2, C, E, flavonoids, carotenes (in orange, yellow, and dark green vegetables), and salicylates. Flavonoids that are particularly eye-friendly include proanthocyanidins (in blue and black berries) and quercetin (in onions and tea).
Food supplements
◆ Vitamins C and E.
◆ Quercetin.
Herbal remedies Take bilberry extract twice a day.

✚ WHAT ELSE DOCTORS MAY SUGGEST

Cataract removal is successful and quick. A surgeon makes a tiny cut, breaks up the inside of the lens with ultrasound, then removes this material and substitutes an artificial lens.

The operation is often done under local anesthetic and needs no stitches.

Bilberries contain proanthocyanidins, substances that can reduce the harmful effects of smoking and UV light.

Make some chamomile tea and allow it to cool. Soak two cotton pads in the liquid and place on your eyes for ten minutes.

ANEMIA

❓ WHAT IT IS AND WHAT CAUSES IT

There are several different types of anemia, but iron-deficiency anemia is the commonest. As many as one woman in 25 is short of iron and some children are anemic too. We need iron to make hemoglobin, the red pigment in red blood cells that transports oxygen and carbon dioxide around the body. Mild anemia causes few, if any, problems, so it's often unrecognized until someone has a routine blood test. However, severe anemia can make a person tired, pale, and even breathless on exertion. She may have a sore tongue and soreness of the corners of the mouth. Her nails may be thin and brittle, without the normal side-to-side convexity. She may also notice that her periods are heavier than normal.

Common causes include a diet lacking in iron, and a reduced absorption of iron. The lack of iron sometimes results from unusual bleeding due, for example, to heavy periods or continued low-level blood loss from the gut (perhaps from an irritated intestinal lining such as with gluten intolerance; *see page 164*). The effect on periods means there's a vicious cycle. Anemia causes heavy periods that, in turn, worsen the anemia. Poor digestion and absorption of iron can be caused by stress. Rapid growth may be responsible for anemia in children.

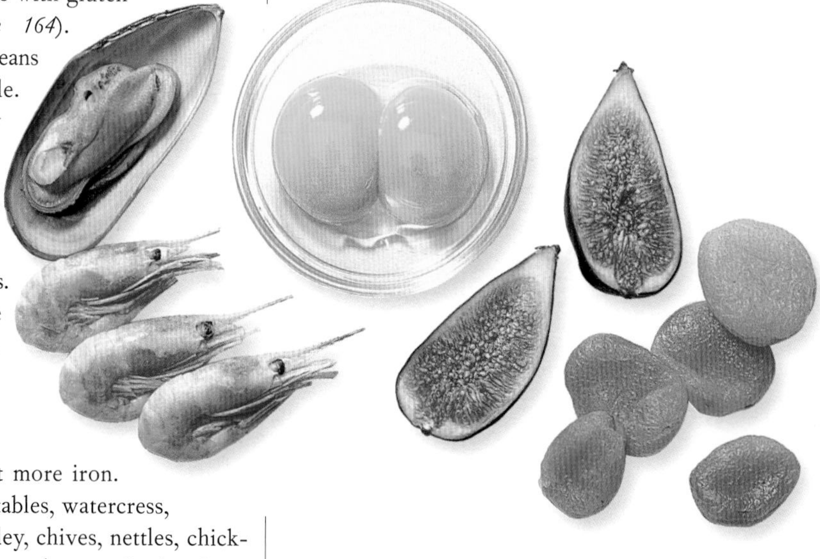

Copper is needed for the proper absorption of iron into your body. Add shellfish, egg yolks, figs, and apricots to your diet.

�֍ TREATMENT

Food and drink Eat more iron. Dark green leafy vegetables, watercress, and herbs such as parsley, chives, nettles, chickweed, and dandelion leaves also contain vitamin C, which aids iron absorption. Copper-containing foods (cheese, egg yolk, seafood, liver, green vegetables, apricots, cherries, and figs) do the same. Avoid coffee, tea, cola, and alcohol with meals, as they reduce iron absorption. Instead, drink vitamin C-rich orange juice. Consider cooking in stainless steel or non-enamel-coated cast-iron pans to raise your iron intake.

Stress management Use effective strategies to make mealtimes more relaxed occasions.

Light and color therapy Some color therapists believe that people with iron-deficiency anemia benefit from red light on their legs, and orange light on their spleen (in the left upper abdomen). They also recommend breathing red light. They claim that this breaks down iron salts, releasing ferric ions that are more easily used to make hemoglobin. This sounds interesting but as yet there is little or no scientific evidence to support such claims.

However, you will lose nothing by getting more exposure to sunlight (taking care not to burn), or even bathing in red light (from a red light bulb, or a bulb shielded with a red gel sheet) for half an hour each day.

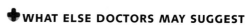

✚ WHAT ELSE DOCTORS MAY SUGGEST

Your doctor will work with you to discover and treat the cause. You may benefit from iron-containing medicine. Some formulations are better tolerated than others, so if yours causes any problems (such as stomach upsets or constipation), tell your doctor.

VARICOSE VEINS

❂ WHAT THEY ARE AND WHAT CAUSES THEM

Lumpy, bumpy varicose (permanently distended) veins can lead to aching, throbbing, ankle swelling, night cramps, and restless legs. They sometimes become inflamed, causing phlebitis (*see page 174*). Any back-pressure on the blood as it travels from the legs to the heart can weaken the veins' valves. This allows blood to pool in the veins by stretching their thin, elastic walls. Constantly, or repeatedly stretched, veins eventually become varicose. The pressure may come from sitting for long periods, especially with legs crossed, from being pregnant, from constipation, or from obesity. Other causes include a poor diet; high levels of certain hormones during pregnancy, before a period, or around the menopause; standing still for a long time; and a family history of varicose veins.

❂ TREATMENT

Exercise and posture Make a daily half-hour of aerobic exercise a priority. When standing, tighten and relax your calf muscles frequently. When sitting down check that the edge of your chair does not cut into the backs of your thighs; and don't cross your legs. Rest tired legs by sitting or lying with your feet above hip level. Slow down gradually after aerobic exercise to avoid blood pooling in your leg veins.

Food and drink Try to lose excess weight. Eat more foods rich in essential fats and have at least five daily helpings of fruit and vegetables to provide vitamins C and E, silica, and flavonoid plant pigments to help keep vein walls strong and flexible. Eat berries, cherries, and black grapes (rich in jewel-colored proanthocyanidins); buckwheat (rich in an antioxidant called rutin) and onions and, in moderation, red wine (rich in vein-strengthening quercetin).

Food supplements

◆ Vitamin C.
◆ Proanthocyanidins.
◆ Quercetin.
◆ Rutin.
◆ Silica.

Hydrotherapy Soothe aching veins by putting your legs up and covering the veins with a cold compress (*see page 130*) twice a day.

Herbal remedies Add four drops of marigold (*Calendula*) tincture to a tablespoonful of witch-hazel, and smooth over aching veins at the end of the day. A daily dose of tincture made from the nuts or bark of the horse-chestnut (*Aesculus*) tree is as likely to reduce leg swelling as elastic stockings (*see below*); take 20 drops in water once or twice daily after meals.

Daily supplements of butcher's broom (*Ruscus aculeatus*) and ginkgo may also help.

Aromatherapy Each day put your feet up and soothe your legs with upward strokes, lubricating with a mixture made from two teaspoonfuls of sweet almond oil, two drops of wheatgerm oil and four each of parsley and cypress oils. (*Warning*: Avoid cypress oil if you know you are, or might become, pregnant.)

✚ WHAT ELSE DOCTORS MAY SUGGEST

Elastic support stockings relieve symptoms by compressing the veins. If necessary, injections of sclerosing fluid make the vein walls stick together, or, as a final option, an operation can remove varicose veins completely.

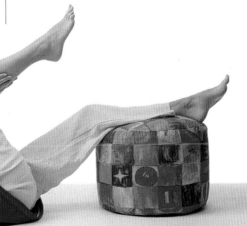

Encourage the return of blood to your heart by sitting with your feet raised if you have been standing all day.

173

THROMBO-PHLEBITIS

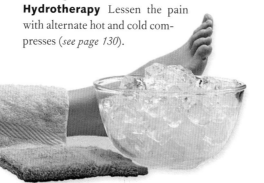

Wear gloves outside in cold weather and consider wearing fingerless mittens if you need your fingers free.

❓ WHAT IT IS AND WHAT CAUSES IT

Phlebitis (superficial thrombophlebitis) is inflammation of part of a vein beneath the skin that makes the blood inside form a clot (thrombus). The vein becomes hard, swollen, and tender and the overlying skin red, itchy, and – after repeated attacks – discolored. The problem is most common in people with varicose veins (*see page 173*) and is especially likely after sitting more than usual, for example, on a long journey. A knock or other injury can also set it off, as can, occasionally, an intravenous drip, varicose vein injections, and the contraceptive Pill.

✳ TREATMENT

The inflamed vein usually improves spontaneously within seven to ten days. Use the treatment plan outlined for varicose veins in addition to the following therapies.

Exercise and rest Take daily exercise. Have frequent exercise breaks if you have to sit down on long journeys. And put your affected leg up as much as possible.

Hydrotherapy Lessen the pain with alternate hot and cold compresses (*see page 130*).

Support the affected leg and apply hot and cold compresses alternately to relieve inflammation.

✚ WHAT ELSE DOCTORS MAY SUGGEST

Non-steroidal anti-inflammatory drugs can help reduce the inflammation. Put on elastic stockings before a long, seated journey, and walk around for five minutes every half-hour, if possible – for example, on an airplane. Taking a small daily dose of aspirin can help prevent phlebitis recurring, but talk to your doctor about this first.

Warning: Unusual leg swelling and pain need urgent attention because they can be signs of a coincidental deep vein thrombosis (*see facing page*); If untreated, this can be fatal.

COLD HANDS AND FEET

❓ WHAT CAUSES THEM

Chilled extremities are caused by a cold environment, poor circulation, or limited heat production – from inactivity, depression (*see page 202*), or an underactive thyroid (*see page 181*). Raynaud's phenomenon is a common artery disorder in women. Cold weather, stress, or a sudden change of temperature make artery walls constrict. Affected fingers or toes become purplish-blue, then white, then, as they warm up, red and painful.

✳ TREATMENT

Keeping warm Wear several thin layers rather than one thick one; use high-tech fabrics; heat the air; avoid chilling when inactive; pre-warm your bed; and bathe before retiring. Prevent Raynaud's with hand-warmers (microwaved or button-activated) in gloves. Keep wrists warm and draft-free.

Exercise Split your daily half-hour of aerobic exercise into two 15-minute sessions. This speeds up your circulation, warms you for hours, and encourages your muscles to grow and produce more heat.

No smoking Stop smoking (*see page 37*), with help if necessary. If you can't, then cut down.

Stress management Use more effective stress-management strategies to widen arteries narrowed by stress hormones.

Food and drink Eat more foods rich in magnesium (for its blood-vessel dilating effect), and flavonoids – including berries and cherries (for proanthocyanidins), buckwheat (for rutin), and onions and garlic (for quercetin). And have oily fish three times a week.

Food supplements
◆ Multivitamin and mineral supplements.
◆ Proanthocyanidins.
◆ Rutin.
◆ Quercetin.
◆ Fish oil.
◆ Ginkgo.
◆ Ginger – this helps one person in three with Raynaud's after a few weeks.

✚ WHAT ELSE DOCTORS MAY SUGGEST

Artery-dilating drugs sometimes help Raynaud's. Other treatments available for certain other causes of cold hands and feet include surgery.

HEMORRHOIDS

❓ WHAT THEY ARE AND WHAT CAUSES THEM

Hemorrhoids are swollen veins in the anal canal. You may feel them outside the anus as little knobs or balls, or they may be hidden inside. Hemorrhoids may itch or ache, and a large one hurts badly if trapped in the back passage. They are encouraged by inactivity, pregnancy (because of the pressure of the baby on the bowel), and constipation (*see page 162*).

✳ TREATMENT

Food and drink Drink more to make bowel movements softer and easier to pass. Eat brightly colored flavonoid-rich fruits (especially berries and cherries) and vegetables to strengthen vein walls. Buckwheat is useful because it contains a helpful flavonoid called rutin. Onions contain another called quercetin. Other helpful foods are those rich in vitamin C and silica.

Food supplements
- Vitamin C.
- Proanthocyanidins.
- Quercetin.
- Rutin.

Exercise Take a daily half-hour of exercise.

Skin care Ease itching by washing with soap and water after opening your bowels; finish with a cold rinse. Alternatively, use a moist wipe.

Hydrotherapy and aromatherapy Sit in some cold water containing four drops of cypress or juniper oil for four minutes each day to help shrink hemorrhoids

Herbal remedies Either dab with some tea (*see page 137*) made from a teaspoon of grated or powdered bistort root, or apply some cream containing an extract of lesser celandine (pilewort).

✚ WHAT ELSE DOCTORS AND PHARMACISTS MAY SUGGEST

Don't use laxative suppositories regularly as your bowel may learn to rely on them. See the doctor if hemorrhoids become troublesome or bleed. Treatments include injections, freezing therapy, or even surgery.

Seek medical help if you notice dark blood, feel ill, lose weight, or have an unexpected change in your bowel habit.

DEEP VEIN THROMBOSIS

❓ WHAT IT IS AND WHAT CAUSES IT

A deep vein thrombosis (DVT) is a clot in a deep vein, usually in a leg. It may cause aching, swelling or an ulcer. The biggest problem is a piece breaking off and traveling in the bloodstream to a lung. A lung clot (pulmonary embolism) can cause breathlessness, coughing up of blood, and even death. Blood clots occur more readily in smokers; during inactivity (especially during surgery and on prolonged seated journeys); during and just after pregnancy; when taking the estrogen-containing Pill or HRT (hormone replacement therapy) or certain other drugs; and in older people, individuals with certain cancers, and those who are overweight or stressed.

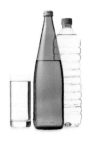

Drink plenty of water throughout the day to keep your digestive system active.

✳ PREVENTION AND TREATMENT

If you are inactive, help prevent a DVT by moving your legs frequently, even if only by wiggling your toes, or ask someone to bend your ankles and knees. Walk as soon as possible.

Foods rich in monounsaturates, such as avocados, olives, and olive oil, will help reduce your chances of developing a DVT.

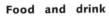

Food and drink
Eat more fruit and vegetables, for their salicylates, and more oily fish, nuts, seeds, avocados, and olive oil (and other monounsaturate-rich oils), for their fatty acids.

Food supplements
- Fish oil (*Warning*: Avoid this if you are on anticoagulant drugs).

✚ WHAT ELSE DOCTORS MAY SUGGEST

If you smoke, eat unhealthily, or have phlebitis (*see facing page*) or any other illness, ask about taking daily low-dose aspirin before and during a long journey; if you've had a previous clot, discuss a heparin injection. If you're having surgery, ask for "compression" stockings, inflatable bags, or a vein pump. Some people benefit from anticoagulant drugs and many surgeons use such drugs routinely before certain operations.

Warning: Watch out for DVT symptoms for two weeks after a long flight or a long bus trip.

HIGH BLOOD PRESSURE

❓ WHAT IT IS AND WHAT CAUSES IT

Your blood pressure (BP) is recorded with two figures, one over the other, measured in millimeters of mercury (mmHg) – for example, 120/80. The upper figure (the systolic pressure) represents the maximum arterial blood-flow pressure created by each heartbeat. The lower (diastolic pressure), the minimum. Most experts agree that the normal systolic pressure should be below 140, and the diastolic below 90.

The BP generally rises with age, and may rise temporarily with lifting, stress, cell phone use, pre-eclampsia and, perhaps, food sensitivity. The causes of continued high BP (hypertension) include arterial or kidney disease, and obesity (when the heart has to work too hard to push blood around the body). However, often there is no obvious reason. Hypertension is particularly likely in overweight people who had a low weight and were short or thin as newborns. And a history of pre-eclampsia in pregnancy encourages high BP later.

Headaches, blurred vision, breathlessness, or chest pain occur only with very raised blood pressure. But any high BP encourages angina, heart attacks, strokes, and kidney disease, though only in a few people (seemingly those with too little nitric oxide – broken down from arginine, an amino acid in peanuts, chocolate, seeds, and cereal grains). Experts recommend treating everyone with high BP until there is a test to identify those at risk.

✺ TREATMENT

Lose excess weight: for each kilogram (2.2lb) lost, BP falls by 2.5 mmHg (systolic) and 1.5 (diastolic). This is especially important if you're "apple-shaped." Most important, stop smoking or, at least, cut down.

Exercise Combining a daily half-hour's exercise – even walking, t'ai chi, or other non-vigorous exercise – with weight loss lowers the BP more than either alone.

Stress management Feeling continuously stressed raises the BP as much as does an extra 20 years or 40lb of body weight. Visualization and progressive muscular relaxation are useful; transcendental meditation is effective. The Alexander technique (*see page 135*) reduces stress from muscle tension.

Food and drink Eat more foods rich in vitamins B6 and C, flavonoids, potassium, magnesium, calcium, and omega-3 fatty acids, including five (some experts say nine) daily helpings of vegetables and fruit, and oily fish two or three times a week. Avoid salted foods as these may raise your BP. A test is being developed to identify salt-sensitive people. Go easy on coffee and alcohol. In moderation, alcohol may lower the pressure, but overindulgence does the opposite. Note that beer is surprisingly salty.

Food supplements

◆ Calcium and magnesium (*Warning*: Avoid magnesium if you have kidney disease).
◆ Vitamin C.
◆ Proanthocyanidins.
◆ Rutin.
◆ Quercetin.
◆ Fish oil.
◆ Taurine and arginine (amino acids that may reduce high blood pressure).

Light exposure Get some unfiltered daylight each day; UVB light helps lower high blood pressure; this may be because of the calcium-regulating effect of vitamin D, or because ultraviolet light is at the blue end of the light spectrum, and exposure to blue light has been proven to reduce high blood pressure (*see page 18*).

Herbal remedies Black cohosh (*Cimicifuga racemosa*) contains a substance called acteine which can help lower the BP. Dong quai (*Angelica sinensis*) lowers the BP, and yarrow (*Achillea millefolium*) and motherwort (*Leonurus cardiaca*) help reduce tension in the blood vessels. Take half a teaspoon of tincture made from a combination of these herbs twice a day. Better still, get personal advice on remedies from a herbalist.

✚ WHAT ELSE DOCTORS MAY SUGGEST

If six months of natural treatments do not work, or your BP is very high, doctors generally recommend BP-lowering drugs (such as beta blockers, diuretics, or calcium channel blockers).

ANGINA, HEART ATTACKS, STROKES

WHAT THEY ARE AND WHAT CAUSES THEM

Angina is a pain that warns of a patch of heart muscle being starved of oxygen. A heart attack is pain and breathlessness triggered by such a patch actually dying. A mini-stroke (transient ischemic attack) warns of a patch of brain cells being starved of oxygen. A stroke ("brain attack") is a collection of symptoms such as numbness, weakness, or paralysis, perhaps with a loss of speech or eyesight, triggered by such a patch dying.

The main culprit is a layer of fatty material called atheroma that forms on the lining of arterial walls, thus narrowing the blood channel. Atheroma contains low-density lipoprotein (LDL) cholesterol. Substances called free radicals in the blood oxidize LDL cholesterol, making artery walls inflamed, torn, scarred, and rough. Blood clots readily form on roughened artery walls, especially if the blood is abnormally sticky. This narrows the artery further and may even cut off the blood-flow completely.

Risk factors include high blood pressure, obesity, diabetes, smoking, stress, and an unhealthy diet (with insufficient antioxidants and other important nutrients, too much fat, and an unhealthy balance of blood fats). Gum disease and certain other chronic infections may increase the risk.

TREATMENT

Most important, stop smoking. This halves the likelihood of having a second heart attack. Treat high blood pressure. And lose excess weight.

Food and drink Eat plenty of foods rich in fiber, vitamins A, C, and E, flavonoids, salicylates, and essential fatty acids. Fats should provide no more than 30 percent of your daily calories; saturated fats should form no more than a third of your total fat intake per day; and you should have no more than five times as much omega-6-containing food as omega-3-containing food (*see page 25*) and preferably only three times as much.

Have three helpings of oily fish (such as salmon, sardines, herring, mackerel, pilchards) each week for their protective omega-3 fats. Spice your food with turmeric and ginger, rich in powerful antioxidants. A little alcohol may be good for your arteries but too much is unwise.

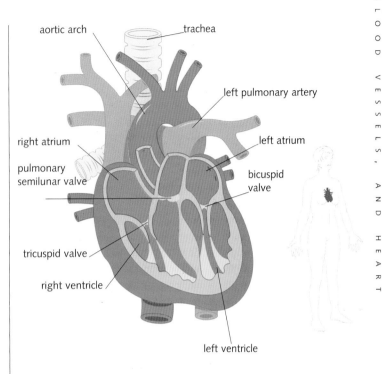

aortic arch
trachea
left pulmonary artery
right atrium
left atrium
pulmonary semilunar valve
bicuspid valve
tricuspid valve
right ventricle
left ventricle

Food supplements
◆ Vitamin E.

Stress management Two personality styles are particularly associated with arterial disease. The first is a gloomy outlook, with a tendency to feel unhappy and irritable and to mull over difficult feelings. The second is a penchant for hostile feelings, attitudes, or behavior. Arteries are more likely to clog up if you either hold anger close to your chest or get angry easily. So think positively, treat any depression, and polish your conflict-resolution and other stress-management skills.

WHAT ELSE DOCTORS MAY SUGGEST

A small daily dose of aspirin helps protect some people by reducing inflammation of the artery lining and making blood less sticky. Some experts hoped hormone replacement therapy would be protective, but recent studied suggest not. Other drugs may be necessary for continued symptoms. Various techniques using instruments passed through blood vessels can improve the heart's blood supply, reducing the need for major surgery.

The heart beats on average about 70 times every minute. To keep it healthy, take regular exercise, don't smoke, eat a sensible diet with plenty of antioxidants, and use effective stress management to help keep your blood pressure healthy.

ARTHRITIS

❓ WHAT IT IS AND WHAT CAUSES IT

Arthritis means pain and stiffness in the joints.

OSTEOARTHRITIS (OA)

This usually affects the neck, lower back, hips, knees, fingers, and toes. It often appears or worsens at the menopause, and is encouraged by a hysterectomy for heavy periods. The problem is roughening of the joint cartilage from aging, overuse, or other damage. Contributory factors include an unhealthy diet, and certain foods (particularly tomatoes, potatoes, bell peppers, eggplant – perhaps because they contain certain lectins, substances that can damage joints in some people).

RHEUMATOID ARTHRITIS (RA)

This begins in wrists, fingers, or toes and young women are most likely to be affected. The Pill lowers the risk; childlessness increases it, and some people inherit a high risk. Pregnancy can improve RA for up to three months after childbirth.

Associated problems include anemia, a poor circulation, and trouble with the tendons, eyes, and thyroid gland. RA is an autoimmune disease – one that results from abnormal immune cell behavior (*see page 210*). Triggers include certain foods (wheat, meat, dairy produce, eggs, animal fat, sugar, coffee), stress, infections, and certain chemicals (such as leaking domestic gas).

✳ TREATMENT

Food and drink Reduce your intake of saturated fat. Have more raw leafy vegetables (including parsley) and foods rich in essential fats (with a good balance of omega-3 and omega-6 fats, *see page 25*). Eat more foods rich in flavonoids (especially proanthocyanidins), beta carotene, vitamins C, D, and E and selenium. Identify any food sensitivity with an elimination diet (*see page 164*). Have half a tablespoon of apple cider vinegar with a teaspoon of honey in hot water twice a day, and a daily glass of vegetable juice (choose from from beets, carrot, cucumber, and celery). Drink a cup of ginger tea twice a day – ginger contains powerful antioxidants.

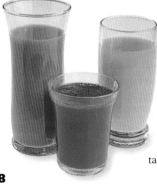

Vegetable juices – particularly those made from carrots, celery, beets, or cucumber – can be helpful for arthritis sufferers.

Food supplements

◆ Beta carotene.
◆ Vitamins C, D, and E.
◆ Selenium.
◆ Fish oil (for polyunsaturated fatty acids – PUFAs) or cod liver oil (for PUFAs and vitamins A and D). *Warning*: If you take cod liver oil, then avoid other vitamin A and D supplements.
◆ Proanthocyanidins.
◆ Glucosamine – an amino-sugar that is a great help to some people with arthritis.

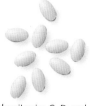

Take vitamins C, D, and E as supplements.

Exercise Balance rest and exercise without overstressing joints. Move painful joints frequently to prevent stiffening. Strengthen the muscles around the joints.

Light exposure Daylight exposure helps by warming joints and stimulating vitamin D, estrogen, and endorphin production.

Heat and cold therapies Help to ease joint pain with warm, cold, or alternating warm and cold treatments.

Breathing exercises If you are prone to hyperventilating (*see page 13*), practice breathing using breathing exercises (*see page 141*) to counteract a high body-acidity level.

Stress management Use effective anti-stress strategies to reduce inflammation and pain.

Massage and aromatherapy Massage around painful joints with carrot seed oil.

Herbal remedies Try a daily cup of tea or dose of a tincture made from one or more of the following: frankincense (Boswellia), celery seed, yarrow, ginger, coriander, black cohosh, buckbean, wild yam (rheumatism root), prickly ash, burdock, feverfew, willow bark, poplar bark, elderflowers, clivers (goosegrass), uva ursi (bearberry), and stinging nettle. Or consult a medical herbalist.

✚ WHAT ELSE DOCTORS MAY SUGGEST

Painkillers and hormone replacement therapy may help. (*Warning*: Avoid long-term non-steroidal anti-inflammatory drugs.) Specialist treatment can help prevent permanent damage from RA. The newest treatment for RA is regular filtering of the blood to remove antibodies.

OSTEOPOROSIS

❓ WHAT IT IS AND WHAT CAUSES IT

One in three women develops osteoporosis, but only 1 in 12 men. Affected bones are thinner, lighter, and more fragile and likely to fracture. Several things encourage osteoporosis:

◆ An early natural menopause.

◆ An early menopause induced by medical treatment. A hysterectomy makes the menopause arrive on average two years earlier than otherwise expected, partly because it may damage ovarian function by interrupting the ovaries' blood supply. Some treatments cause an abrupt early menopause due to the cessation of ovarian hormone production. These include removal of the ovaries, radiotherapy to the ovaries, and any anticancer chemotherapy.

◆ A long time without periods (for example, from an eating disorder leading to a very light body weight, or from habitual overexertion). The absence of periods during pregnancy and while breastfeeding is proven not to be a problem.

◆ Smoking. This advances the menopause by an average of two years, and contributes to a raised risk of osteoporosis after the menopause.

◆ A poor diet.

◆ Too much alcohol on a regular basis.

◆ A sedentary lifestyle.

◆ A light build.

◆ Long-term steroid treatment.

◆ Cancer.

◆ A liver or thyroid disorder.

◆ Osteoporosis in the family.

◆ Too little exposure to natural light.

Our bones normally stay strong and resilient because their frameworks of collagen are flexible and interlaced with mineral salts. Bones are an important mineral depot. This means their minerals are in a constant state of flux, continually entering and leaving bone according to the body's needs. They become stronger when more minerals enter than leave, and vice versa.

Bone mineral-density normally peaks in the late 20s, starts falling in the 30s, and drops faster as hormone levels decrease after the menopause. But at any age, simple lifestyle measures can help strengthen your bones or, at least, prevent any further weakening.

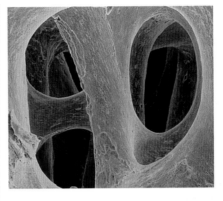

❀ TREATMENT

Most important, stop smoking.

Food and drink Eat plenty of foods rich in calcium, magnesium, zinc, vitamins C and K, flavonoids, and plant hormones. Adults need 1,200mg of calcium each day, preferably from food. Cut out added salt and sugar, and carbonated drinks, and reduce your intake of coffee, animal protein, and processed foods. Avoid drinking excessive alcohol.

Food supplements

◆ A multimineral (including calcium, magnesium, boron, silica, and zinc) supplement.

◆ Vitamin D.

◆ Vitamin K.

◆ Glucosamine – an amino-sugar.

◆ Plant hormones such as isoflavones.

Exercise Take regular weightbearing exercise, such as walking, dancing, or tennis, to raise the bone mineral density in your leg, hip, and spinal bones.

Light Get some natural daylight on your bare skin each day to boost your vitamin D production and aid calcium uptake by the bones.

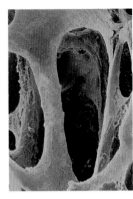

A scan of a healthy bone (above left) and one showing the bone-destroying effects of osteoporosis (above right). Protect your bone density by having a healthy diet and daily exercise and sunshine.

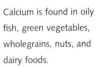

Calcium is found in oily fish, green vegetables, wholegrains, nuts, and dairy foods.

✚ WHAT ELSE DOCTORS MAY SUGGEST

After the menopause your doctor may recommend HRT (hormone replacement therapy), raloxifene (one of the new selective estrogen reuptake modulators known as SERMs; this reduces the osteoporosis risk without increasing that of breast cancer), or, if necessary, a drug called etidronate.

DIABETES

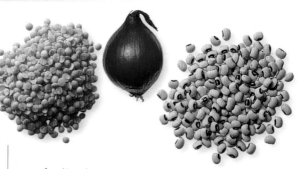

❓ WHAT IT IS AND WHAT CAUSES IT

When someone has diabetes, her pancreas makes little or no insulin, so her blood-sugar level rises. There are two types of diabetes, and both can run in families. Type 1 is less common and usually begins rapidly between the ages of 10 and 16, with weight loss, thirst, and a frequent need to urinate.

RIGHT: Including onions, beans, and lentils in your diet is a good idea if you have diabetes.

Type 2 begins slowly after the age of 40. Early signs include thirst, tiredness, blurred vision, and frequent urination. Sometimes this is provoked by infection, drugs (such as steroids), or pregnancy. Risk factors include being overweight, especially with fat around the middle; high blood pressure; Asian or Afro-Caribbean ancestry; and heavy smoking. A continuing high blood-sugar level may cause cataracts, kidney damage, leg ulcers, pins and needles, and arterial disease.

✳ TREATMENT

Stop smoking and lose excess weight.

Exercise Take a daily half-hour of aerobic exercise to help stabilize your blood-sugar level.

Food and drink Eat more vegetables (including onions, garlic, beans, and lentils); salads; foods rich in vitamins B, C, and E; chromium (go for beans, mushrooms, brown basmati rice), and zinc. Reduce your saturated fat intake and eat a good balance of essential fats (*see page 25*).

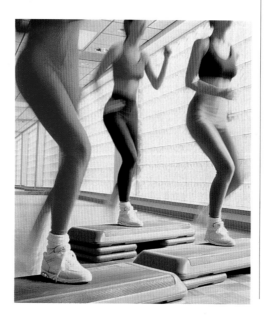
Regular aerobic exercise such as a step class will help stabilize blood-sugar levels.

A food's glycemic index (GI) indicates how rapidly the food releases sugar and ranges from 0 to 100. The higher a food's GI, the more rapidly does eating that food raise the blood-sugar level. People with diabetes need to keep their blood sugar relatively stable. So:

◆ Favor foods whose GI is below 50.

◆ Combine foods whose GI is 50–70 with some low-GI food.

◆ Avoid foods whose GI is over 70, or eat them only in small amounts and together with protein, green vegetables, or other low-GI food. For examples of the GI of various foods, *see page 216*.

Food supplements

◆ Vitamin B complex – to aid sugar metabolism.

◆ Vitamins C and E – for their antioxidant properties.

◆ Quercetin – for antioxidant protection of the eyes' lenses.

◆ Chromium picolinate – to stabilize the blood-sugar level if you have type 2 diabetes.

Herbal remedies A daily 25g (under an ounce) dose of powdered fenugreek seeds may help prevent arterial disease by lowering a high level of LDL cholesterol (*see page 177*) and of triglyceride blood fats.

✚ WHAT ELSE DOCTORS MAY SUGGEST

People with type 1 diabetes require daily insulin injections, and a healthy diet that is carefully balanced with activity. The risk of celiac disease (*see page 164*) is raised, so your doctor may recommend tests to rule this out.

Type 2 diabetes doesn't cause problems for a long time, so have an annual test if your risk is raised. If lifestyle measures don't keep your blood-sugar level down, you may need antidiabetic tablets, or even insulin injections. Discuss with your doctor whether your arteries could be protected with a small daily dose of aspirin.

UNDERACTIVE THYROID

❓ WHAT IT IS AND WHAT CAUSES IT

The thyroid gland lies in the neck, is controlled by the pituitary and hypothalamus, and produces two hormones. These are called thyroxine and tri-iodothyronine. They help regulate the body's oxygen consumption, heat production, and growth. An underactive thyroid (hypothyroidism) is ten times commoner in women than in men, and affects almost one woman in ten at some time. It can cause heavy periods; weak, aching muscles; fatigue; coldness; and weight gain. The skin may be dry and pale, with puffiness around the eyes. Some people develop anemia, constipation, bloating, swollen ankles, and depression. A croaky voice, unsteadiness, and insomnia are possible; fertility problems, numb and tingling fingers, rheumatoid arthritis, and heart disease are more common; and the gland may swell in the neck.

Triggers include antibody attack (Hashimoto's thyroiditis, *see page 210*), a poor diet, treatment for an overactive thyroid, and certain drugs. Hypothyroidism after childbirth can mimic postpartum depression. Smoking, stress, and inactivity encourage thyroid underactivity.

✳ TREATMENT

The problem sometimes corrects itself. It's important to stop smoking, to manage stress effectively, and to take regular exercise.

Food and drink Eat more foods rich in iodine, selenium, and essential fatty acids. Avoid piped water (as its fluoride and chlorine content can block iodine receptors in the thyroid gland) and drink distilled water.

Food supplements
◆ Kelp (a type of seaweed).
◆ Vitamin B complex.

✚ WHAT ELSE DOCTORS MAY SUGGEST

Some people need treatment with thyroid extract or thyroxine.

---

hypothalamus

pituitary gland

parathyroid glands

thyroid gland

The thyroid is a ductless gland in the neck controlled from the brain.

OVERACTIVE THYROID

❓ WHAT IT IS AND WHAT CAUSES IT

The thyroid gland in the neck is the "energy gland," because its hormones, thyroxine and tri-iodothyronine, regulate how fast the body burns energy. The increased hormone production resulting from an overactive gland causes abnormal sweating, feeling hot, hunger, shaky hands, and a rapid heartbeat. The gland may swell and the person may feel anxious, restless, and exhausted. There may be muscle wasting and irregular periods. Sleep becomes difficult, the heartbeat rhythm may be irregular, and the eyes can take on a startled, staring appearance. The commonest cause of thyroid overactivity (thyrotoxicosis) is Graves' disease. This mostly affects young and middle-aged women. It results from antibody attack but the trigger is unclear, though stress sometimes plays a part. Other causes include inflammation, infection, a tumor (benign or cancerous), and certain drugs.

✳ TREATMENT

Graves' disease often disappears spontaneously in time. However, it's wise to check that your stress-management strategies are effective.

Food and drink Eat more foods rich in vitamin C, and more thyroid-suppressing foods. The latter include cabbage, turnips, brussels sprouts, cauliflower, spinach, and broccoli. Cut down on dairy products. And avoid stimulating, caffeine-containing drinks such as coffee, tea, and cola.

Food supplements
◆ A multivitamin and mineral supplement — to make up for the overactive cells' increased nutrient intake.

✚ WHAT ELSE DOCTORS MAY SUGGEST

Antithyroid drug treatment helps prevent unpleasant symptoms. A few people need surgery or radio-iodine treatment.

LEFT: If the thyroid gland is over or underactive it can cause unpleasant symptoms and health problems. Occasionally it improves on its own, but adjusting your diet, and perhaps having drug treatment, can help.

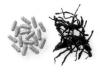

Kelp supplements made from seaweed provide iodine for an underactive thyroid gland.

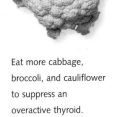

Eat more cabbage, broccoli, and cauliflower to suppress an overactive thyroid.

181

LOW SEX DRIVE

❓ WHAT IT IS AND WHAT CAUSES IT

Too little time or expertise spent on becoming aroused before intercourse itself is probably the commonest cause of a lack of sexual pleasure. However, there are many things that may reduce a woman's capacity to be interested in sex and become genitally aroused.

Psychological causes include depression; anxiety; fear of pregnancy; disappointment because pregnancy isn't possible; a reaction to genital surgery; fear of criticism, loss of control, or of being overheard; dislike of the man; perceiving the man as a parent; identifying with a mother-figure who should be sexless; or any environmental discomfort or other turn-off.

Physical causes include an underactive thyroid, arterial disease, diabetes, anorexia nervosa, other illness, overindulgence in alcohol, a hormone deficiency, aging, and certain drugs.

Behavioral causes include having been conditioned out of sexuality in childhood, child sexual abuse, insufficient foreplay, and poor methods of masturbation.

✳ TREATMENT

Exercise Take regular aerobic exercise to increase hormone levels.
Food and drink Eat more foods rich in vitamins B and E, zinc, and plant hormones. Include brown rice and whole rye or wheat grains; these contain histidine, an amino acid that aids sexual arousal.
Food supplements
◆ Histidine (on an empty stomach).
◆ Vitamin B complex.
Herbal remedies Potentially helpful remedies include catuaba, ginseng, schizandra, dong quai, muira puama, and astragalus.
Aromatherapy Experiment with ylang ylang, jasmine (*Warning*: Not if you are pregnant or breastfeeding), benzoin, ginger, sandalwood, and rose oils by putting three drops of any two in your bathwater. Alternatively, ask your partner to massage you, using three drops of any two oils in two teaspoons of sweet almond oil.

✚ WHAT ELSE DOCTORS MAY SUGGEST

Some women who have had their menopause find hormone replacement therapy useful.

Eat foods that are rich in vitamin B such as brown rice, whole wheat and rye grains.

FAR RIGHT: Black cohosh is the source of a herbal remedy for a dry vagina.

DRY VAGINA

❓ WHAT IT IS AND WHAT CAUSES IT

A dry vagina and vulva can cause itching, soreness, and discomfort during intercourse, and the symptoms of cystitis (*see page 196*). The production of one of the parts of vaginal moisture, mucus, rises around ovulation and during sexual arousal, and may fall for some months after childbirth. If prolonged this can encourage antibodies to attack mucus glands (*see page 210*). A lack of vitamin A can dry the vagina too and aging and falling hormone levels reduce mucus production after the menopause.

✳ TREATMENT

Vaginal care After childbirth or the menopause, take time when becoming sexually aroused, and use either saliva, a commercial vaginal lubricant, or sweet almond oil, if necessary. The more often you become aroused, the moister you'll be. Regular orgasms help as well. Some women benefit from inserting a tampon coated in plain yogurt for half an hour twice a week, or a capsule of vitamin E each day.
Food and drink Eat foods rich in plant hormones and vitamins A and E.
Food supplements
◆ Plant hormones – such as isoflavones.
◆ Vitamin E.
Aromatherapy Add two drops each of geranium, lavender, and fennel oils to your bathwater. These are relaxing and believed to stimulate female hormone production.
Exercises Take regular exercise and do pelvic floor exercises (*see page 136*).
Herbal remedies Drink a daily cup of fennel or sage tea. Take a teaspoon of black cohosh (*Cimicifuga racemosa*) once or twice a day. This contains plant hormones, and studies show it is as effective as taking estrogen (such as that in HRT).

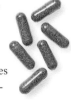

✚ WHAT ELSE DOCTORS AND PHARMACISTS MAY SUGGEST

Your doctor may check that there is no infection causing the itching, and may suggest estrogen-containing vaginal cream or suppositories or, if necessary, hormone replacement therapy.

PAIN DURING INTERCOURSE

❓ WHAT CAUSES IT

The first few times a woman has sex may hurt because of anxiety, being insufficiently aroused, and having a tight vaginal entrance. Women who are used to making love may find that their vagina tightens when they're stressed or tired. This makes them less able to relax and enjoy sex, so they don't become sufficiently aroused for their vagina to produce enough moisture or expand as normal. Tightness can also occur when a woman doesn't feel like sex for other reasons (*see facing page*). Dryness (*see facing page*) can make sex painful, and an episiotomy scar may be uncomfortable. Painful

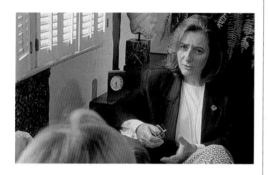

sex may result from an infection (*see below*), irritation of the bladder (*see page 196*), or pelvic inflammatory disease (*see page 188*). A vagina that's sensitive to condoms, or spermicidal and lubricating creams or jellies can hurt during sex, as can an irritable bowel (*see page 161*) or patch of endometriosis (*see page 191*) outside the vagina. Occasionally sex is painful after a hysterectomy, possibly because of the presence of scar tissue at the top of the vagina.

❀ TREATMENT

Relaxation, taking time over foreplay, and using a vaginal lubricant can ease discomfort. At other times, you need to identify and treat the underlying cause (*see above*).
Food and drink During times of hormonal change, be sure to eat plenty of foods rich in plant hormones, vitamin E, and essential fatty acids.

✚ WHAT ELSE DOCTORS MAY SUGGEST

You may need help from a psychosexual therapist for stress, or for relationship-related discomfort.

SEXUALLY TRANSMITTED INFECTIONS

❓ WHAT THEY ARE AND WHAT CAUSES THEM

Several types of infection can be passed from an infected person to a sexual partner. The microorganisms responsible for such infections include: *Candida* (a yeast-like fungus), *Trichomonas* (a one-celled organism), *Chlamydia* (a bacterium), *Herpes* (a virus), gonococci (bacteria), genital warts (caused by certain human papillomaviruses – HPV types 6 and 11), and HIV (human immunodeficiency virus). For the possible early symptoms, *see page 72*. However, these aren't all. Many women experience infertility as the first symptom (*see page 195*). Continued infection with certain other types of HPV encourages cancer of the cervix and vulva (*see page 208*), especially as you get older. HIV infection depresses the immune system and can progress to potentially fatal AIDS (acquired immunodeficiency syndrome) or a related AIDS-like condition.

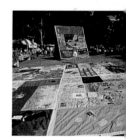

If you have any concerns about sex, don't be embarrassed to talk to your doctor.

Many people still believe AIDS only affects homosexual men. It doesn't, so be sensible.

❀ PREVENTION AND TREATMENT

Protect yourself during sex with someone who might be harboring an infection by ensuring that your partner uses a condom. Alternatively, only ever have sex with one faithful and non-infected partner. See a doctor without delay if you suspect a sexually transmitted infection. You'll need tests to reveal the nature of the infecting organism and then, perhaps, treatment with antibiotics. Your partner and any other sexual contacts should also be seen by doctors and then treated if necessary.
Other treatments Boost your immunity by eating a healthy diet with plenty of foods rich in beta carotene, vitamins C and E, folic acid, flavonoids (especially the proanthocyanidins in berries, cherries, and grapes), selenium, zinc, and essential fatty acids.
Food supplements
◆ Beta carotene.
◆ Vitamin C with flavonoids.
◆ Vitamin E.
◆ Folic acid.
◆ Proanthocyanidins.

PAINFUL PERIODS

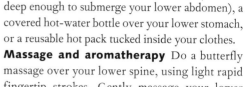

❓ WHAT THEY ARE AND WHAT CAUSES THEM

One woman in two sometimes has period pain. This is felt low in the stomach, or in the thighs or lower back, and lasts, on average, for 12 hours. It's most common in the late teens and early 20s. Some women feel sick and faint, and have diarrhea. The pains are similar to labor pains and result from a reduced blood flow in the womb's muscular wall as it contracts to dislodge its lining. The chemical culprits are increased levels of antidiuretic hormone and oxytocin (from the pituitary), noradrenaline (from nerves and adrenal glands) and endothelins, nitrous oxide, and certain prostaglandins (produced locally). A poor diet, a coil, fibroids (*see page 189*), pelvic inflammatory disease (*see page 188*), endometriosis (*see page 191*), or ovarian cysts (*see page 193*) can be to blame, as can chemicals inhaled from cigarette smoke.

✳ TREATMENT

Take an early dose of a non-steroidal anti-inflammatory painkiller such as ibuprofen. And consider having an orgasm, as this sometimes helps.

Food and drink Help balance prostaglandins in the week before your period by choosing more foods rich in omega-3 essential fatty acids and monounsaturated fatty acids (*see page 25*), calcium, magnesium, and vitamins C and E. Minimize your consumption of refined carbohydrates, animal protein, fat, alcohol, and caffeine-containing drinks. Add a lot of parsley to your food when you have the pain, as parsley stimulates menstruation.

Food supplements
◆ Magnesium.
◆ Calcium.

Exercise Try the pelvic tilt: kneel on all fours and rock your lower spine repeatedly up and down. Deep breathing exercises (*see page 141*) may make your pain easier to bear.

Heat therapy Relax in a hot bath (with water deep enough to submerge your lower abdomen), a covered hot-water bottle over your lower stomach, or a reusable hot pack tucked inside your clothes.

Massage and aromatherapy Do a butterfly massage over your lower spine, using light rapid fingertip strokes. Gently massage your lower stomach with slow sweeping strokes, lubricating with two teaspoons of sweet almond oil plus three drops of lavender, rose, cypress, sage, or Roman chamomile oil.

Herbal remedies Alternate drinking a cup of cramp bark (*Viburnum opulus*) tea with a cup of raspberry leaf, ginger, or jasmine tea every two hours. (*Warning*: Don't drink jasmine tea if you're breastfeeding.)

Alternatively, two or three days before your period is due, take a twice-daily teaspoon of herb tincture; when the pain begins, increase the dose to two hourly. For pain that's relieved when bleeding increases, take either blue cohosh (*Caulophyllum halictroides*) for acute cramps, or mugwort (*Artemisia vulgaris*) for dull pain, together with valerian (*Valeriana officinalis*). And have some ginger tea every two hours.

Acupressure Place your thumb tip four finger-widths above your inner ankle, just behind your large lower leg-bone. Press for two minutes with small circular movements.

✚ WHAT ELSE DOCTORS MAY SUGGEST

Stronger non-steroidal anti-inflammatory painkillers such as mefenamic acid may help, as may the Pill, or a progestogen pill for 20 days each month. If you have unfamiliar, uncontrollable, or worsening pain, or a coil, your doctor may check for other conditions (such as endometriosis, *see page 191*, a twisted fibroid, *see page 189*, or pelvic inflammatory disease, *see page 188*).

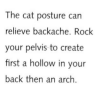
Applying pressure to the acupoint above your inner ankle can relieve painful periods.

The cat posture can relieve backache. Rock your pelvis to create first a hollow in your back then an arch.

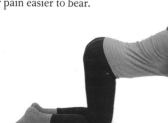
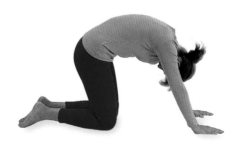

HEAVY PERIODS

❓ WHAT THEY ARE AND WHAT CAUSES THEM

One woman in three sometimes has periods heavy enough to be disruptive, perhaps with clots and flooding. The blood loss can cause fatigue and, eventually, iron-deficiency anemia.

The culprit is often a poor diet, with an imbalance of omega-3 and omega-6 fatty acids (*see page 25*) leading to an imbalance of prostaglandins and other important substances that affect your blood vessel tone. Eating insufficient food containing plant hormones to help maintain a good balance of your own estrogen and progesterone may make the problem worse.

There may be one of several womb problems (fibroids, polyps, infection, inflammation from a coil, or adenomyosis – endometriosis, *see page 191*, in the wall of the womb). Pelvic inflammatory disease (*see page 188*) may be the culprit.

Iron deficiency anemia (*see page 172*) is a frequent cause. For while heavy periods can cause anemia, in turn anemia causes heavy periods. An inherited blood disorder sometimes encourages bleeding too.

Stress, food sensitivity (*see page 164*), an underactive thyroid (*see page 181*), and certain drugs can be responsible. And smoking makes heavy bleeding worse, because the inhaled chemicals interfere with the ability of the womb's arteries to stop bleeding.

If heavy periods are also irregular, there may be a hormone imbalance (estrogen dominance – *see pages 187 and 216*) associated with the absence of ovulation. For similar reasons, periods may become heavier and cause flooding as the menopause approaches.

Sometimes what seems like a heavy period is actually a miscarriage. And occasionally womb cancer (*see pages 208–9*) is to blame.

✳️ TREATMENT

Food and drink Eat more salads, vegetables, and fruits to provide calcium, magnesium, zinc, and essential fatty acids; check that you have a good balance of the latter (*see page 25*). Make sure you eat plenty of plant hormones, especially those called lignans (in sunflower and sesame seeds, cracked flaxseeds, wholegrains, beans, and peas). Some people find eating too much meat makes periods heavier. However, cinnamon-spiced food reputedly eases heavy bleeding, as do citrus fruits. Liquidize whole lemons, oranges, or pink grapefruit for a thick juice containing blood vessel-conditioning flavonoids and vitamin C. Add fresh or dried thyme to one of your meals each day. And use a food elimination diet (*see page 164*) to identify any food sensitivity.

LEFT: Drink citrus fruit juices, as these are reputed to ease heavy bleeding.

Herbal remedies Many herbs can be useful and because there are so many causes of heavy periods, there's understandably a lot of controversy over which ones are best. However, beth root (*Trillium erectum*) is a good one. Take a cup of tea or teaspoon of tincture twice a day. Even better, see a herbalist for personal advice.

Aromatherapy A daily stomach massage (using three drops each of geranium, cypress, and rose oils in two teaspoons of sweet almond oil) may help ease stress-related heavy periods. You can also put six drops of any of these essential oils in your bathwater.

➕ WHAT ELSE DOCTORS MAY SUGGEST

Having blood tests, an ultrasound scan and a womb biopsy gives a 50:50 chance of discovering the cause. If there's no treatable cause and six months of home treatments don't help, consider medication with a non-steroidal anti-inflammatory drug. Mefenamic acid, for example, reduces bleeding by up to 30 percent by rebalancing prostaglandins. It's also especially useful if you have a coil. Alternatively, consider tranexamic acid, a progestogen-releasing contraceptive coil, the combined Pill or, if approaching your menopause, hormone replacement therapy. If necessary your doctor may recommend removal of the womb lining (endometrial ablation) with heat, laser-light, or microwaves; or as a last resort, hysterectomy.

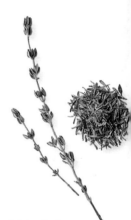

Dried or fresh thyme can be helpful for heavy periods.

PREMENSTRUAL SYNDROME

WHAT IT IS AND WHAT CAUSES IT

Many women notice physical and emotional changes in the two weeks after ovulation; these correspond with cyclical changes in hormones and other body chemicals. Increased creativity and energy are welcome; other changes are unwanted – or even incapacitating, in which case a woman is said to have premenstrual syndrome (PMS). This is commoner after a first child, after coming off the Pill, and in the 30s and 40s.

Some women feel irritable, with mood swings and sleep disturbances. Others experience depression, forgetfulness, easy weeping, and insomnia. Fluid retention causes tender swollen breasts, weight gain, bloating, and ankle and finger swelling. And some women crave carbohydrates; feel hungry, dizzy, tired, and faint; and have headaches and palpitations.

An extract from yams, applied daily in a cream, relieves PMS for some women.

TREATMENT

Exercise Take daily aerobic exercise in your two premenstrual weeks, even if you don't feel like it.

Stress management Pamper yourself, prioritize tasks and say "no" when necessary.

Aromatherapy You may find a daily massage with lavender or other relaxing essential oils (*see page 133*) particularly helpful.

Food and drink Eat small, regular meals, favoring foods rich in chromium, iron, magnesium, zinc, vitamins A, B, C, and E, and plant hormones. Eat a good balance of fats, including essential fats (*see page 25*). The amino acid tryptophan may be helpful, but only if from a low-protein source such as bananas, cauliflower, potatoes, nuts, dates, pumpkin seeds, or wholegrain foods, such as oatmeal made with whole oats. Cut out added salt and reduce your intake of alcohol and caffeine-containing drinks.

Eat low-protein foods that contain tryptophan, such as dates and bananas.

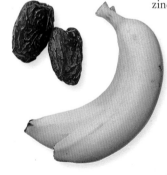

Food supplements

◆ Vitamin B6.
◆ Magnesium.
◆ Plant hormones.
◆ Evening primrose oil.

FAR RIGHT: Evening primrose is available as a supplement and in creams.

Light therapy Exposure to two hours of bright light in the evening may help. Some women benefit from a battery-operated mask with red lights programmed to flash in sequence. Wear this with your eyes closed for 15 minutes a day for two weeks before a period. Researchers suggest it helps by resetting a disturbed body clock, altering neurotransmitter levels, or speeding slow brainwaves.

Herbal remedies Apply a teaspoon of yam cream over your thighs or abdomen twice daily in the premenstrual two weeks. This provides beta carotene, vitamin C, and diosgenin, and other plant hormones. Plant hormones are not converted into human hormones by the body, but may help balance disturbed hormone levels by occupying hormone-receptors on cells. (Manufacturers add synthesized progesterone to some yam creams. In some countries – such as the USA – these are on sale to the public; in others, including the UK, any cream containing progesterone requires a prescription.)

Alternatively, take a twice-daily cup of tea or a daily teaspoon of tincture containing the hormone-balancing herbs *Vitex agnus castus* (chasteberry), black cohosh, and dong quai (Chinese angelica, *Angelica sinensis*). Continue for three months.

Warnings: Don't take *Vitex* if you're on the Pill, HRT, or other hormones. Don't take black cohosh if you could be pregnant.

Ginkgo tablets may ease sore breasts.

Hydrotherapy and aromatherapy Have a warm sitz bath every other day in the two weeks before your period is due. Add to the main bath two drops each of rose, geranium and lavender oils to help relax you and balance your hormone levels.

WHAT ELSE DOCTORS MAY SUGGEST

Medical treatments include the Pill, antidepressants and diuretics. Many doctors are reluctant to prescribe progesterone-containing cream, as proof of progesterone absorption through the skin is lacking.

IRREGULAR PERIODS

❓ WHAT CAUSES THEM

Normal menstrual cycles last from 20 to 35 days. Regular ovulation and periods depend on a balance of hormones from the hypothalamus, pituitary, and ovaries. Irregular ovulation is common for several years after a girl's periods start, and near the menopause. It can also occur after stopping the Pill or when breastfeeding. Damage to the ovarian arteries during sterilization can prevent ovulation. Hormones may be unbalanced by rapid weight loss, being very underweight, bingeing or obesity (sometimes associated with polycystic ovaries, *see page 193*). Up to nine women in ten with infrequent periods have polycystic ovaries. A hormone imbalance called estrogen dominance, associated with polycystic ovaries (or stress, excitement, depression, overexercising, changes in time zones, or other conditions or lifestyle factors, *see pages 187 and 216*), disrupts periods by stimulating the womb lining unevenly. Other causes include a vitamin B deficiency; diabetes (*see page 180*); anemia (*see page 172*); an overactive thyroid (*see page 181*); and certain drugs (including the Pill and some high blood pressure medications). Women who live together may develop irregular periods; later these synchronize as pheromones from their skin affect each other's hormonal cycles.

Early pregnancy or miscarriage may give the impression of irregular periods. Bleeding between periods can mimic irregular periods. Causes include fibroids (*see page 189*); womb polyps; certain ovarian cysts; pelvic inflammatory disease (*see page 188*); and cervical or womb cancer (*see pages 208–209*).

🌸 TREATMENT

Food and drink Eat more foods rich in plant hormones (to balance hormone levels), vitamin B (if feeling stressed), and vitamin E and essential fatty acids (to aid hormone production). Also, have a good balance of essential fats (*see page 25*) to reduce inflammation. Lower your estrogen level (especially if you are overweight) by eating less fat, especially saturated fat, and more fiber.

Food supplements
- Vitamins B and E.
- Evening primrose oil.
- Plant hormones such as isoflavones.

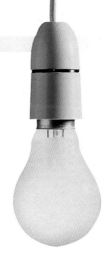

Irregular ovulation and periods can be stimulated by light therapy. Try it for six months, then if there is no improvement, replace it with a different therapy.

Herbal remedies Ideally, take personal advice from a medical herbalist.

If you wish to use herbs yourself, and if blood-hormone tests (arranged by your doctor) reveal a low level of progesterone after ovulation, take half a teaspoon of *Vitex agnus castus* (chasteberry) tincture each morning. Start the course as close as possible to the first day of a period and continue for three months.

If the tests reveal that you aren't ovulating, take half a teaspoon of false unicorn root (*Chamaelirium luteum*) tincture twice a day instead. (This is expensive because it's in short supply.) Alternatively, for unexplained irregularity, take half a teaspoon of tincture containing both herbs each morning.

Warnings: If under 20 years old, take *Vitex* only if advised by a qualified herbalist. Don't take *Vitex* if on the Pill, HRT, or other hormones.

Aromatherapy Aid relaxation and hormone balance with two drops each of rose, geranium, and lavender oils in your bathwater. Alternatively, add them to two teaspoons of sweet almond oil and use for a massage.

Light therapy For a six-month trial, sleep, from days 14–17 of your cycle, with a 100-watt light turned on to encourage ovulation.

✚ WHAT ELSE DOCTORS MAY SUGGEST

Tests may reveal what's wrong. Treatments include the progestogen-only Pill, or progesterone suppositories (proof of absorption from cream is lacking) for one to three months, or an ovulation-stimulating drug (clomiphene).

Warning: See your doctor if you bleed after sex, between periods, or after the menopause; or haven't had a period by 16 or 17 years old.

PELVIC INFLAMMATORY DISEASE

The first attack of PID can be very stressful. Talk to your doctor and in the meantime rest and boost your intake of beta carotene, vitamins C and E, flavonoids, selenium, and zinc.

❓ WHAT IT IS AND WHAT CAUSES IT

Microorganisms occasionally gain access to the womb and may even pass through the fallopian tubes into the peritoneal space around the womb, bladder, and bowel. Infected areas can become inflamed and tender. This is known as pelvic inflammatory disease (PID); womb infection is also called endometritis, and infection of the fallopian tubes, salpingitis.

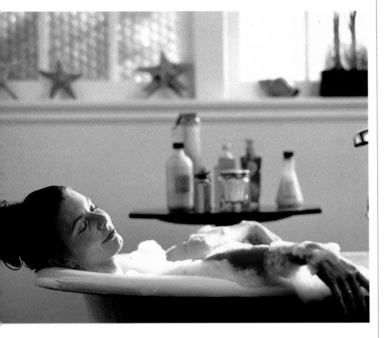

The first attack is often the worst. You may have a fever and feel nauseated, with aching and tenderness low in your abdomen, and pain in your thighs, bottom, and lower back that's worse before a period. You may find you're most comfortable on your back with knees bent. Periods and sex are usually painful, and you may have symptoms of cystitis, and even pain in your back passage. There may be a slight but smelly vaginal discharge. Salpingitis in the right fallopian tube mimics appendicitis; symptoms in either tube can be difficult to distinguish from an ectopic pregnancy (one occurring in a tube instead of the womb).

Signs and symptoms of persistent PID may be more vague. In addition, perhaps, to having some of those listed above, periods may become frequent, irregular, or heavy. Inflamed tubes can eventually become kinked, blocked, and scarred. This can impede the passage of eggs as they try to travel from one of the ovaries toward the womb.

Without prompt and adequate treatment, PID can lead to blocked tubes, an abscess in a tube or ovary, infertility, or, in pregnancy, a high risk of an ectopic pregnancy.

Causes include having a coil or a sexually transmitted infection (*see page 183*). Infecting organisms occasionally enter during pregnancy (when they can encourage premature birth), or during or after childbirth, miscarriage, termination or other surgery.

◆ Pain from endometriosis (*see page 191*) readily mimics that from PID.

❀ TREATMENT

Pamper yourself with plenty of rest and do what you can to ease your symptoms.

Food and drinks Eat more foods rich in beta carotene, vitamins C and E, flavonoids, selenium, zinc, and essential fats. Drink enough to keep your urine very pale.

Food supplements

◆ Beta carotene.
◆ Vitamins C and E.
◆ Flavonoids.
◆ Selenium.
◆ Zinc.

Exercise Take some gentle exercise each day (*Warning*: Not if you have a fever.) Boost your pelvic circulation twice a day with some pelvic tilt exercises: kneel on your hands and knees, and rapidly rock your lower back up and down for a minute or so.

Hydrotherapy and aromatherapy Stimulate your pelvic circulation with a daily contrast sitz bath (*see page 130*), with warm water in the bath and hotter water in the smaller container.

✚ WHAT ELSE DOCTORS MAY SUGGEST

Cervical swabs and, perhaps, a laparoscopy (an examination under anesthetic via a tube inserted below your umbilicus into your abdomen) and womb biopsy can confirm the diagnosis. Treatment is with antibiotics. A few women need surgery to remove damaged tubes or scar tissue from around their organs.

FIBROIDS

❓ WHAT THEY ARE AND WHAT CAUSES THEM

One woman in four develops fibroids – gristly white non-cancerous growths in the wall of the womb. They sometimes run in families, are most common between age 30 and the menopause and usually go unnoticed. After the menopause, they tend to shrink. A large one can cause heavy periods (*see page 185*) or bleeding between periods. Fibroids sticking out from the womb can press on the bowel or bladder and lead to constipation or frequent urination. They occasionally trigger low backache and painful periods and sex.

No one knows the cause but estrogen dominance (*see pages 187 and 216*) makes fibroids enlarge. Fibroids are more likely in very overweight women because their fat cells manufacture so much estrogen.

✳ TREATMENT

It's possible – though unproven – that regular orgasms might help prevent or shrink fibroids by increasing the pelvic circulation.

Food and drink Eat more foods rich in plant hormones, vitamins A and B (including inositol) from fruits, beans, peanuts, chickpeas (garbanzo beans), lentils, vegetables, and wholegrain foods; methionine, from plant sources such as beans, garlic,

Beans, garlic and onions contain inositol and methionine which improve circulation and can reduce fibroids.

lentils, onions, and seeds; and choline, from plant sources such as beans, peanuts, lentils, chickpeas (garbanzo beans), and wholegrain foods. Methionine is an amino acid that helps prevent a build-up of fat; together with inositol and choline it helps lower a high estrogen level. Eat less saturated fat and animal protein, and eat a good balance of essential fatty acids (*see page 25*).

Food supplements
- Vitamin B complex.
- Methionine.
- Choline.
- Magnesium.
- Plant hormones such as isoflavones.

Exercise When possible, boost the circulation in your womb by taking a half-hour's aerobic exercise each day.

Hydrotherapy Boost your womb's blood supply with a daily contrast sitz bath (*see page 130*) with cool water in the bath and fairly hot water in the other container.

Herbal remedies Each morning, take a teaspoon of tincture containing *Vitex agnus castus* (chasteberry) and false unicorn root (*Chamaelirium luteum*). If this doesn't help after two months, change to lady's mantle (*Alchemilla vulgaris*). This counteracts a high estrogen level and reduces heavy bleeding. Take a teaspoon of tincture, or have a cup of tea, twice a day. For other herbs that reduce heavy periods, *see page 185*.

Warning: Don't take *Vitex* if on the Pill, HRT, or other hormones.

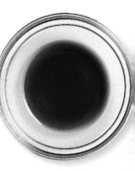

A teaspoonful of chasteberry tincture each morning can help balance hormone levels.

✚ WHAT ELSE DOCTORS MAY SUGGEST

A scan or hysteroscopy (viewing of the womb lining via a viewing tube passed through the vagina and cervix) can reveal fibroids. Treatments include the progestogen-only Pill, a progestogen-releasing contraceptive coil, hormones that provoke an artificial menopause, and surgery.

A surgeon may remove the fibroid or womb lining via the vagina, or use keyhole or traditional surgery to remove either the fibroid or the whole womb. Embolization is a promising new treatment. This involves injecting tiny particles into the womb's blood supply to starve and shrink the fibroid.

189

PROLAPSE OF THE WOMB

WHAT IT IS AND WHAT CAUSES IT

A prolapsed womb (uterus) means that the ligaments, muscles, and other tissues supporting the womb have become so slack, inelastic, and weak that the womb "drops" into the vagina. A minor prolapse means the cervix protrudes a little lower into the vagina than normal – the more serious the prolapse, the lower the cervix and the womb. At worst and, thankfully, rarely, the womb pulls the vaginal walls inside out like a sock.

A woman can feel a prolapsed womb as a lump inside or, if it's serious enough, even outside the vagina. A prolapse usually becomes bigger the longer a woman is upright, or when she raises the pressure in her abdomen by straining to open her bowels, coughing, sneezing, or lifting a heavy weight. When she lies down, her womb disappears back up toward its normal position. Some women with a prolapse have backache or a dragging sensation, especially after standing for some time, but many have no pain.

Occasionally the rectum or bladder prolapses too. The rectum may bulge into the back wall of the vagina, and the bladder into its front wall, either being sensed as a lump in the vagina. A prolapsed rectum may lead to difficulty with opening the bowels, and a prolapsed bladder to urinary problems, such as leaking, frequent urination, and a burning sensation when passing water.

Anything that weakens the womb's supporting tissues makes a prolapse more likely. Repeated, difficult or prolonged childbirth is a major culprit. Aging makes tissues slacker; smoking weakens supportive structures; a falling level of estrogen after the menopause may play a part; and being overweight or constipated puts extra stress on the womb's supports.

PREVENTION AND TREATMENT

When you give birth don't push until the urge to bear down is overwhelming, and your attendant gives you the all clear because your cervix is fully dilated and smooth-rimmed. It's also wise to maintain a normal weight; prevent constipation (*see page 162*); treat any cough promptly (*see pages 168 and 170*); and stop smoking.

Food and drink Eat more foods rich in vitamin C, flavonoids, calcium, and silica to strengthen the womb's supporting structures.

Exercise The most important thing is to do regular pelvic floor exercises (*see page 136*) every day to strengthen the tissues that support your womb and improve their circulation. It's also wise to take a daily half-hour of aerobic exercise to improve the blood flow in your pelvis.

WHAT ELSE DOCTORS MAY SUGGEST

Wearing a ring-shaped polythene pessary fitted by a doctor and changed every three to 12 months helps support a small prolapse. Hormone replacement therapy can help prevent weakening of the womb's supports. Surgery, if necessary, cures the problem.

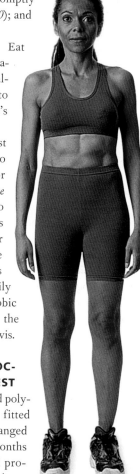

ABOVE LEFT: Take some exercise each day to improve pelvic circulation.

ABOVE: Include pelvic floor exercises in your daily half-hour aerobic workout to help strengthen the pelvic muscles.

ENDOMETRIOSIS

🌀 WHAT IT IS AND WHAT CAUSES IT

Endometriosis means there are patches of womb-lining cells outside the womb. It may affect up to 44 percent of women. The patches are most common on the ovaries, womb, cervix, bladder, and bowel, but can occur anywhere. Endometriosis in the womb's muscular wall is called adenomyosis.

Monthly bleeding from the patches can inflame nearby tissues, which, in turn, causes scarring and makes organs stick together. The commonest symptom is pain, either continuous, or during periods or around ovulation. Sex, passing water, and opening the bowels may hurt. And fertility problems are common. Occasionally a patch becomes a painful blood-filled cyst, but such a cyst usually corrects itself.

The cause is unclear, though endometriosis can run in families. One suggestion is retrograde menstruation, in which some womb-lining cells, shed during a period, exit the womb from the fallopian tubes. Another is damage by the body's immune cells. One study found that women who had at some time taken the Pill had twice the risk of endometriosis than those who had not. Patches are more troublesome with a hormone imbalance leading to estrogen dominance (*see pages 187 and 216*)

The pain of endometriosis generally clears during and for some years after pregnancy, and disappears after the menopause.

🌸 TREATMENT

Use sanitary napkins, not tampons, especially at the height of your period, when a saturated tampon could encourage retrograde menstruation. Be sure to take regular exercise.

Food and drink Eat more foods rich in essential fatty acids, vitamins B, C, and E, magnesium, flavonoids, salicylates, plant hormones, and fiber to counteract inflammation. Have less saturated fat, and a good balance of essential fats (*see page 25*). Include vegetables of the cabbage family, as well as bitter foods and drinks, such as watercress, chicory, young dandelion leaves, rosemary, and tonic water; these encourage the breakdown of estrogen in the liver. Have three helpings a week of oily fish, as omega-3 fatty acids shrink the patches. And eat wholegrain foods to lower your estrogen level further.

Stress management Balance stimulation from work and other activities with rest and relaxation, and use more effective stress-management strategies if necessary. Feeling stressed worsens pain and inflammation.

Herbal remedies Ideally, consult a medical herbalist for personal advice. Alternatively, twice a day, take a teaspoon of tincture containing peony (*Peonia lactiflora*) to reduce your estrogen level and relieve pain; dandelion root (*Taraxacum officinale*) to boost the breakdown of estrogen in the liver; dong quai (*Angelica sinensis* – Chinese angelica) to reduce pain; mugwort (*Artemisia vulgaris*) to counteract scanty periods; and feverfew (*Tanacetum parthenium*) to relieve pain from inflammation. Do this for no longer than three months. Drink ginger tea twice a day.

Heat therapy Relieve pain with a warm bath or a covered hot-water bottle, hot compress, or electrically heated pad.

Massage and aromatherapy A gentle stomach massage with relaxing essential oils may relieve pain. Add three drops of lavender oil to three teaspoons of sweet almond oil. Warm this by partly immersing its container in hot water. Use the flat of one lubricated hand to sweep slowly around your stomach with a smooth, continuous, clockwise stroke for several minutes.

Peony extract can help reduce your estrogen levels and relieve the pain of endometriosis.

✚ WHAT ELSE DOCTORS MAY SUGGEST

Endometriosis is confirmed by a laparoscopy, in which the surgeon passes a viewing-tube through the abdominal wall. Destroying patches with laser light is increasingly popular. Drugs can counteract estrogen, or reduce or prevent menstruation. Possibilities include the combined Pill; continuous progestogens or the combined Pill; or drugs such as danazol that prevent the pituitary from stimulating the ovaries. Some doctors recommend progesterone cream; others are holding back as there is no reliable proof that the skin absorbs progesterone.

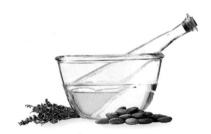

Lavender oil dropped into sweet almond oil can be used to give a pain relieving massage.

VAGINAL DISCHARGE

🔍 WHAT CAUSES IT

It's perfectly normal for the lining of the vagina to produce its own moisture, and for this to increase during sexual arousal. The cervix produces mucus and this production increases around the time of ovulation. However, an abnormally profuse, smelly, or colored discharge can indicate an infection. This can result from an overgrowth of certain microorganisms that are normally present in the vagina, or from infection with foreign organisms. The symptoms of an infection can include an abnormal discharge, itching, soreness, pain during sex, and — if the infection spreads to the womb and beyond, causing pelvic inflammatory disease (see *page 188*) — a fever, stomachache, and other symptoms.

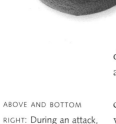

Intense itching with a creamy-white discharge and soreness may be due to infection with the yeast-like fungus *Candida*. A fishy-smelling, grayish-white discharge is probably due to bacterial vaginosis. This is more common than *Candida* infection, results from an overgrowth of various organisms, and is sometimes triggered by the presence of a coil. If you are pregnant, the presence of bacterial vaginosis may encourage premature labor. Other causes of vaginal discharge include a forgotten tampon or diaphragm, a foreign body, and sexually transmitted infections (*see page 183*) such as *Chlamydia*, genital *Herpes*, trichomoniasis, and gonorrhea.

✳ TREATMENT

If *Candida* symptoms continue, or recur, it may help to wear cotton underwear and to avoid tight trousers, as yeasts thrive in hot, moist, airless conditions. Use only unperfumed soap and don't use vaginal deodorants. Unfortunately, studies show that neither inserting a yogurt-soaked tampon for a few hours a day nor eating yogurt combats thrush.

Food and drink For *Candida*, avoid alcohol and foods containing added sugar and white flour, as

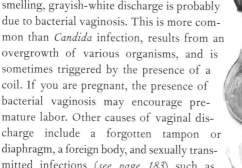

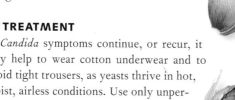

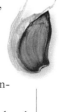

ABOVE AND BOTTOM RIGHT: During an attack, boost your intake of vitamin C.

these organisms thrive on a high blood-sugar level. Benefit from garlic's bactericidal action by adding six raw garlic cloves to your food each day. And eat more foods rich in beta carotene, vitamins C and E, flavonoids, and zinc. Each day, liquidize and drink a whole grapefruit, complete with peel, pith, and seeds.

Food supplements
◆ Vitamin A.
◆ Vitamin C with flavonoids.
◆ Vitamin E.
◆ Zinc.
◆ Grapefruit seed extract.

Herbal remedies Try a daily cup of tea or dose of tincture made from mahonia and (but not if pregnant) echinacea.

Aromatherapy Add six drops of tea tree oil to your bathwater.

✚ WHAT ELSE DOCTORS MAY SUGGEST

If symptoms continue, or recur, your doctor can arrange tests to check what's causing them, and then recommend treatment. If you have *Candida*, it's wise to have your blood tested for sugar, as *Candida* is more common in women with diabetes. Your partner may need treatment too. For *Candida* infection you may need antifungal medication (from a drugstore) such as clotrimazole suppositories and cream, or a capsule of fluconazole (with a doctor's prescription; but not to be taken if you are pregnant, under 16, or over 60). Medical treatment is advisable for bacterial vaginosis so as to avoid problems such as pelvic inflammatory disease and, if pregnant, miscarriage or preterm birth. Sexually transmitted diseases require medical treatment for both you and your partner.

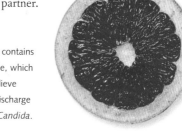

LEFT: Garlic contains a bactericide, which can help relieve excessive discharge caused by *Candida*.

OVARIAN CYSTS

❓ WHAT THEY ARE AND WHAT CAUSES THEM

Ovarian cysts are common, usually problem-free and can come and go within hours or days.

Single cysts mostly develop from egg follicles and are commoner after the menopause. They sometimes cause pelvic pain, painful sex, frequent urination, weight gain, and swelling. Occasionally one bursts, bleeds, twists, or becomes infected.

One woman in five has multiple small cysts brought about by an imbalance of certain of the hormones produced by fat cells, ovaries, hypothalamus, pituitary, or adrenals. Symptoms caused by such cysts are called the polycystic ovary syndrome (PCOS).

Women with PCOS usually make high levels of ovarian androgens (hormones such as testosterone), estrogen (mostly estrone, made by fat cells from androgens), and luteinizing hormone (LH – a pituitary gonadotrophin that stimulates ovaries). A high testosterone level (or an abnormal sensitivity to testosterone) encourages acne and excessive body hair. Four in five hairy women have PCOS. Ovulation often stops, leading to infrequent or absent periods, and infertility. There's likely to be an early menopause. And the risk of womb cancer rises. This is because estrogen dominance – *see pages 187 and 216* – causes continued stimulation, unopposed by progesterone, of the womb lining, and because the lining isn't shed each month if there are no periods.

Stress, obesity, and bingeing can unbalance hormones, and over a third of women with PCOS are overweight. Most women with bulimia (*see page 206*) have polycystic ovaries. And one woman in three with PCOS often binges.

The body cells of many women with PCOS are relatively insensitive to insulin. This "insulin resistance" leads to high blood-sugar and low cell-sugar levels, with a raised risk of diabetes and arterial disease. PCOS can be hereditary and therefore may run in families.

✳️ TREATMENT

Help balance hormones by taking regular exercise and using effective stress management. Losing weight helps many women with PCOS become less hairy and more fertile.

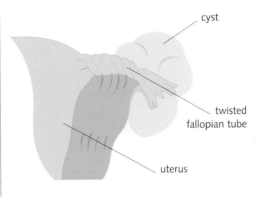

cyst

twisted fallopian tube

uterus

Food and drink Eat regularly and favor foods rich in plant hormones, chromium, magnesium, manganese, zinc, and fiber. Avoid refined carbohydrates and other high-glycemic-index foods (*see page 216*); eat less saturated fat, and have a good balance of essential fats (*see page 25*).

Herbal remedies Consult a medical herbalist for personalized advice. Alternatively, twice daily, and for no longer than three months, take a teaspoon of tincture containing:

◆ False unicorn root (*Chamelirium luteum*) – its plant estrogens counteract a high estrogen level without suppressing ovulation.
◆ Black cohosh (*Cimicifuga racemosa*) – particularly useful for stress.
◆ Peony (*Peonia lactiflora*), and either licorice (*Glycyrrhiza glabra*) or sarsaparilla (*Smilax*, wild licorice) – helpful for acne and excess body hair.

Light therapy Experiment to see if exposure to bright light helps.

➕ WHAT ELSE DOCTORS MAY SUGGEST

An ultrasound scan and blood tests reveal the nature of the cysts. Monthly bleeding induced by the combined Pill reduces the womb-cancer risk. Surgery may be advised. Having only one ovary decreases fertility, so if you need surgery and want to become pregnant in future, ask the surgeon to remove only the cyst if possible, rather than the whole ovary.

The treatment of PCOS depends on a woman's size, age, and fertility hopes. Cyproterone acetate (an anti-androgen) reduces hairiness. The combined Pill reduces symptoms by preventing ovulation. And clomiphene or electrical stimulation can trigger ovulation. *Warning*: See a doctor if you have a fever or severe pain.

Abdominal pain or discomfort might result from ovarian cysts. If self-help remedies do not quickly relieve the pain, consult a doctor.

BREAST PAIN AND LUMPS

WHAT THEY ARE AND WHAT CAUSES THEM

Breast discomfort is common just before a period. This sort of pain (cyclical mastalgia) makes breasts painful, heavy, and tender when unsupported or touched. It is related to the high progesterone level after ovulation. Once your period starts, your breasts will rapidly return to normal. Sometimes pain is associated with lumps (*see below*). Sometimes breast pain increases on the Pill, or appears around the menopause or when starting hormone replacement therapy.

Many women with painful breasts fear cancer. However, cancer doesn't usually hurt. If it does, it's very unusual for pain to be the only sign. However, 1 woman in 11 in westernized countries will eventually get breast cancer (*see pages 208–209*), so it's very wise to be "breast-aware." This means being sensitive to the way your breasts feel and look so you can recognize unexpected changes that could indicate cancer. Being breast-aware is an art because breasts constantly change in shape, size, and consistency. They change at puberty and during the teens. They grow and shrink with menstrual cycles; vary according to diet, exercise, and weight; alter on the Pill and during pregnancy and breastfeeding; and change again with the menopause and hormone replacement therapy.

Some women's breasts normally feel lumpy, especially just before a period. This is called diffuse nodularity, or benign breast change. The lumps tend to be of a similar size.

TREATMENT

Breast-awareness Look at your breasts in a mirror, feel them and visit your doctor if they seem different from usual for that time of the month. Otherwise, feel again after your period and see your doctor if you are still anxious. Keep a diary of your periods, pain, and lumpiness to see whether pain and lumps are always related to periods.

See your doctor if one lump is bigger, harder, or otherwise different from the others; if a lump develops unexpectedly; or if you have a hard or puckered area of skin, an abnormally colored patch, eczema, or an unusual nipple discharge or

bleeding. Although most lumps are benign, if a lump were to be cancerous you must get treatment as early as possible.

Food and drink Eat foods rich in a good balance of essential fatty acids (*see page 25*), but cut down on your total fat intake, especially saturated fats.

Food supplements
◆ Evening primrose oil – this contains gamma linolenic acid, an omega-6 fatty acid that sometimes eases breast pain. The body normally produces this from an essential fatty acid (*see pages 25 and 216*) called linoleic acid; but stress and aging can reduce this production. Take full doses for at least four months.

WHAT ELSE DOCTORS MAY SUGGEST

PAIN

Coming off the Pill may help the pain. If necessary your doctor may recommend a three-month trial of danazol or bromocriptine.

LUMP

The doctor may advise a mammogram or ultrasound scan. You may need a needle aspiration or biopsy to check what's in the lump. Cancer should be treated without delay. If there is a simple cyst, the fluid can be drawn off through a needle. A fibrous lump (fibroadenoma) may be best removed if you are over 30 or if your mother, sister, or daughter has had breast cancer.

A supplement of evening primrose oil can ease breast pain. If it persists consult your doctor.

Examine your breasts regularly and get to know what is normal for you. Anything unusual, including any discharge, should be investigated further, so don't delay in seeing a doctor.

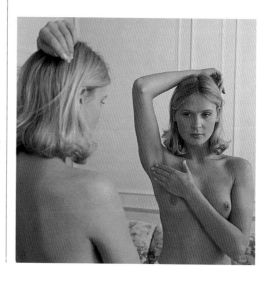

FERTILITY PROBLEMS

❓ WHAT THEY ARE AND WHAT CAUSES THEM

A couple's infertility has a 40 percent chance of stemming from the woman, and 30 percent chance of stemming from the man. The causes of female fertility problems include: repeated early miscarriage (*see page 81*); polycystic ovary syndrome (*see page 193*); endometriosis (*see page 191*); being over- or underweight; no sex around ovulation; smoking; stress; excessive exercise; a poor diet; sensitivity to cereal gluten; and blocked fallopian tubes from pelvic inflammatory disease (*see page 188*).

The average woman ovulates on day 14 (the first day of her period being day one) and is most fertile on days 10–15. An egg must be fertilized within 24–36 hours, and sperms usually survive up to 72 hours. So the best time for sex is from 72 hours before to 36 hours after ovulation.

Seek medical help if you are over 30 and have not conceived after a year of regular, frequent sex, or if you're over 35 and have been trying for six months without success.

✳ TREATMENT

The week before ovulation have sex daily on waking (most women ovulate in the afternoon and it helps for sperms to arrive first). Having an orgasm helps sperms to reach the egg. And lying down on your back after sex with your hips raised on a pillow for half an hour helps this too.

To work out when you ovulate:

◆ Keep a period diary.

◆ Check your vaginal mucus. Fertile mucus is thin, clear, plentiful, slippery, and stretchy and forms a string when stretched between the finger and thumb. Ovulation occurs within 24 hours of peak production.

◆ Use an ovulation-predictor kit, or an electronic ovulation-predictor monitor.

Lose excess weight, stop smoking, and use effective stress management.

Food and drink Limit alcohol as this encourages early miscarriage. Eat foods rich in vitamins B, C, and E, folic acid, selenium, and zinc, all important for nourishing eggs. Avoid foods to which you are sensitive. When possible, choose organic vegetables and fruits, as certain pesticide residues encourage miscarriage.

Food supplements

◆ A mineral and vitamin supplement especially formulated for preconception.

◆ Evening primrose oil.

✚ WHAT ELSE DOCTORS MAY SUGGEST

A blood test on day 21 will indicate whether you are ovulating. Other investigations include an ultrasound scan, laparoscopy (examination of ovaries, tubes and womb via a viewing tube through the abdominal wall), X-rays of womb and tubes, a look inside the womb (hysteroscopy), and a womb-lining biopsy. A blood test indicates the likelihood of gluten sensitivity. Treatments include:

◆ Gonadotrophin or clomiphene to stimulate ovulation. But this could raise your future risk of ovarian or breast cancer.

◆ Removal of eggs, test-tube fertilization (IVF), and embryo transfer (ET) to the cervix or womb (IVF-ET).

◆ Micro-surgery on blocked tubes.

◆ Destruction of patches of endometriosis.

◆ Removal of eggs, test-tube fertilization, and embryo transfer to a fallopian tube (ZIFT – zygote intra-fallopian transfer).

◆ Removal of eggs, and egg-transfer to a fallopian tube (GIFT – gamete intra-fallopian transfer).

◆ Test-tube fertilization of donated eggs, and embryo transfer to the womb (egg donation or donor IVF).

◆ Embryo donation – as above but with a donated embryo.

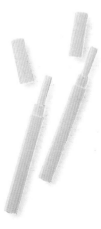

Kits are available to help you predict the day you are likely to ovulate. Use in conjunction with careful observations of your body.

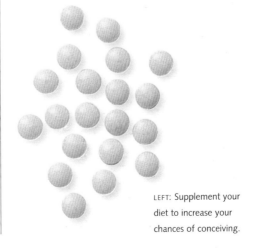

LEFT: Supplement your diet to increase your chances of conceiving.

CYSTITIS

❓ WHAT IT IS AND WHAT CAUSES IT

Cystitis is an inflammation of the bladder lining. This makes a woman want to pass water urgently and frequently, even with little to pass, and causes burning and a low stomachache. One woman in two with these symptoms has a urinary tract infection. Infected urine may be cloudy, bloodstained, or smelly. Infection which reaches the kidneys causes a fever and low backache. Women have a 50:50 chance of getting cystitis at some time in their lives, and some have it repeatedly. Honeymoon cystitis is triggered by sex. The penis physically irritates the bladder-neck or urethra and encourages bacteria from the vulva to enter the bladder. A contraceptive diaphragm can irritate the bladder and prevent it from emptying properly, encouraging bacteria to breed.

Other cystitis triggers include pressure from a tampon or fibroid (*see page 189*); tight underwear, hose, or trousers; getting chilled; or wearing a sanitary napkin for too long. Some women are sensitive to bubble-bath, soaps, deodorants, spermicide, or swimming-pool chlorine. Some women develop cystitis after the menopause because the low estrogen level encourages infection by causing dryness and inflammation around the urethral opening in the vulva (*see page 182*), and colonization of the vagina with *E.coli* bacteria instead of lactobacilli.

✿ TREATMENT

If your cystitis usually follows sex, try to make sure you are highly aroused before penetration, or use a commercial lubricant. Avoid positions that seem to encourage cystitis.

Hygiene Wipe your bottom from front to back and wash afterward if possible. Use unperfumed soap and avoid other toiletries on your vulva. Wash before sex. Empty your bladder before sex and within half an hour afterward. Ask your partner to wash his penis. Favor showering instead of bathing. Urinate every two hours during the day.

Clothing Avoid tight trousers and hose and don't use biological laundry detergent.

Food and drink Drink plenty (though not coffee, tea, carbonated drinks, and alcohol, as these irritate the bladder) until your symptoms disappear. Start with a pint of water, then have a glass

every 20 minutes for three hours. Homemade lemon barley water is a good alternative: boil pot barley in water for 45 minutes, strain, and flavor the liquid with lemon juice and honey. Make urine less acid with a teaspoon of baking soda in every third glass of fluid, or buy a flavored cystitis remedy. Cranberry juice (or cranberry extract tablets) is good for infection because its proanthocyanidin flavonoids prevent bacteria from sticking to the wall of the bladder.

Eat asparagus, beets, and raw garlic to counteract infection, as well as foods rich in beta carotene, vitamins C and E, selenium, zinc, and flavonoids.

Heat and cold Keep warm, and ease stomachache with a covered hot-water bottle or electrically heated pad.

Hydrotherapy Stimulate your pelvic circulation to counter inflammation with a ten-minute soak in a hot bath, then a brief cold shower.

Massage and aromatherapy Massage your stomach with two drops each of juniper and lavender oils in two teaspoons of warmed sweet almond oil.

Herbal remedies Have a cup of tea three times a day made from an anti-inflammatory herb such as uva ursi, and one of the diuretic herbs, buchu, cornsilk, or couchgrass.

✚ WHAT ELSE DOCTORS MAY SUGGEST

See your doctor if home treatment doesn't ease symptoms, or you have a fever or recurrent cystitis. If a urine test reveals infection, you will need to take antibiotics.

Drink plenty of fluids, particularly cranberry juice, to flush out your bladder and soothe inflammation.

Lemon barley water is simple to make, very palatable, and can soothe an irritated bladder.

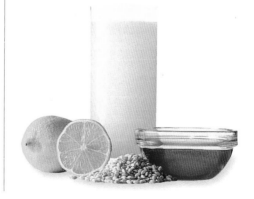

INCONTINENCE

❓ WHAT IT IS AND WHAT CAUSES IT

Many adults sometimes wet themselves. This can be frustrating and embarrassing, but with the right help many become dry or discover how to manage better. Fifty percent of people with this problem have what's called stress incontinence, 30 percent have urge incontinence, and 20 percent have both stress and urge incontinence.

STRESS INCONTINENCE

This results from weakness of the muscle around the top of the urethra (which normally keeps urine in the bladder) and of the pelvic floor muscles (which support the bladder neck and urethra). People with stress incontinence tend to leak when their bladders are stressed by a rise in the pressure inside their abdomens. This can happen when coughing, jumping, or laughing. Having a difficult delivery or several pregnancies in rapid succession weakens the pelvic floor muscles and encourages stress incontinence, as does being overweight, eating a poor diet, repeated coughing, aging, having a low estrogen level after the menopause, and being severely constipated.

URGE INCONTINENCE

With this, the muscle in the bladder wall becomes unreliable and overactive, giving little warning of when it needs to be emptied. An individual may wet the bed and find she can't get to the lavatory in time by day. This is most likely if the person also has a urine infection. Other triggers include stress, smoking, strong tea, coffee, cola, or alcohol, and certain drugs. The unreliability may result from a problem with those nerves in the lower spine that control the bladder.

✳ TREATMENT

Lose excess weight and stop smoking. Highly absorbent sanitary pads are available to cope with leaks, but if possible it's better to prevent the problem from occurring.

Food and drink Eat foods rich in plant hormones and a good balance of essential fats to help incontinence that develops after the menopause. Avoid eating or drinking anything that irritates your bladder, including coffee, tea, spicy foods, alcohol, fruit juice, sugar, and dairy products.

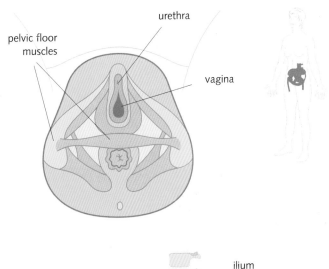

pelvic floor muscles / urethra / vagina

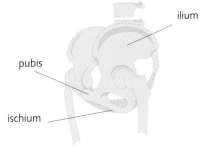

ilium / pubis / ischium

Exercise For stress incontinence, do several sets of pelvic floor exercises (*see page 136*) each day. This is the best way of strengthening the muscles. Another way is with "vaginal weight training". This involves putting a special cone-shaped weight in your vagina and contracting the muscles to hold it in place. As your muscles become stronger, use increasingly heavy weights.

Training your bladder to hold urine for progressively longer intervals can help if you have urge incontinence. Start by going once every hour, then as your bladder becomes more reliable, make the interval gradually longer day by day.

✚ WHAT ELSE DOCTORS MAY SUGGEST

Other treatments include electrostimulation of the nerves supplying the pelvic floor muscles or bladder, and collagen injections around the urethra. A ring-shaped estrogen-releasing vaginal suppository can counteract a low estrogen level. A u-shaped suppository or surgically implanted sling can hold the bladder neck in place.

Incontinence can be caused by weak muscles, poor diet, or infection but it can be treated successfully at home. If your symptoms do not improve, your doctor can offer supplementary therapies.

BACKACHE

❓ WHAT CAUSES IT

Backache usually results from muscle tension; sometimes muscles or ligaments are inflamed too. Only rarely does the gel inside one of the intervertebral disks ooze out (as a prolapsed or "slipped" disk). Tension usually results from overworking or overstretching muscles. Damage to a facet joint by a sharp twisting movement makes muscles tighten up to protect the joint. Other causes include arthritis (*see page 178*), osteoporosis (*see page 179*), period pain (*see page 184*), labor (*see page 84*), endometriosis (*see page 191*), urine infection (*see page 196*), prolapse (*see page 190*), and pelvic inflammatory disease (*see page 188*). To help prevent backache:

◆ Exercise regularly.
◆ Stretch your long back muscles each day. Lie with hands clasped on your stomach; stretch, gradually raise your straight arms (hands still clasped), then lower them behind your head. Relax into

1. Breathe in as you raise your arms above your head, then out as you stretch them behind you.

2. After a few breaths, raise your arms vertically, while breathing in.

3. Breathe out as you bring your arms down to rest on your stomach. Relax and repeat.

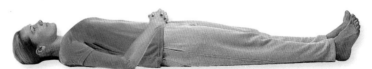

the stretch, then slowly return your arms to their starting place. Repeat several times.
◆ Keep fit.
◆ Maintain a good posture, using the Alexander technique (*see page 135*) if necessary.
◆ Choose a comfortable chair that supports your back and elbows.
◆ Lift and carry skillfully: bend your knees when picking something up; lift without twisting; keep heavy objects close to your body; and distribute weight equally across shoulders.
◆ Don't stay in the same position for long.
◆ Avoid being overweight.

◆ Eat more foods rich in calcium, magnesium, silica, vitamins C and E, flavonoids, plant hormones, and essential fats.

✻ TREATMENT

Rest, exercise, and relaxation When backache begins, try not to rest for more than 48 hours at most, as inactivity weakens muscles. Start exercising as soon as possible; gradually increase the amount, and include muscle-strengthening and stretching exercises. Try the pelvic tilt – kneel on all fours and gently rock your pelvis up and down.

When swimming, people with facet-joint trouble are usually more comfortable doing back stroke; this is because front stroke tends to worsen irritation by closing up the joints.

Massage and aromatherapy Ask someone to massage you with four drops of relaxing lavender oil in a tablespoon of sweet almond oil. You may be more comfortable sitting up. You may like firm pressure on tender points, but tell your helper what feels best.

Sleeping habits Put a pillow or two between your knees and lower legs if you sleep on your side, and beneath your knees if you sleep on your back. Some people prefer a firm mattress or specially shaped pillow.

Heat and cold therapies See whether heat or cold therapy (*see page 131*) helps.

Heat is usually preferable for muscle tension, cold for inflammation. Alternatively, alternate heat (for three minutes) with cold (for one minute), and repeat four or five times.

✚ WHAT ELSE DOCTORS MAY SUGGEST

Discuss painkillers. Diazepam relaxes tension (but take this for no longer than seven days). Your doctor may recommend an osteopath, chiropractor or physiotherapist. Treatments include massage, stretching, manipulation, mobilization, and an electrical treatment called interferential therapy. Surgery is a last resort.

CRAMP

🕐 WHAT IT IS AND WHAT CAUSES IT

Cramp is a sudden painful tightening of the muscles. It causes period pain (*see page 184*) and labor pains (*see page 84*), angina (*see page 177*), irritable bowel syndrome (*see page 161*), tension headaches (*see page 204*), and repetitive strain injury (*see page 201*). But here we'll discuss calf cramp.

Cramp in the lower leg is commoner in older people. Among its triggers are: being cold, dehydration, alcohol, sweating, a poor diet, insufficient UV-light exposure, and not warming up and cooling down properly when exercising.

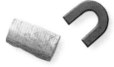

✳ TREATMENT

Some people swear by putting a cork or magnet beneath the mattress although the origin and usefulness of this remedy are unclear.

Food and drink Eat plenty of foods rich in calcium, magnesium, potassium, zinc, vitamins C and E, and essential fatty acids. Eat oily fish three times a week, and benefit from the calcium in their bones by choosing canned fish with soft edible bones, or marinating fish in vinegar for 48 hours.

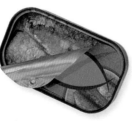

Food supplements
- ◆ Calcium.
- ◆ Vitamin B3.
- ◆ Vitamin D.
- ◆ Fish oil.

Exercise Stretch the cramped muscle to ease it. Help prevent cramps by doing similar stretches three times daily.

Massage and heat Rub the muscle for two minutes, then keep it warm.

Herbal remedies Put a thermos flask of cramp bark (guelder rose) tea by your bed. To ease cramp lay a hot compress made with the tea (*see page 131*) on your muscle.

✚ WHAT ELSE DOCTORS MAY SUGGEST

Drugs such as quinine may help.

RESTLESS LEGS

🕐 WHAT THEY ARE AND WHAT CAUSES THEM

One person in 20 sometimes has restless legs. The legs may feel heavy, swollen, uneasy, itchy deep inside, tired, achy, or twitchy. The condition is worse when relaxing, may prevent sleep, and sometimes affects the arms too.

Restless legs can run in families and is commoner in pregnancy. One in four people with rheumatoid arthritis (*see page 178*) has restless legs, and they're also more likely with varicose veins (*see page 173*), lung disease, fibromyalgia (*see page 200*), and diabetes (*see page 180*). One person in four suffering from restless legs has iron-deficiency anemia (*see page 172*). Other triggers include smoking, alcohol, coffee, food sensitivity and a lack of vitamins B, B12, and E, and folic acid. (Kidney failure, nerve damage, and certain antidepressants and tranquilizers can cause a different type of restlessness.)

✳ TREATMENT

Help prevent restless legs with regular exercise. Some people find relief from earthing the body's static electricity by standing on a cold floor with bare feet, or holding faucets with wet hands.

Food supplements
- ◆ A daily multivitamin and mineral supplement.

Massage Firmly massage the legs with long, upward strokes.

Heat and cold therapy Try cooling muscles with a cold compress or bath, heating with a hot compress or bath, or applying hot (for two minutes) then cold (for one minute) compresses.

✚ WHAT ELSE DOCTORS MAY SUGGEST

A blood test can rule out anemia. Drugs such as a benzodiazepine, clonazepam, or carbamazepine can help but may have side effects.

LEFT: Some people find that putting a cork or magnet underneath their mattress relieves cramp.

LEFT: The bones found in canned fish, such as sardines, are rich in calcium – a vital nutrient for healthy muscles and bones.

Alternate hot and cold compresses can relieve the irritation of restless legs.

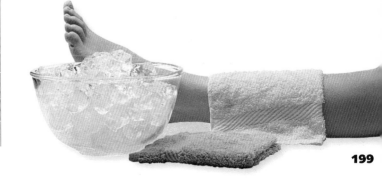

199

FIBROMYALGIA

❓ WHAT IT IS AND WHAT CAUSES IT

People who suffer from fibromyalgia have muscle pains and stiffness, often with hard knots and cords in the shoulders and back. To be diagnosed with fibromyalgia, a person must have tenderness in any 11 of the following 18 points (myofascial trigger points):

◆ Either side of the base of the skull.

◆ Either side of the neck (between the fifth and seventh vertebrae).

◆ The middle of each upper trapezius muscle (between neck and shoulder).

◆ One end of either supraspinatus muscle (along the shoulder blade's upper edge).

◆ Either pectoral muscle (over where the second rib meets the breastbone).

◆ The outer part of either elbow.

◆ Deep in either buttock.

◆ Behind either hip (where the piriformis muscle is inserted).

◆ The inside of either knee.

Fatigue is common. Indeed, people with fibromyalgia share many symptoms with those who have chronic fatigue syndrome (*see page 211*). Most sufferers are women and up to nine in ten have disturbed sleep, with more light dreaming sleep than usual. Activity level, stress, and weather may affect symptoms. Several other problems are more likely. These include: headaches, Raynaud's phenomenon (*see page 174*), period pain (*see page 184*), a poor memory or concentration, depression (*see page 202*), restless legs (*see page 199*), and irritable bowel syndrome (*see page 161*).

Fibromyalgia sometimes begins after a shock. Increased sensitivity to pain, and a low level of the neurotransmitter serotonin may be partly responsible. Older terms for it include muscular rheumatism and fibrositis.

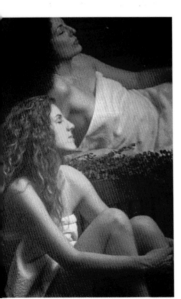

Frequent steam baths or saunas may help fibromyalgia.

✴ TREATMENT

Rest and exercise Discover the combination of rest and exercise that best relieves your pain and stiffness.

The 18 myofascial trigger points which can feel tender in people who have

Heat therapy Try heat treatments (*see page 131*), or alternate steam bath or sauna sessions with a cold shower or swim. (*Warning*: Not if you have heart disease.)

Food and drink Eat foods rich in vitamin B, calcium, and magnesium. Benefit from anti-inflammatory substances in cabbage and lemons. Have three helpings a week of salmon or tuna (for their omega-3 fatty acids); unlike other oily fish these are low in purines which produce uric acid that can irritate muscles. Avoid offal, beef, pork, chocolate, herrings, mackerel, shellfish, fish roe, sherry, and port (which contain purines), and refined carbohydrates (which encourage fluid retention). Cut down on caffeine-containing drinks.

Food supplements

◆ Calcium and magnesium – to help muscles relax.

Massage and acupressure Ask someone to massage you. Firm pressure over the tender points may be most helpful.

Tens Using a TENS (trans-cutaneous electrical nerve stimulation) machine may block pain.

✚ WHAT ELSE DOCTORS MAY SUGGEST

Acupuncture and osteopathy are of proven success. Certain antidepressant drugs may help, partly by improving the quality of sleep. Other possibilities include non-steroidal anti-inflammatories, steroids, and tranquilizers.

REPETITIVE STRAIN INJURY

❓ WHAT IT IS AND WHAT CAUSES IT

Frequent repetitions of any movement without adequate respite can affect the muscles and nerves involved, and lead to a collection of symptoms known as a repetitive strain injury (RSI). This, in turn, causes fatigue and irritability from interrupted sleep. One common type occurs in those whose work involves hours at computer keyboards. This can cause a variety of symptoms, including pain, weakness, and cramp in the hand and arm. Some individuals also develop the carpal tunnel syndrome, with pain, numbness, and tingling in the index and middle fingers and thumb; the fingers may also feel swollen, although they aren't. This condition is more common in women and results from pressure on the median nerve as it runs through a structure called the carpal tunnel in the wrist.

Repetitive strain injury of the hand and arm is more likely when the hands are used with the wrists bent up or down. Carpal tunnel syndrome in particular is commoner in those who have fluid retention (*see page 211*), diabetes (*see page 180*), thyroid problems (*see page 181*), or are overweight, pregnant, premenstrual, on the Pill, or in the first year after their menopause.

❋ TREATMENT

Most important, take frequent and adequate breaks from the activity responsible for your symptoms. A guide is to cease that movement for five minutes every half-hour. Check the position in which you work and the way in which you move so as to minimize the strain on your muscles. For example, you may need to change your typing position; use a chair with arms and an adjustable-height seat, support your wrists on a foam block in front of the keyboard; and invest in a track-ball mouse that requires much less movement than an ordinary mouse.

Exercise For hand and arm symptoms, do the following simple exercises once every half-hour while working to improve the circulation and reduce fluid retention. Swing your arms for one minute. Then stretch them forward at shoulder height, clench your fists with the fingers over the thumbs, tighten your arm and shoulder muscles, and slowly rotate your wrists first one way, then the other; repeat 20 times.

Heat Keep uncomfortable arms, wrists, or hands warm, and soothe them once or twice a day by covering them with a hot compress.

Food and drink Improving your diet can help prevent repetitive strain that is made worse by fluid retention (*see page 212*). Eat more foods rich in vitamin B, calcium, and magnesium to encourage overworked muscles to relax.

✚ WHAT ELSE DOCTORS MAY SUGGEST

Wearing a wrist splint at night can help hand and arm symptoms. Sometimes an injection of steroids into the wrist is necessary for carpal tunnel syndrome. A few people need an operation.

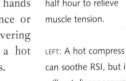

If you can't take a complete break, at least have a drink and do some exercises every half hour to relieve muscle tension.

LEFT: A hot compress can soothe RSI, but it will not disappear unless you eliminate its triggers.

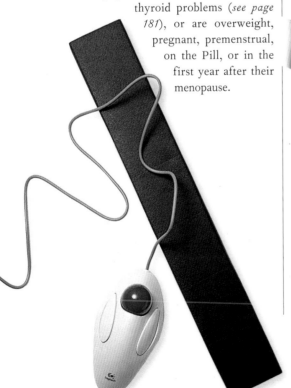

The prolonged use of a computer mouse can cause RSI.

201

DEPRESSION

❓ WHAT IT IS AND WHAT CAUSES IT

Everyone feels unhappy sometimes. But true depression is deeper than this. It can cause illness, poor sleep, and weight loss (or, for mild depression, weight gain). Triggers include illness; job loss and relationship problems; an unhealthy diet; food sensitivity; sensitivity to low light levels in winter (seasonal affective disorder, or SAD); loneliness; and a lack of social support.

Sometimes there is no obvious cause. Some women are particularly prone to depression before their periods (*see page 186*), during their first years after childbirth (*see page 89*), and around the menopause (*see page 104*). Depression is associated with an imbalance of neurotransmitters in the brain; and is two to three times as likely to occur in women.

✳ TREATMENT

Exercise Take a half-hour's brisk exercise every day, come rain or shine. This boosts the levels of "feel-good" chemicals called endorphins. Help lift low spirits by walking tall, using tips from the Alexander technique (*see page 135*).

Food and drink Look after yourself by preparing nutritious, attractive, regular meals rich in vitamins B and C, calcium, iron, magnesium, and zinc, and with a good balance of essential fats (*see page 25*) and three helpings of oily fish a week.

The brain needs an amino acid called tryptophan to make serotonin, a neurotransmitter that relays messages between nerves. Although proteins contain tryptophan, it is those foods that are rich in tryptophan but not other amino acids that boost the brain's tryptophan level. This is because tryptophan is lowest in the hierarchy when it comes to amino acids being able to enter the brain. So have snacks of baked potatoes, bread, beans, hazelnuts, pumpkin seeds, dates, or bananas. Also, make sure you eat enough fat. Having too little can lower the cholesterol level so much that it prevents brain cells using serotonin (a neurotransmitter) and encourages depression. Finally, track down any suspected food sensitivity (*see page 164*).

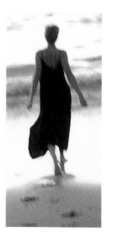

Whatever the weather a walk will lift your spirits because it encourages the release of endorphins. For maximum benefit walk briskly, let your arms swing freely by your sides, and breathe deeply.

Food supplements

◆ A multivitamin and mineral supplement.
◆ Fish oil.

Light exposure Go outside each day to get some bright light in your eyes. And use a brighter light in the room where you spend the most time. If winter depression is a big problem, buy a light box containing fluorescent tubes that supply intense light. Sit close by for half to two hours a day. Consider drinking some water twice a day that has been solarized (*see page 129*) in a red glass.

Herbal remedies Take a twice-daily cup of tea or a teaspoon of tincture made from St. John's wort (hypericum). This is often more effective than antidepressant drugs.

Warning: Avoid if you are taking antidepressant drugs, tetracycline (an antibiotic), or piroxicam (a painkiller). If you have postpartum depression, a herbalist may recommend a daily teaspoon of *Vitex agnus castus* (chasteberry) tincture for one to three months.

Flower essences Choose the flower essences whose descriptions best match your feelings.

Heat, cold, and hydrotherapy Try lifting your spirits by having a warm bath or shower for ten minutes, then a quick cold shower, then repeating this cycle.

Mind work Discover (with a friend, or a counselor if necessary) what makes you feel low, what – if anything – you can do about it, and how to manage your reactions in a way which is effective rather than damaging. Force yourself to laugh and smile as this should make you feel more like laughing and smiling spontaneously. Program into each day things you know you would normally like. If nothing gives you enjoyment, do something that used to give you pleasure. And at the end of each day, write down at least one and preferably three good things that have happened, however small they may be.

✚ WHAT ELSE DOCTORS MAY SUGGEST

See your doctor if your depression is severe or long-lasting, or if you feel suicidal. Antidepressant drugs may take a while to work.

ANXIETY AND PANIC ATTACKS

❓ WHAT THEY ARE AND WHAT CAUSES THEM

Any worry or anxiety that is bad enough can make muscles tense and breathing shallow and fast (see hyperventilation, *page 13*). You may be short of breath and have chest pain. Your heart beats faster and within seconds you look pale and feel dry-mouthed, sick, sweaty, shaky, and faint. The ears ring and you feel hot or cold, have butterflies in your stomach, stomach-rumbling, diarrhea, or keep wanting to pass water. At worst the feeling becomes one of panic, and your symptoms may be so frightening that you think you are going to die.

Some people experience panic attacks like this in particular situations, such as when flying, performing, taking tests, at heights, with spiders, or when outdoors. Many have other stressful problems in their lives. Anxiety is associated with altered levels of certain hormones and neurotransmitters. Certain foods encourage anxiety by influencing the levels of these substances, or by producing a low blood-sugar level. The body's blood-sugar level normally changes relatively slowly and remains within a certain fairly constant range, but it may dive to a low level after strenuous exercise, a missed meal, or too much food made with sugar or white flour (which send it plummeting after an initial rapid rise). Eating too few foods containing calcium, magnesium, and vitamins E and B – needed for healthy nerve function – can also cause anxiety.

❀ TREATMENT

Some people react to anxiety by drinking too much alcohol, bingeing on comfort foods, or doing other things which, though offering short-term relief, can also be damaging.

There are nearly always more effective, non-harmful solutions.

Food and drink Choose more naturally calming foods, rich in vitamins B and E, calcium, and magnesium. Steady your blood-sugar level between meals by eating whole foods – wholegrains and foods made with wholegrain flour (such as wholewheat bread), legumes (such as peas, beans, lentils, and peanuts), fruit, vegetables, nuts, and seeds. Boost your level of the "feel-good" neurotransmitter serotonin with a high-carbohydrate, low-protein snack that is rich in readily available tryptophan. Examples include wholewheat bread, bananas, dates, hazelnuts, pumpkin seeds, and beans. Don't eat too much protein, as this has the opposite effect. Track down suspected food sensitivity (*see page 164*). Avoid caffeinated drinks.

Herbal remedies Drink a cup of chamomile or lemon balm tea several times a day. Lemon balm is particularly good for anxiety affecting the stomach.

Exercise and relaxation Plan in a daily half-hour's exercise, and check that you get enough relaxation and sleep. Use breathing exercises (*see page 141*) and other stress-management techniques to help you feel more in control of your symptoms.

Mind work Avoid bottling up anxiety by unburdening to friends, or writing down how you feel. Consider counseling to help you understand what triggers your fear and help deal with your reactions. It may help to confront in your mind what is the worst that could happen; facing the possibility can make it seem less monstrously frightening.

✚ WHAT ELSE DOCTORS MAY SUGGEST

Your doctor may recommend tranquilizers to tide you over while you deal with the causes of your anxiety and your reactions to it.

Lemon balm tea can calm an anxious stomach.

A peanut butter sandwich is calming because it stabilizes the blood sugar level, and is high in carbohydrates.

203

HEADACHE AND MIGRAINE

❓ WHAT THEY ARE AND WHAT CAUSES THEM

Tension headaches result from tight muscles in the scalp or neck. Triggers include anxiety (*see page 203*), drafts, bad posture, and a poor diet.

Migraine is a severe one-sided headache sometimes associated with nausea, vomiting, or even temporary one-sided paralysis. It is often preceded by an "aura" such as a visual disturbance or a feeling of elation. The many triggers include stress, bright or flashing light, loud noise, the Pill, premenstrual hormone changes, certain weather, hunger, and food sensitivity (most often to chocolate, cheese, milk, oranges, alcohol, or wheat).

Cluster headaches occur in groups over two months, last about an hour, and occur up to ten times a day. Each causes burning pain in and around one eye; the affected eye may look red and watery, and have a drooping lid. The nose may be congested. Triggers include cigarette smoke and drinking alcohol or coffee.

Chronic daily headache occurs most days. There is an almost constant background headache, punctuated by worse pain. These headaches often result from painkillers taken for migraines, tension headaches, or a neck or head injury.

Other causes of headaches include a fever, a hangover, toothache, sinus infection, food sensitivity, noise, a stuffy room, dehydration, very high blood pressure, and, rarely, a brain tumor.

Warning: Consult your doctor urgently for pain in the temple or neck: pain in the temple may indicate a potentially dangerous condition called temporal arteritis; pain in the neck may indicate meningitis. Both need treatment at once.

Locate the acupressure points at the base of the skull and press each for 15 seconds to relieve a headache. For a migraine, press between the eyebrows for 15 seconds.

Ginger tea can also help treat migraine.

✳ TREATMENT

Massage Relieve a tension headache by kneading and smoothing your scalp and neck muscles, particularly any tender lumps or points. Try a reflexology treatment: press along the sides and top of each big toe with both thumbs for five minutes.

Acupressure To help relieve a migraine, press between your eyebrows for 15 seconds. For any headache, press in the hollows at the base of the skull between the front and back neck muscles, behind the bony prominence behind the ear for 15 seconds each.

Hot and cold therapies A cold shower, compress or ice pack on the head may relieve migraine. You could also buy a special plastic hood that you fill with water and keep ready in the refrigerator. Some headaches respond better to heat.

Food and drink Ease tension headaches with more foods rich in calcium and magnesium. To help prevent migraine, eat a good balance of omega-3 and omega-6 fats (*see page 25*), have oily fish three times a week, and drink a cup of ginger tea once or twice a day. Also, identify any food sensitivities (*see page 164*).

Biofeedback Use a biofeedback gadget (*see page 207*) as a relaxation training aid to help you relax .

Eye care Glasses with lenses of an individually chosen colored tint (such as certain blues, greens, or oranges) prevent some migraines. Visit an optometrist who has the necessary equipment (the "Intuitive Colourmeter", *see page 219*) to choose as appropriate.

Herbal remedies For migraine, eat a few feverfew leaves in a sandwich, or take feverfew tablets (in the dose recommended on the pack).

Warning: Avoid if you are taking non-steroidal anti-inflammatory painkillers.

✚ WHAT ELSE DOCTORS MAY SUGGEST

Drugs for cluster headaches include inhaled ergotamine, verapamil tablets, and sumatriptan injections. Breathing pure oxygen for 10 to 20 minutes may also help. (You need a firm plastic mask without holes, and a valve to regulate the oxygen-flow at seven liters a minute.)

If you have fewer than four migraines a month, try painkillers such as aspirin, with a metoclopramide tablet 15 minutes earlier if you feel sick. Daily aspirin or propanolol may relieve more frequent attacks. If necessary your doctor can prescribe tablets, injections, or a nasal spray of a serotonin-boosting drug such as sumatriptan or the newer narotriptan. Menstrual migraine often responds to an estrogen patch.

SLEEP PROBLEMS

❓ WHAT CAUSES THEM

Being unable to get to sleep can result from anxiety, depression, overexcitement, indigestion or other pain, certain foods or drinks, feeling too hot or cold, environmental noise or light, or an uncomfortable bed. Waking soon after you've gone to sleep is often due to underlying anxiety, or to a disturbance such as a loud or irritating noise. Disturbed sleep may result from a partner snoring. Nightmares are often associated with stress; other triggers include hunger, feeling overfull, indigestion, and taking caffeine-containing drinks before bedtime. Waking unrefreshed usually means you haven't spent enough time either dreaming or sleeping deeply. A light bedroom, young children, or depression can encourage early waking too.

❀ TREATMENT

Check that your bed, bed covers, and bedroom are comfortable. Invest in earplugs if a partner's snoring or a noisy road keeps you awake. Avoid falling asleep in front of the TV in the evening.

Food and drink Eat more foods rich in calcium, magnesium, manganese, zinc, and vitamin B. Lettuce is renowned for making people feel soporific. Flavoring your supper with rosemary and thyme could also help. Foods containing the amino acid tryptophan may aid sleep by boosting your brain's serotonin level. However, they do this only if they contain very little protein, as other amino acids compete with tryptophan for access to the brain. So eat low-protein, high-carbohydrate foods such as bread, pasta, cereal, rice, dates, bananas, or potatoes half an hour before retiring. Don't have milk, as this contains a lot of protein. This said, some people find a hot malted milky nightcap helps. Avoid cocoa, cola, coffee, and tea (unless decaffeinated) after 4p.m. Alcohol relaxes muscles, so a small drink in the evening may help if you're tense. A small glass of beer is especially good as hops encourage drowsiness, but if you overindulge, you may find it difficult to sleep. Have your last meal relatively early and keep later snacks small, light, carbohydrate-rich, and cheese-free.

Food supplements
◆ Vitamin B taken in the morning.
◆ Calcium and magnesium taken in the evening
◆ Zinc taken in the morning.
◆ Tryptophan, an amino acid, and melatonin, a hormone produced at night (both available by import only in the UK), taken in the evening.

Exercise Take half an hour's exercise around five or six hours before you go to bed.

Herbal remedies Drink chamomile, lemon balm or linden (lime) blossom, vervain, or hop tea in the late afternoon and evening. Take a teaspoon of tincture containing valerian root and passiflora an hour or so before you go to bed.

Aromatherapy Before bedtime enjoy a warm bath scented with a camomile teabag or a few drops of lavender oil.

Homeopathy Try out the homeopathic remedy coffea, which can help with sleep problems.

Relaxation and stress management If worry is stopping you from sleeping, consider discussing effective problem- and stress-management strategies with a friend or counselor. If you simply cannot sleep, it could be that you are not sufficiently tired, so get up and read or relax with some soothing music.

✚ WHAT ELSE DOCTORS MAY SUGGEST

See your doctor if you have slept badly for more than two weeks, and are exhausted, depressed, desperate, or unable to cope with everyday life. You may benefit from a course of drugs to relax you or to aid sleep.

Add rosemary or thyme to your evening meal.

Ear plugs can eliminate virtually all invasive noise.

Lettuce is one of many foods that might make you drowsy. Add some to your final meal of the day.

ANOREXIA NERVOSA

❓ WHAT IT IS AND WHAT CAUSES IT

When a person who isn't overweight drastically reduces her food intake for no apparent reason, she is said to have anorexia nervosa (*see also page 66*). Most people with this disease feel hungry, though continued weight loss may reduce their appetite. Such a girl or woman quickly becomes much too light for her height and bone-span. She looks gaunt. Her periods stop if her weight falls too low. And she may feel cold and develop a hairy back and, eventually osteoporosis.

Around 1 teenager in 100 suffers from anorexia nervosa at some time, and most are girls. Many stop eating because it is the only way they can manage stress. Rigidly controlling and limiting their food intake may help them blot out emotional pain and feel more in control. However, this does nothing to help them manage stress effectively and also greatly endangers their health.

Peer pressure causes some young women to diet to extremes. Stress is another reason. Talk to people if your self-esteem is low and you are losing a lot of weight.

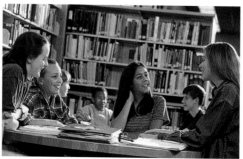

FAR RIGHT: Take control of your life by introducing regular exercise, as this will give both physical and psychological benefits.

✴ TREATMENT

A multivitamin and mineral supplement, more daylight, and gentle exercise may be beneficial. What you most need, though, is an understanding of your problem and help in learning effective and non-damaging stress-management techniques.

✚ WHAT ELSE DOCTORS MAY SUGGEST

The doctor will rule out other causes of weight loss and refer you for specialized help, perhaps to an eating disorders unit. Here they'll help you use food for pleasure again, rather than to control or punish yourself (or others), or as a cry for help. Treatment generally includes one-to-one or group counseling (with counseling or group work for parents, too). Your eating may need to be carefully supervised to save your life.

BULIMIA

❓ WHAT IT IS AND WHAT CAUSES IT

Having bulimia means being in the habit of bingeing and vomiting or taking laxatives (*see also page 66*). Bulimia affects around 1 in 100 girls and usually starts in the late teens or early 20s. The late Princess Diana overcame this debilitating illness and helped to publicize it. The trigger is generally a family or other problem. The individual longs to improve matters and cope with her sadness, loneliness, anger, or fear. Yet she feels powerless to control these matters. So instead, she may eat compulsively or go on a diet. Either of these causes intense hunger for sweet, starchy, fatty food. She then binges on these foods and feels out of control again. Afterward she reasserts control (and, perhaps, punishes herself too) by secretly vomiting or taking laxatives.

Bingeing and vomiting, or laxative abuse, disrupt the body chemistry, which makes recognizing hunger and fullness difficult. A woman with bulimia may have stomach pain, corroded teeth, frequent throat infections, absent periods, bloating, fatigue, and ovarian cysts (*see page 193*). More serious medical problems or other compulsive behaviors sometimes develop.

✴ TREATMENT

Take daily aerobic exercise to make you feel better.

Food and drink Most important, talk to someone about your problem, treat yourself to healthy, appetizing meals rich in low-glycemic-index foods (*see page 216*), as well as calcium, magnesium, zinc, vitamins B and C, and essential fatty acids.

Stress management See a therapist for help in managing stress in a non-damaging way. Ideas include learning to deal with feelings, keeping a diary to pinpoint binge triggers, and finding activities to replace the need to binge.

SEIZURES

? WHAT THEY ARE AND WHAT CAUSES THEM

A seizure is an uncontrollable movement of all or part of the body, together with a loss of consciousness or an altered state of consciousness. During a seizure, certain areas of the brain fire a sudden burst of chaotic electrical activity. Other names for a seizure are a fit or convulsion; epilepsy is the name for certain types of seizure. Many people about to have a seizure experience a warning such as a feeling of restlessness or irritability.

Seizures result from an oversensitivity of part of the brain to one or more of many triggers. Two possible early triggers are damage to part of the brain from an accident, an abnormality, or a lack of oxygen before, during, or after birth. Others include: a loud noise; anxiety or anger; fatigue; flickering or patterned light (from a flickering fluorescent tube, TV or VDU screen, or strobe light); foods (such as wheat); a nutrient deficiency; alcohol; changing hormone levels; certain drugs; certain pesticides; and exposure to certain electromagnetic frequencies.

✽ TREATMENT

Food and drink Eat foods rich in vitamins B6 or E, copper, magnesium, and selenium.

Aromatherapy For stress-induced seizures, choose an essential oil you find relaxing or, for fatigue-induced seizures, choose one you find stimulating. Ask someone to massage you regularly with this oil (six drops in a tablespoon of sweet almond oil). As you relax or become more alert during these massages, you'll learn to associate these feelings with the scent of the oil. Keep a small bottle with you. Then, when a seizure seems imminent, simply smell the oil, as research indicates that this alone may prevent it.

Biofeedback Learn to relax when you want – and so, perhaps, prevent a seizure – with biofeedback. This involves using one of a variety of electrical gadgets (bought from specialist medical supply stores) that provide feedback on how relaxed you are. If this indicates you are stressed, use deep breathing or other relaxation methods to improve the feedback. Such gadgets measure skin temperature or electrical resistance, muscle tension, brainwave activity, or the heart or breathing rate.

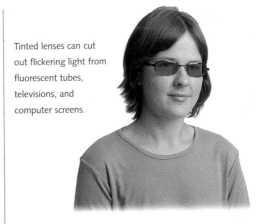

Tinted lenses can cut out flickering light from fluorescent tubes, televisions, and computer screens.

Tinted lenses If you have light-sensitive seizures, ask an optometrist with a colourimeter to prescribe glasses with tinted lenses for seizures (*see page 219*). Tints cut out flickering light of certain wavelengths that irritate the brain.

✚ WHAT ELSE DOCTORS MAY SUGGEST

Identify the trigger if possible. This is easier before beginning medication; but never stop your medication without your doctor knowing. If you can't discover or avoid the trigger, the right amount of antiepilepsy medication will probably suppress your seizures. Certain medications make the Pill less reliable, so you may need to discuss contraception. One new treatment is with an electronic gadget implanted in the chest. This can prevent seizures by stimulating the vagus nerve in the neck every five to 15 minutes.

A tailor-made aromatherapy massage can reduce the frequency of seizures.

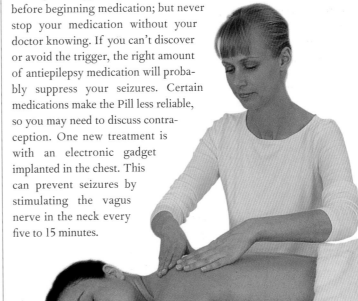

CANCER

❓ WHAT IT IS AND WHAT CAUSES IT

Cancer results from damage to a cell's DNA (genetic material). This allows it to multiply in an uncontrolled way instead of dying at its allotted time. Individual cancer cells arise continually throughout our lives. Most either die or are quickly destroyed by the immune system. If they are not destroyed, they can grow into a cancer.

As a cancer grows it destroys adjacent tissues. And it may eventually cause more widespread damage, or even kill. This is because cancer cells can break away, travel in the blood or lymph, and, unless destroyed by well-functioning immune cells, settle elsewhere, causing more growths ("secondaries" or metastases).

Simple lifestyle factors such as an unhealthy diet, smoking, stress, too little exercise, and too much or too little exposure to daylight, can lower immunity. Researchers say that half of all fatal cancers are linked to such factors, and suspect that a better diet could prevent up to four in five breast cancers. The likelihood of getting a cancer increases with age. A variety of factors encourage individual cancers.

The following list, for example, shows some of the triggers for "women's" cancers:

BREAST

◆ Starting periods early.
◆ Being overweight.
◆ The high estrogen level known as estrogen dominance (*see pages 187 and 216*). Four in five breast cancers are estrogen-sensitive.
◆ The combined Pill (the risk is slight and may normalize once off the Pill for ten years).
◆ Never having children, or having children late.
◆ Drinking more than one unit of alcohol a day.
◆ A family history of breast, ovarian, or colon cancer.
◆ A late menopause.
◆ HRT (the risk normalizes once off HRT for five years; death from breast cancer may perhaps be less likely in women who develop it while on HRT than in those who get it when not on HRT).
◆ Using dark hair dye.
◆ Previous breast lumps with unusual cells ("atypical hyperplasia").

WOMB

◆ The high estrogen level known as estrogen dominance (*see pages 187 and 216*).
◆ Estrogen-only HRT.
◆ Being overweight.
◆ Tamoxifen (a hormonal treatment for some breast cancer).
◆ Irregular periods.
◆ Infertility from ovarian failure.
◆ A late menopause.

CERVIX

◆ Starting sex very young.
◆ Many sexual partners.
◆ Human papillomavirus infection.
◆ Smoking.
◆ Abnormal cervical cells (dyskaryosis), or pre-cancerous ones.

OVARY

◆ Not having children.
◆ A Western lifestyle.
◆ A family history of ovarian cancer.

SCREENING

Routine screening for breast cancer and cervical cancer is advisable at certain ages (*see pages 72, 95, 107, 113*). Breast screening is done with an X-ray called a mammogram and, if necessary, a physical examination, ultrasound scan, and biopsy.

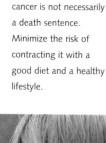

Being diagnosed with cancer is not necessarily a death sentence. Minimize the risk of contracting it with a good diet and a healthy lifestyle.

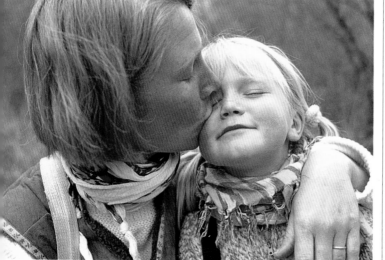

Cervical screening is done with a Pap (cervical) smear and, if necessary, colposcopy (direct viewing of the cervix via the vagina) and biopsy.

Researchers are investigating whether ovary screening (with, for example, a blood test and ultrasound scan) is useful for women with a raised risk of ovarian cancer.

To help prevent any cancer, lead a healthy lifestyle (*see Part 1*), minimize controllable risk factors, have any recommended screening, and report unexplained symptoms early.

❀ TREATMENT

Home treatments sometimes slow the progression of cancers that haven't already spread, and can occasionally reverse or cure them. For people with advanced cancer, treatments may prolong life and improve its quality.

Food and drink Eat more foods rich in plant hormones. These substances can occupy hormone receptors on cells, which may discourage estrogen-sensitive cancers. Eat more foods rich in calcium (to discourage breast cancer) and fiber (to lower a raised estrogen level). Have a good balance of essential fats (*see page 25*). This boosts immunity by encouraging a healthy balance of prostaglandins. Eat three helpings a week of oily fish because one of its omega-3 fatty acids, eicosapentanoic acid, can reverse the weight loss that kills one in four people with cancer. Eat more foods rich in natural salicylates (to inhibit the production of prostaglandins that stimulate cancer growth and suppress immunity). And have more foods rich in antioxidants such as beta carotene, vitamins C and E, selenium, and flavonoids (to fight the free radicals – *see page 216* – which encourage new cancers to begin).

Include at least five – preferably more – helpings of fruit and vegetables each day for a variety of cancer-fighting substances. Tomatoes cooked in olive oil have high amounts of lycopene, a potent flavonoid. Garlic contains S-allomercaptocysteine, a natural breast-cancer inhibitor; onions contain similar substances. Cruciferous vegetables (cabbage, broccoli, brussels sprouts) offer glucosinolates which help kill genetically damaged cells. The oil in citrus fruit peel contains anticancer substances. Drink a whole citrus fruit liquidized with its peel each day. Grapeskins contain resveratrol, which can inhibit all stages of cancer growth. Cherries contain ellagic acid, which blocks an enzyme that cancer cells need for growth. Ginger and turmeric supply helpful antioxidants.

Each day drink several cups of green tea; its polyphenols encourage the death of cells with damaged DNA.

Identify any suspected food sensitivity (*see page 164*). Though the research into substances in food called lectins is in its infancy, some cancers may improve when no longer exposed to those lectins (*see page 217*) to which an individual is sensitive.

Visualization Imagine your immune cells successfully destroying the cancer.

Laughter, enjoyment, stress management Boost immunity by finding things to laugh at and enjoy, and using effective stress management.

Change your perspective Live your life to the full and you may find you have reason to thank your cancer for improving the quality of your life and relationships.

Light exposure Get some unfiltered daylight each day to lift your spirits and raise your level of vitamin D (which is sometimes low in women with breast cancer).

Warning: Take care not to burn.

✚ WHAT ELSE DOCTORS MAY SUGGEST

Treatments may include anticancer drugs (chemotherapy); other medications; surgery; and laser destruction of cancer cells (perhaps after sensitizing them with light-attracting pigment).

The polyphenols in green tea encourage the death of cells that contain damaged DNA.

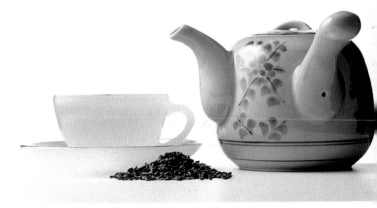

AUTOIMMUNE DISEASES

❓ WHAT THEY ARE AND WHAT CAUSES THEM

We expect our immune system to help protect us from invasion by antigens such as infecting organisms, foreign particles, and cancer cells. But sometimes our immune cells can "change sides" and attack our own cells as if these were invaders. This mistake results from a mutation of certain antibodies embedded in the immune cells. These are known as antigen-receptors. Their usual task is to destroy antigens. Normally, immune cells with mutated antibodies self-destruct. But if the immune system isn't working properly, they can attack normal tissue and cause autoimmune diseases.

Among these are rheumatoid arthritis (*see page 178*) and lupus erythematosus, which has many possible symptoms including arthritis, skin rashes, kidney damage, and frequent miscarriages due to blood clots in the placenta. Other auto-immune disorders include insulin-dependent diabetes (*see page 180*), an under- or overactive thyroid due to Hashimoto's thyroiditis or Graves' disease (*see page 181*), systemic sclerosis (with various symptoms due to thickening and tightening of the connective tissue in the skin, arteries, and elsewhere), Sjögren's syndrome (dry eyes, *see page 171* and a dry vagina, *see page 182*), glomerulonephritis (a type of kidney inflammation), and AIDS (*see page 183*). It is possible that autoimmune attack also causes endometriosis (*see page 191*), and infertility (*see page 195*) due to unexplained ovarian failure before the age of 40.

Three in four people suffering from an autoimmune disease are female and such diseases are more likely after an early menopause. The cause is not clear. But it is possible that anything that reduces immunity – such as stress, a nutritionally poor diet, a lack of exercise, and too much sunshine – may play a part. New research implicates lectins found in certain foods (*see page 216*).

✸ TREATMENT

Following the healthy lifestyle advice given in Part 1 may help you recover.

Food and drink Eat more foods rich in beta carotene and other plant pigments, vitamins C and E, folic acid, copper (in liver, nuts, seeds, beans, fish, wholegrains), magnesium, selenium, zinc and, most important, omega-3 fatty acids. Identify any food sensitivity (*see page 164*) and remember that eating common foods such as wheat and milk, either too frequently or in large amounts, can often be to blame.

Protect your immune system by adopting a healthy lifestyle. This means a balanced diet, exercise, fresh air, and stress management. Be careful not to overexpose yourself to the sun as this may compromise your immunity.

Food supplements

◆ Glucosamine – it's suspected that this amino-sugar may protect against diseases induced by lectins (*see page 217*).

Relaxation and stress management Get any help you need to identify and then avoid or otherwise deal with your main sources of stress. Work on more effective stress-management strategies. Being assertive, rather than passively accepting events, could boost your immune system. Biofeedback (*see page 207*) may help you relax. Enough good quality sleep is important. And rewarding intimate relationships with your friends and partner can boost immunity.

Herbal remedies Boost your immunity with a three-month course of echinacea and astragalus. Take a teaspoon of tincture containing these herbs twice a day.

✚ WHAT ELSE DOCTORS MAY SUGGEST

Treatment with steroids and powerful immuno-suppressant drugs may be recommended.

CHRONIC FATIGUE SYNDROME

❓ WHAT IT IS AND WHAT CAUSES IT

Feeling tired or fatigued from time to time is a universal experience. Fatigue usually results from working hard – physically or mentally – or feeling stressed, excited, or upset. The solution is normally to take time to recuperate and, perhaps, to program in more opportunities for relaxation, emotional restoration, and other ways of recharging your batteries.

However, a few people develop prolonged fatigue that doesn't respond to these measures. They have chronic fatigue syndrome. This used to be called ME – for myalgic encephalomyelitis – but isn't anymore because we know there is no brain inflammation.

People with chronic fatigue syndrome (CFS) have inexplicable and disabling exhaustion lasting six months or more. They may also have muscle aches, headaches, and sleep problems. Some have poor concentration, memory, and temperature control; others are breathless or faint, or have slurred speech. People with CFS are three times as likely to develop irritable bowel syndrome (*see page 161*).

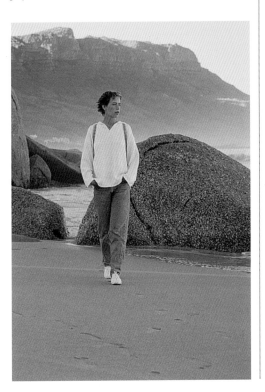

The cause of CFS is still unknown, though it sometimes follows an infection or a time of stress. Attacks last for four years on average; but four people in five have a relapse later. One sufferer in two is depressed, and one in four has some other mental health problem. While depression and anxiety may, of course, be caused by the illness itself, they are also the strongest known risk factors for CFS. This isn't surprising because our minds and bodies are intimately linked by body chemicals such as neurotransmitters (which carry nerve messages) and hormones.

✳ TREATMENT

There is no proof that nutritional supplements or complementary therapies cure CFS, but a healthy diet and anything that makes you feel better without doing harm are well worth trying.

Exercise Try to strike the right balance between rest and exercise. Too much rest will weaken your muscles and may be depressing, while too much exercise may encourage muscle pain and fatigue. Start an exercise program by taking a short walk each day. Then gradually increase the amount of exercise that you do.

Mind work Consider seeing a psychotherapist for cognitive-behavioral therapy. This will help you deal with the limitations your symptoms impose on your daily life, and with your reactions to the illness. Such therapy also sometimes helps cure the underlying cause.

Herbal remedies Try a three-month course of St. John's wort (*Hypericum perforatum*). You can take this as a cup of tea twice a day, or as a tincture (one teaspoon once or twice a day), or tablets (take according to the instructions on the pack). Other herbs to consider include Siberian ginseng and ginger root (as tablets, tea, or tincture).

✚ WHAT ELSE DOCTORS MAY SUGGEST

If you've been inexplicably exhausted for a long time, your doctor will consider conditions that can mimic CFS – such as anemia, or a lack of estrogen or thyroid or pituitary hormone – before diagnosing CFS itself. However, there is no specific test. Your doctor or a physiotherapist will help you to work out your own personalized program of graduated exercise.

Take gentle exercise when your body feels up to it. The fresh air and sunlight will make you feel better.

FLUID RETENTION

❓ WHAT IT IS AND WHAT CAUSES IT

Around three-fifths of our body weight is usually made of water. So the body of a person who weighs 140 pounds (10 stones) contains 84 pounds (6 stones) of water. The amounts of water in the blood and the tissue fluid that bathes the body's cells are normally delicately balanced. However, certain conditions create a surplus of water in the tissue fluid and it's then that we are said to suffer from fluid retention.

Fluid retention is obvious if the tissue fluid increases by more than 15 percent, because the ankles swell. However, one of the commonest signs is frequent weight change. The weight may, for example, sometimes rise or fall by many pounds in a short time. Some women have headaches or a sensation of fullness in the head, or feel moody, "muzzy-headed" (less mentally acute than usual), irritable, low, or slow. Others are accident-prone. Many have tight rings from swollen fingers, puffy eyelids, deeply indented marks on their skins when they remove their underwear, tense painful breasts, bloating (*see page 162*), or carpal tunnel syndrome (*see page 201*). Some pass water more often at night. A very large water surplus causes swelling of the abdomen from fluid around the organs and intestines, or difficulty in breathing because of fluid in or around the lungs.

Fluid retention may result from being over-weight, exercising too little, or having varicose veins. Other causes include: food sensitivity (to wheat and other grains, milk, eggs, and yeast, *see page 164*); the premenstrual syndrome (*see page 186*); pregnancy; protein deficiency (most likely in people in developed countries if they have an alcohol problem); certain drugs (including steroids); and heart, liver, and kidney disease.

Carrots are a natural diuretic and so can help expel excess fluid.

✿ TREATMENT

Take steps to identify and treat the cause, with help from your doctor (*see below*) if necessary. Take regular exercise, and lose excess weight with a combination of exercise, a healthy diet, and effective stress management.

Food and drink For unexplained fluid retention, eat more fruit and vegetables (especially carrots and celery, which have natural diuretic qualities, meaning they encourage urine production). Eat foods rich in vitamin B6 (which also has diuretic qualities). Cut out added sugar, white flour, salt, and animal fat.

Herbal remedies Discuss your problem with your doctor before taking herbal remedies with diuretic properties. Such remedies include dandelion leaf, buchu, bladderwrack (a seaweed), couch grass, and squaw vine (*Mitchella repens*). Take them as tea, tincture, or tablets two or three times a day when necessary.

Aromatherapy Add three drops each of geranium and rosemary oils to your bathwater. Their inhaled vapor is claimed to counteract fluid retention.

✚ WHAT ELSE DOCTORS MAY SUGGEST

Your doctor will do an examination and tests, if necessary, to discover why you are retaining fluid. The treatment depends on the cause.

Warning: If you are pregnant it's important to report ankle swelling, as this might be a sign of pre-eclampsia (*see page 74*).

FAR RIGHT: If you are prone to fluid retention, try adding a few drops of geranium and rosemary oils to your bath.

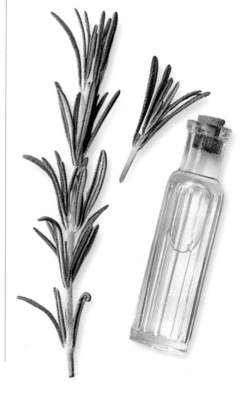

PAIN

WHAT CAUSES IT

Pain results from stimulation of specialized nerve fibers that carry messages to the brain. This stimulation can be from inflammation, pressure, or something very hot or cold. Experiencing pain is always unpleasant and persistent pain can be extremely dispiriting. Chronic pain has many causes, including muscle tension in the back (*see page 198*), arthritis (*see page 178*), a stroke, a leg ulcer, and the aftermath of shingles – postherpetic neuralgia. Then there are the complications of diabetes (*see page 180*), such as painful feet because of poor circulation and damage to the nerves. And, not as rare as some might think, is the feeling of a painful "phantom limb" after losing an arm or leg in an operation or accident.

TREATMENT

The most important thing is to identify and treat the cause of the pain. If it continues, try to find ways of reducing it or, at least, of learning to manage your reaction to it. There are tips on pain relief for specific conditions throughout this book.

Mind control It's surprising how powerful our brains can be at overcoming pain. This isn't to say the pain is imagined, but that many people find they notice it less if they do certain things. These include relaxing, because while muscle tension may result from pain, it then makes the pain worse. Use more effective stress management, and biofeedback (*see page 207*) to help if necessary. You may find a technique called "targeting" useful. You decide on and aim for achievable goals each day, rather than having your hopes repeatedly dashed by wanting to do more than you can.

Exercise Doing exercise of an appropriate level boosts the level of naturally occurring morphine-like substances called endorphins. These act as painkillers and mood enhancers. Even gentle exercise such as t'ai chi or yoga may be effective.

Heat and cold therapies Some pains respond to the application of heat or cold (*see page 131*).

Massage This relieves some pains either by encouraging muscular and mental relaxation, or by preventing pain messages from reaching the spinal cord (*see TENS, below*).

TENS Using a TENS (trans-cutaneous electrical nerve stimulation) machine helps many painful conditions. This provides electrical stimulation via electrodes stuck to the skin, which can prevent pain messages from gaining access to the spinal cord (and traveling to the brain).

WHAT ELSE DOCTORS MAY SUGGEST

Your doctor will search for the cause of your pain, treat it if possible, and suggest painkillers. If necessary you can visit a pain clinic to benefit from the expertise of doctors and nurses who specialize in pain control and, perhaps, other practitioners offering such things as physiotherapy, acupuncture, hypnosis, and electrotherapy. Blocking pain transmission by freezing, anesthetizing, or even destroying a nerve is sometimes necessary.

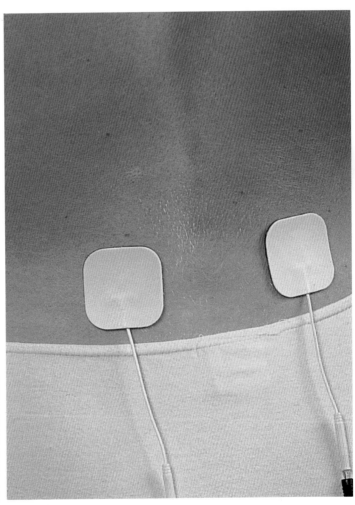

Many women use a TENS machine to relieve labor pains, but it can be used for other pain too. It is easy to control and has no adverse side effects.

AFTERWORD

Each of us is unique, which is why the most effective health-care plan for any woman is one that is tailored to meet her needs. Some health information and advice is right for every man, woman, and child, but if you are to maximize your health and wellbeing, you have to know how best you can do this at your precise age and stage of life, and in your particular circumstances.

The good news is that working out a health-care plan that matches the complexity of your life can be not only challenging, but also fascinating and rewarding. To that end, the wealth of reliable, up-to-date information in this book has been arranged in a way that aims to be very user-friendly.

Part 1 offers the basic ways of encouraging and maintaining good health. Part 2 gives particular information and advice for each age or stage of life. Part 3 teaches the rudiments of some useful complementary healing therapies. And Part 4 suggests ways of treating any health problems you may have with a mix of complementary and orthodox healing methods. Together, the four parts should enable you to work out – with professional help if necessary – your own personalized health-care plan.

This plan will include making those health choices and adopting those behaviors that are particularly important for you right now.

Women are mostly very interested in information about encouraging good health and wellbeing. This interest allows them to form carefully considered health beliefs and to make sensible choices about their lifestyles and behaviors. A continuing interest enables them to modify their beliefs and their behaviors as new findings concerning health emerge.

It can be frustrating when things you thought were right are turned on their heads by new findings. One moment, for example, you are told to eat more carbohydrates, the next you are told that carbohydrates make you fat. But knowledge from medical research usually builds up only slowly, and sometimes it changes completely as more information becomes available.

However, science is certainly not the only thing – or even the main thing – which affects our health beliefs and behaviors. More often such changes result from altered personal circumstances. Ordinary, everyday influences concerning our roles, relationships, and socio-economic status can be vitally important to our health. Such influences include being single or having a partner; being employed or unemployed; becoming pregnant; and having more or less money. Changing circumstances may mean that we suddenly have to face our vulnerability and discern the best way forward for health and happiness.

Whatever your circumstances, I hope this book helps you to develop your own understanding of what it means to feel well and be well. I hope it helps you learn how to boost your health and that of your family and, perhaps, even your community. And I hope it teaches you how to use lifestyle changes, and natural remedies and therapies, to look after yourself and those you love during particularly challenging stages of life, or during a time of illness.

If you have, or someone close to you has, a permanent physical problem, it helps to remember that physical health, while obviously good to have, certainly isn't everything. Health can come in many forms, physical, mental, and spiritual. Someone with paralyzed legs can be just as healthy in the rest of her body and in her mind and spirit as a top-class athlete. And an individual with severe learning difficulties can be just as healthy (with her own particular brain power, the rest of her mind, and her body and spirit) as a Nobel prize-winning mathematician.

But regardless of bodily health, a person's spirit is the most important thing of all. With a free spirit that can help you transcend the mundane and enjoy the beauty in life, it is possible to live peacefully with even a serious health problem. Each of us has only a limited time on earth, so it's wise to enjoy, care for, and make the most of your body, mind, and spirit while you are here. And apart from making your life more pleasant, it will help you to prepare for what lies ahead.

You are a very special person. Whatever your age, stage, or circumstances, I wish you all the very best as you look after yourself and those whom you love.

And may you always go well as you continue your journey through life.

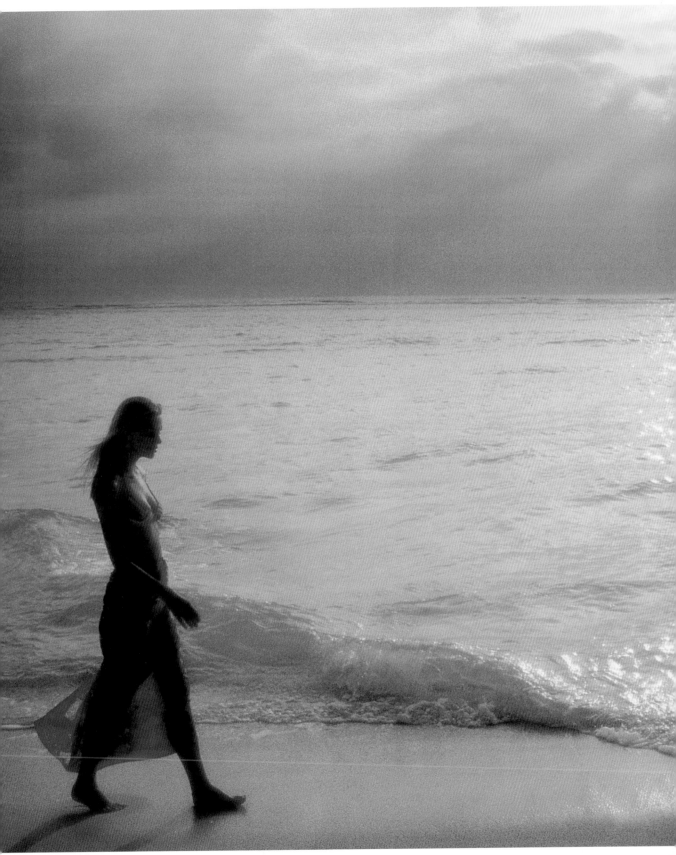

GLOSSARY

adrenaline – a hormone that is known in the USA as epinephrine. Similarly, noradrenaine is called norepinephrine.

aerobic exercise – moderate to vigorous exercise that raises the heart rate and, unlike very intense exercise, can be continued for some time.

allergen – any substance that triggers a rapid allergic response that is mediated by the immune system, and involves the production of immunoglobulin E (IgE) antibodies.

allergy – symptoms resulting from the interaction between an allergen (*see above*) and IgE antibodies that have been presensitized to that allergen. Examples include certain types of asthma, eczema, and allergic rhinitis (hay fever being the best-known example).

antibody – a small particle, attached to an immune cell, which can destroy an antigen.

antioxidants – substances that suppress the damaging effects of free radicals (*see below*).

body mass index (BMI) – a figure based on an individual's weight and height, and used to determine whether her weight carries any health risk.

"cardio" exercise – aerobic exercise sufficiently intense to raise the heart rate to 50–75 percent of its maximum rate, and to be of particular benefit to the cardiovascular system (heart and blood vessels).

colposcopy – an examination of the cervix through a viewing tube in the vagina.

complementary medicine – a healing system based on natural therapies or remedies that can be used alongside orthodox medicine (*see below*).

compress – a pad of material soaked in hot or cold water (perhaps containing herbs or essential oils) and placed on part of the body to soothe certain local symptoms.

essential fatty acids – linoleic acid and alpha-linolenic acids. These are the "parent" PUFAs (*see below*) of the omega-6 and omega-3 groups of fatty acids from which the body makes many body chemicals, including prostaglandins (*see below*). We need only five times as much linoleic as alpha-linolenic acid, but most of us eat very much more. To improve the balance, eat more foods rich in omega-3 (*see page 25*) and monounsaturated fatty acids (*see below*), but fewer omega-6 rich foods (*see page 25*).

estrogen – a group of hormones (with several similar sub-types varying in strength) produced mainly by the ovaries, but also by the adrenal glands and fat cells. Estrogens are responsible for female sexual characteristics and ovulation.

estrogen dominance – an upset in the hormone balance that allows estrogen to be too powerful, perhaps because its level is too high in itself, or in relation to that of progesterone. It can result from a diet low in fiber and plant hormones; the Pill or HRT; or xenestrogen exposure (*see below*). Alternatively, it may follow an abnormal failure to ovulate (for example, because of stress, eating too much or too little, a high or low body weight, or over-exercising).

fatty acids – the constituents of fats.

fish oil – oil from the muscles of cold-water fish, rich in docosahexenoic and eicosapentanoic acids. The body normally produces these omega-3 PUFAs (*see below*) from an essential fatty acid (*see above*) called alpha-linolenic acid; if anything (such as aging, smoking, or stress) prevents this, fish oil supplements can be helpful.

flavonoids – plant pigments that act as antioxidants (*see above*).

free radicals – active oxygen particles that, unless mopped up by antioxidants (*see above*), can damage fats and encourage arterial disease, infection, arthritis, and certain other inflammatory diseases.

glycemic index (GI) – a figure from 0–100 assigned to each food to indicate how rapidly it raises the blood-sugar level after being eaten. The higher its GI, the more rapidly a food raises this level. Habitually eating a lot of high-GI foods encourages diabetes and obesity. Moderate-to high-GI foods include root vegetables, bread (especially French), most breakfast cereals (except pure bran cereals), and white rice. Low-GI foods include proteins, fats, nuts, and most vegetables and fruits (except bananas, grapes, pineapple, and watermelon).

HRT – hormone replacement therapy, used to help counteract any adverse effects of naturally lowered levels of estrogen and progesterone. HRT is usually with estrogen and, for women who haven't had a hysterectomy, synthetic progestogen (progesterone is better but isn't well absorbed orally, and we don't yet know if it's reliably absorbed through the skin).

hypothalamus – part of the brain that helps control the pituitary gland. It is sensitive to hormone levels, emotional and physical stress, body weight, and the amount eaten.

integrated medicine – the combination of orthodox medicine (*see below*) and complementary medicine (*see above*).

lectins – natural substances in many foods, including wheat, tomatoes, potatoes, and peanuts. Large amounts can cause illness. And it's suggested that individual sensitivity can cause a wide variety of adverse reactions including, for example, autoimmune diseases (*see page 210*).

monounsaturated fatty acids – fatty acids that are less saturated with hydrogen than saturated fats (*see below*), and more saturated than PUFAs (*see below*). Examples of sources include peanuts and olives and their oils, canola (rapeseed) oil, and avocados.

naturopathy – a gentle system of medicine based on a healthy lifestyle, hydrotherapy, herbal (and, sometimes, homeopathic) remedies, and massage. One treatment most doctors think unnecessary is colonic irrigation (the washing of the large bowel with water via a tube passed through the anus); this removes valuable bowel bacteria and other microorganisms.

orthodox medicine – the system of medicine mainly used in Westernized countries and, increasingly, in others too. It provides excellent diagnostic facilities, and its treatments include drugs, surgery, and a wide variety of therapies that are carried out by paramedics such as physiotherapists. (*See also* Integrated medicine, *above*.)

Pap (cervical) smear – a sample of cells taken from the cervix to check for abnormalities that indicate a raised risk of cervical cancer.

pituitary gland – a gland in the brain that controls the levels of many hormones, including those that stimulate the ovaries. It responds to information from the hypothalamus (*see above*).

plant hormones – substances in many vegetables (especially beans and peas), fruits, grains, nuts, and seeds that can occupy hormone receptors on cells. This can counteract either a high estrogen level, or a low one. It's possible that certain plant hormones may modify the activity of testosterone and certain other human hormones in a similar way.

progesterone – a hormone, made by the ovaries, whose level peaks after ovulation and remains high in pregnancy.

progestogens – synthetic progesterone-like drugs that mimic some actions of human progesterone.

prostaglandins – substances our bodies make from PUFAs (*see below*). A good balance helps regulate blood clotting, insulin and calcium levels, muscle tone, ovulation, periods, and labor, and also helps prevent inflammation. An imbalance of prostaglandins may result from an imbalance of essential fatty acids (*see above*) in the diet. This underlies many common ailments, including period pain, heavy periods, premenstrual syndrome and endometriosis.

PUFAs – polyunsaturated fatty acids. These are fatty acids whose molecules are not, unlike those of saturated fats (*see below*), saturated with hydrogen. Vegetables, nuts, seeds, and oily fish are the best sources. These and monounsaturated fatty acids (*see above*) should provide two-thirds of the calories we obtain from fats.

saturated fats – fatty acids that are saturated with hydrogen (unlike PUFAs and monounsaturated fatty acids, *see above*) and are mainly found in meat, eggs, and dairy products. They should provide only a third of the calories we get from fats.

sitz bath – a treatment taken sitting in a bathtub filled with water of one temperature, with the feet in another container (at one end of the bathtub) filled with water of another temperature.

xenestrogens – synthetic estrogen-like substances. They include nonylphenol; from soft plastic or polystyrene food-packaging; bisphenyl A from the lacquer-coating inside cans; and certain pesticides.

217

FURTHER READING

WOMEN'S HEALTH

Books listing self-help groups and health charities are available in most countries.

Breast is Best by Drs Penny and Andrew Stanway (Pan, 1996).

Coping With Your Premature Baby by Dr Penny Stanway (Orion, 1999).

Crusing Through the Menopause by Maryon Stewart.

Eat Right for Your Type by Dr Peter J D'Adamo (Putnam, 1997).

The Feel-Good Facelift by Dr Penny Stanway (Kyle Cathie, 2000).

First Baby After Thirty … Or Forty? by Dr Penny Stanway (Orion, 1999).

A Little of What You Fancy Does You Good by Dr H B Gibson (Third Age Press, 1997).

Natural Alternatives to HRT by Marilyn Glenville (Kyle Cathie, 1997).

Natural Organic Hair and Skin Care by Aubrey Hampton (Organica Press, 1990).

The Natural Remedy Book for Women by Diane Stein (The Crossing Press, 1992).

New Guide to Pregnancy and Babycare edited by Dr Penny Stanway (UK – Conran Octopus, US – Simon & Schuster, 1999).

The New Natural Family Doctor by Dr Andrew Stanway (Gaia, 1996).

The Pill and Other Forms of Hormonal Contraception by John Guillebaud (Oxford University Press, 1997).

Skin Secrets – the Medical Facts versus the Beauty Fiction by Professor Nicholas Lowe MD and Polly Sellar (Collins & Brown, 1999).

Superyoung by Dr David Weeks and Jamie James (Hodder & Stoughton, 1998).

Women, Hormones and the Menstrual Cycle by Ruth Trickey (Allen & Unwin, 1998).

Women's Bodies, Women's Wisdom by Dr Christiane Northrup (Piatkus, 1998).

THERAPIES AND REMEDIES

Acupressure Step by Step by Jacqueline Young (Thorsons, 1998).

The Alexander Technique by Liz Hodgkinson (Piatkus, 1996).

The Complete Floral Healer by Anne McIntyre (Gaia, 1996).

The Complete Illustrated Guide to Aromatherapy by Julia Lawless (Element, 1997).

The Complete Women's Herbal by Anne McIntyre (Henry Holt, 1994).

Freedom from Asthma by Alexander Stalmatski, with a foreword by Professor Konstantin Buteyko (Kyle Cathie, 1997).

Healing Foods for Common Ailments by Dr Penny Stanway (Gaia, 1994).

LifeLight by Dr Penny Stanway (Kyle Cathie, to be published 2001).

Light – Medicine of the Future by Jacob Liberman OD, PhD (Bear & Co, 1992).

Massage by Stewart Mitchell (Element, 1997).

Natural Medicine by Beth MacEoin (Bloomsbury, 1999).

Not Just a Room with a Bath Dr Keith Souter (CW Daniel Company Ltd, 1995).

Prescription for Nutritional Healing by James F Balch MD and Phyllis A Balch CNC (Avery, 1998).

Yoga for Stress Relief by Swami Shivapremananda (Gaia, 1998).

USEFUL ADDRESSES

USA

American Association of Naturopathic Physicians (601 Valley Street, Suite 105, Seattle, WA 98109. Tel: 206 298 0125.) Has a directory of naturopaths.

American Association of Nutritional Consultants (1641 East Sunset Road, Apr B-117, Las Vegas, Nevada 89119. Tel: 709 361 1132.) Has a list of consultants.

American Herbalists Guild (PO Box 70, Roosevelt, UT 84066. Tel: 435 722 8434.) Has a list of herbalists.

American Holistic Medical Association (4101 Lake Boone Trail, Suite 201, Raleigh, NC 27606.) Has a list of doctors and osteopaths who practice holistic medicine.

Capitol Drugs, Inc (4454 Van Nuys Blvd, Sherman Oaks, CA 91403. Tel:1-800-858-8833.) Supplies nutritional supplements, homeopathic, herbal, and flower remedies.

Simpler's Botanicals (PO Box 2534, Sebastapol, CA 95473. Tel: 1 800 652 7646.) Supplies essential oils and carrier oils.

UK

Aqua Oleum (Unit 3, Lower Wharf, Wallbridge, Stroud, Gloucestershire GL5 3JA. Tel: 01453 753555.) Supplies essential and carrier oils.

Bioforce UK (2 Brewster Place, Irvine KA11 5DD, Scotland. Tel: 01294 277344.)

British College of Naturopathy and Osteopathy (Frazer House, 6 Netherhall Gardens, London NW3 5RR. Tel: 020 7435 6464.) Has a list of naturopaths and osteopaths.

British Association of Nutritional Therapists (c/o SPNT, PO Box 47, Heathfield, East Sussex TN21 8ZX.) Has a list of practitioners.

British Holistic Medical Association (179 Gloucester Place, London NW1 6DX. Tel: 020 7262 5299.) Has a list of doctors who practice complementary medicine.

Bach Flower Remedies (Unit 6, Suffolk Way, Drayton, Abingdon, Oxfordshire OX14 5JX. Tel: 01235 550086.) Supplies flower remedies.

Cerium Optical Products (Cerium Technology Park, Tenterden, Kent, TN30 7DE. Tel: 01580 765211.) Has a list of optometrists who have a Colourimeter.

Institute of Complementary Medicine (PO Box 194, Tavern Quay, London SE16 1QZ Tel: 020 7237 5165.) Has a list of qualified therapists.

National Institute of Medical Herbalists (PO Box 3, Winchester, Hampshire. Tel: 01962 68776.) Has a list of medical herbalists.

Potter's Herbal Supplies Ltd (Leyland Mill Lane, Wigan, Lancs WN1 2BR. Tel: 01942 234761.) Supplies herbal remedies.

Solgar Vitamins (Aldbury, Tring, Herts HP23 5TP. Tel: 01442 890355.) Supplies nutritional supplements.

Women's Nutritional Advisory Service Ltd (PO Box 268, Lewes, East Sussex, BN7 2QN. Tel: 01273 487366)

AUSTRALIA AND NEW ZEALAND

Association of Self-Help Organisations & Groups (39 Darghan Street, Glebe, NSW 2037. Tel: 02 660 6136.) Has a list of self-help organisations and groups.

Australian Natural Therapists Association Ltd (PO Box 308, Melrose Park, South Australia 5039. Tel: 1 800 817 577) Has a list of natural therapists.

Martin & Pleasance Pty. Ltd (123 Dover Stree, Richmond, Victoria. Tel: 03 9427 7422). Supplies Bach flower remedies.

National Herbalists Association of Australia (Suite 305, BST House, 3 Smail Street, Broadway, NSW 2007. Tel: 02 211 6437.) Has a list of herbalists.

USEFUL WEBSITES

American Dietetic Association www.eatright.org
Information on nutrition.

Dr Duke's Phytochemical and Ethnobotanical Databases www.ars-grin.gov/duke/index
An excellent herbal database, funded by the US Department of Agriculture.

The Herb Research Foundation Boulder, CO, US. www.herbs.org
Useful information and links to other herbal sites.

La Leche League www.lalecheleague.org
Breastfeeding information and support.

National Sports Medicine Institute of the UK www.nsmi.org.uk
Useful exercise and fitness tips.

The National Women's Health Information Center www.4woman.gov
Information sponsored by the US Public Health Services on Women's Health.

US Government Healthfinder www.healthfinder.gov
A useful consumer health information website.

INDEX

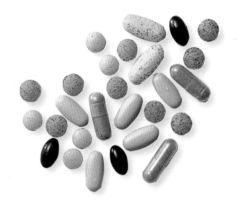

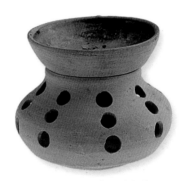

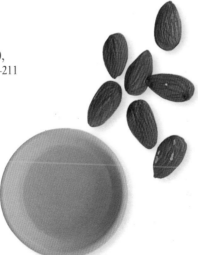

PICTURE ACKNOWLEDGMENTS

Gettyone Stone

pp 3–2, 14 (t), 15, 16 (r), 17 (tl & tr), 18 (tl), 18–19, 21 (br), 36, 40, 41, 42, 48–49, 55 (r), 58, 59, 60, 61 (br), 62 (bl), 63 (r), 64, 81 (t), 85, 89, 90, 91, 93 (t), 95, 97 (t), 100 (bl), 102, 103, 104, 105, 110, 114 (r), 115 (l & r), 116, 118–119, 121, 130 (tr) 142 (tl), 147, 148, 149, 167 (tr), 180 (bl), 183 (l), 188, 191 (t), 200 (b), 202, 206 (l&r), 208, 211, 215

Art Directors/ TRIP

pp. 14 (b), 35, 67 (b), 107 (br), 108–109 (b), 112 (bl), 113 (br), 183 (r)

Garden Picture Library

pp. 156 (br), 171 (tr)

Abode

p. 21 (bl)

Rex Features

pp. 28 (b), 29 (b), 30 (tl & tr), 32 (tr), 92

Image Bank

pp. 6–7, 28 (t), 32 (b), 37, 47, 57, 65 (t), 66 (b), 82 (m), 86, 94, 114 (l)

Corbis

pp. 30 (b), 120 (br)

Science Photo Library

pp. 98, 153 (tr), 179 (tl & tr), 194 (b), 213